MEDICINE
LITERATURE
&
EPONYMS:

AN ENCYCLOPEDIA OF MEDICAL EPONYMS
DERIVED FROM LITERARY CHARACTERS

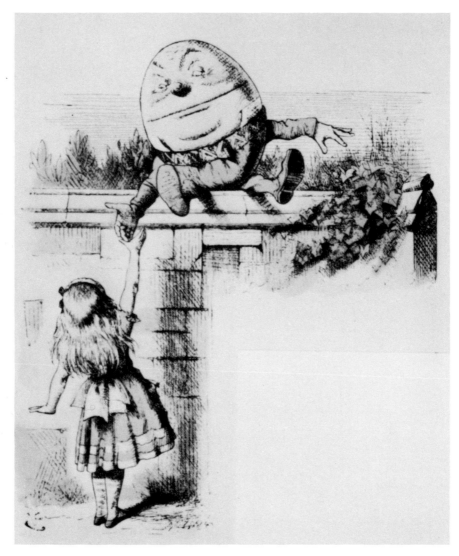

Frontispiece   "When I use a word," Humpty Dumpty said in a rather scornful tone, "it means just what I choose it to mean—neither more nor less." (by John Tenniel) (Dodgson, 1885)

MEDICINE
LITERATURE
&
EPONYMS:

AN ENCYCLOPEDIA OF MEDICAL EPONYMS DERIVED FROM LITERARY CHARACTERS

Alvin E. Rodin, M.Sc., M.D., F.R.C.P.(C)
Wright State University School of Medicine, Dayton, Ohio
and Jack D. Key, M.A., M.S.
Mayo Medical School and Foundation, Rochester, Minnesota

ROBERT E. KRIEGER PUBLISHING COMPANY
MALABAR, FLORIDA
1989

Original Edition 1989

Printed and Published by
ROBERT E. KRIEGER PUBLISHING COMPANY, INC.
KRIEGER DRIVE
MALABAR, FLORIDA 32950

Library of Congress Cataloging-in-Publication Data

Rodin, Alvin E.
    Medicine, literature & eponyms: an encyclopedia
of medical eponyms derived from literary characters /
by Alvin E. Rodin and Jack D. Key.

    p. cm.
bibliography: p.
Includes index.
ISBN 0-89464-277-4
    1. Medicine—Dictionaries. 2. Eponyms—
Dictionaries. 3. Medicine and literature—
Dictionaries. I. Key, Jack D. II. Title. III. Title:
Medicine, literature and eponyms.
R121, R62 1989
610'.3'21—dc19   88-542
                                                   CIP

10 9 8 7 6 5 4 3 2

DEDICATION

To the Librarians of

Wright State University School of Medicine Fordham
  Health Sciences Library
Mayo Clinic and Foundation Medical Library
Dayton and Montgomery County Public Library

without whose expertise, enthusiasm, and indulgence
this project would never have come to fruition.

CONTENTS

*Frequently used references are indicated in each eponym by author's name only or also volume or page numbers where necessary.

List of Illustrations

Frontispiece

Foreword

Authors Al Rodin and Jack Key have done far more than assemble the first encyclopedic listing of medical names derived from literature—though for that immensely useful task alone we should be grateful. They have also produced a book that lures the child in us at the same time that it engages and provokes the adult.

Dip into the book anywhere, an act that does it no disservice, and you will meet arresting images. "Andy Gumps" have no chins. Some retarded children jerk and smile like "Happy Puppets." Sneak a look at any of the pages and discover secret behaviors. Here men desire their mothers. There bearded ladies give birth to bearded babies. Stones melt under an Irishman's buttocks; thus he becomes the patron saint of proctology. Who is proof against such outrageous charm?

Yet reading this book is by no means a game of Trivial Pursuit. The authors have set our oddities in narrative contexts broad enough to mitigate their strangeness. Furthermore, as the stories of the eponyms accumulate, they become a kind of testimony to our humanity. They are evidence of our shared inheritance from the archetypal Adam and Eve. Like them, we are compelled to name everything we see so that we can know it, control it, and cozy up to it, even—as in the case of sickness—to that which is sad or horrible.

But how should we name something? This question the authors inevitably raise through their examination of an eponym's appropriateness. In medicine particularly, should we not provide only names that are emotionally neutral? When recurrent and unexplained staphylococcal skin infections are called "Job's Syndrome," are we not saying a good deal more than we want to? There is no question, on the other hand, that the reference to Job is memorable. It is also simple, playful, and startling enough to motivate our childlike curiosity. Herein lies the first of four provocative tensions underlying this fascinating book.

A tale told by Mark Twain about naming the animals in Eden further illustrates the first point. In Twain's *Papers of the Adam Family*, Adam comes home to Eve from a hard day's work in the Garden.[1] Their conversation goes something like this: "What did you do today?" Eve asks. "Today," Adam says, "I named the four-pronged white squirter." The four-pronged white squirter? "Yes, you know, the animal that . . . ." (here Adam describes in detail how the newly named animal functions). "Oh," says Eve, dismissing his careful work, "you mean the *cow*. Everyone knows that's a cow."

Of course, "Job's Syndrome" is far more logically apt than "cow." Nevertheless, Eve is like the namers in the pages of this book. Her name for the animal in question is inventive. It is capable of attracting connotations. Adam's is descriptive and designed to be useful. He is the scientist. In our times he would be a writer of DSM-

III,[2] the definitive book of psychiatric terminology. Eve would be speaking imaginatively of Oedipus Complexes and, if she were a professor, trailing crowds of wide-eyed students.

She would be morally negligent, however, if she thought that naming an entity fixed our understanding of it forever. Unfortunately, that tendency accompanies any name, especially a name as spirited as a literary eponym. The "Happy Puppet Syndrome," for instance, is so vivid an image that its use may tempt us to look no further for neurological information. A puppet implies an identifiable handler, a brain lesion that controls all movements. But suppose that image prevented investigators from asking whether the smiles present in this syndrome were also socially reinforced? Such a situation is possible, after all, even in severely retarded people. In short, what enchants our imagination may also freeze our understanding.

The opposite is also true. When our rational selves are at work without connection to the vital roots of our imaginations, the results may be deadly: dull lists of four-pronged white squirters. Therefore, insofar as the eponyms in this book rouse our imagination for further work, they do medicine a great service. True creativity in medicine or any other field is always a process uniting rationality and imagination. Call it disciplined imagination. The creative adult drinks regularly from the childlike, intuitive wellspring of fantasy, play, and stark perception. Then he or she returns—that is why creativity is called a process—to disciplined investigation and expression.

A second challenge inherent in the eponyms is their use in communication. Suppose—to return to a previous example—a parent of a newly diagnosed child overhears a physician saying to a colleague, "Come on down to Room 5. I want to show you a Happy Puppet"? There is no way in the world that such a name can encompass the experience of the parent. The parent's and the child's tragedies require a more dignified designation. At such a time, the eponym "Happy Puppet" becomes less a useful image for remembering a neurological condition than a two-dimensional cartoon substituting for a real-life complexity.

Why, then, do medical people reach so often for literary eponyms? The hundreds of examples in this book remind us that communication between physician and patient is extraordinarily difficult. Straightforward scientific descriptions of disease do not always communicate to a patient. Nor, for that matter, do they always satisfy the emotional needs of a physician to place illness in a human context. Every day, therefore, doctors reach for analogies, metaphors, and eponyms to attempt to communicate not only what is known about certain medical conditions, but also—probably the more important function of such imaginative language—what is unknown. So much is still a mystery in medicine, and as such it cannot be scientifically described. But, it can be loosely circumscribed, and thus to some extent controlled, through the use of a figure of speech. "Happy Puppet" can give medical people an image to rest on while they are working out the still unknown neurological details. Physicians who know their patients well might also use the eponym with certain families who can likewise focus their unanswerable questions and roaming terrors through a concrete image.

A third creative tension in this book is that it indirectly reveals certain ambiguities about medicine's understanding of itself. It is easy to forget that at various times in history society assigned some of medicine's current functions to other members. It is not inevitable, for instance, that mental discomfort should be dealt with primarily by people within medicine or even allied to it. Roughly half of these literary eponyms come from psychiatry. That does not mean, as might be assumed by some readers, that psychiatrists necessarily have a deeper education in literature than other physicians do. That may or may not be true. What is certainly true is that society has long allowed, in fact expected, literary people to participate in interpreting mental discomfort.

Literature is a natural resource for psychiatrists as they attempt to name the complexities with which they must deal. Literature dramatizes mental illness, as life does, and as scientific terminology does not. But literary people are more than a resource to medicine. They are fully equal shareholders in the important social task of building perceptions about mental illness. To a lesser extent, literature (together with history, economics, and a range of other perspectives) rightfully participates in the issues that shape all of medical care. However challenging that may be, the fact remains that medicine is simply too big to be left to doctors.

A fourth tension in this book is what it emphasizes about medicine's impact upon literature. Just as eponyms can sometimes misrepresent life, they can also misrepresent literature. That will concern some of us more than others. Readers, after all, have always taken what they want from literature and reinterpreted classics for contemporary needs. Still, the great literary texts—for example, *Oedipus Rex*, the source of the most influential medical eponym—are one of the bases for our concept of civilization. To muddle them is to muddle ourselves. Yet when Freud coined the term Oedipus Complex, he may have left the majority of his intellectual descendants convinced that there was a literary character who desired his mother, hated his father for coming between them, and felt consequent guilt that delayed his development. Sophocles wrote no such play. His Oedipus was led by his fate, not his unconscious, to kill a man and marry a woman who could not possibly have been his parents as far as he knew. In fact, he did what he could to avoid such a tragic outcome, but the fault was there the whole time in his stars. Freud's eponym warped the Greek interpretation of human events so that he could convince people of the role the individual's unconscious motives play in shaping life and history.

Underlying all the issues raised by this fine book, and pervading the valuable lists and tales, is an uneasy awareness that naming has great power. Primitive cultures never confused names with simple labels. A name was thought to give the namer control over people and objects by grasping their essential natures. In some cases, infants were given secret names in addition to everyday ones as protection against those who could bring down malevolent forces upon them if their real names were known. No matter that we have come far from animistic supernaturalism; we can still feel the strength of good and bad names in shaping our reality. It is not going too far to say that the effectiveness of patient care depends upon the seemingly trivial act of naming. In the beginning is the name.

—Joanne Trautmann Banks

Dr. Banks was the first full-time professor of literature and medicine when she was appointed in 1972 at the Pennsylvania State University College of Medicine. She now lives and writes in Florida and is Adjunct Professor of Humanities at Penn State.

1. Twain, M. (S. Clemens): *Letters from the Earth*: ed. Bernard DeVoto, New York, Harper & Row, 1962, pp. 57–114.
2. American Psychiatric Association: *Diagnostic and Statistical Manual of Mental Disorders:* 3rd ed., Washington, D.C., Am. Psychiatric Assoc. 1987.

Preface

Medicine, Literature & Eponyms: An Encyclopedia of Medical Eponyms Derived From Literary Characters provides an interdisciplinary amalgamation that can enrich and interest many different disciplines as well as the general public. The book is oriented to physicians, other health care workers, authors, and the laity—scholars and students alike.

The project began somewhat inauspiciously and insidiously in March 1983 when the authors were brainstorming a medical history project which has since been published. Our long labor of love was serendipitously inaugurated when a literary medical eponym caught our fancy. This seminal eponym was the Mary Poppins Syndrome, derived from a British nanny who could fly with no evident means, and is used, therefore, to describe individuals who have feelings of weightlessness. Much to our embarrassment, the information related to this syndrome has been lost; detailed records were not made in the embryonic stages of enthusiasm for the project. The source of the Mary Poppins eponym has not been recoverable even with expert searches by the ever obliging librarians. To our chagrin, this excellent literary derived eponym cannot be included in this encyclopedia because one of the criteria which we have established is that all entries must be referenced as to source.

Even without the Mary Poppins Syndrome we were hopeful in the initial stages that at least twenty-five literary-derived medical eponyms would be found—enough for a substantial paper. When we eked out fifty, the need to change our orientation to a modest book became evident. Then when one hundred eponyms were uncovered, they proved to be the "critical mass" that opened the flood gates to many more. Factors in obtaining a plethora of further items include an increasing expertise in ferreting out sources, accosting librarians who rapidly became enthused with the subject, and soliciting coworkers for further literary eponyms. As our monomania became generally known, it was fed by well-meaning friends and neighbors who proffered eponyms which they had encountered, an example being Bovarism. Audiences at presentations on the subject provided us with others, such as the Panglossian Paradigm.

At present, over 350 medical eponyms derived from literary characters have been collected and are included in this encyclopedia. But the end may not be in sight. Just before writing this preface, one of the authors was relaxing with a favorite magazine, and came across yet another literary/medical eponym.[1] "Boris and Doris Campbell, famed for decades as the Campbell Soup Kids, died today within hours of each other. Doctors at the scene believe both succumbed to the Smurf Disease, otherwise known as 'acute cuteness.' " Unfortunately, this parody does not meet one of our standards for inclusion in the encyclopedia—a relationship to an actual medical condition or topic.

1. Jacobs, F.: Obituaries of merchandising characters: *Mad*, No. 274, October, 1987, p. 13.

AER
JDK

Introduction

An eponym is one of several linguistic devices in the English language that contribute to its imagery, enrichment, and utility. Among such devices are: *acronyms*, words formed by the initial letters of words in a set phrase (e.g., WAAC, RADAR); *analogies*, comparisons of similar features of two different things (e.g., the heart and a pump); *euphemisms*, mild, indirect, or vague expressions used to replace ones that are considered to be offensive or harsh (e.g., to pass away for to die); *metaphors*, figures of speech in which a term is transferred from the object it ordinarily designates to an object it may designate only by implicit comparison (e.g., God is a mighty fortress); *similies*, figures of speech in which unlike things are explicitly compared (e.g., she is like a rose); and *synonyms*, words having the same or nearly the same meaning as other words in the same language (e.g., glad, elated, joyful).[1]

The *eponym* is not the least of these linguistic devices. It is defined as "a person, real or imaginary, from whom something takes or is said to take its name."[1] The use of personal names for other purposes is considered lightly in civilized societies. It is not so in some primitive tribes in which a name is considered to be a distinct and integral part of the individual.[2] Thus, one could harm an enemy by using his name magically. In our society, names of individuals are used to designate various human or nonhuman conditions, situations, or activities. Usually the transfer of the name immortalizes a positive contribution or characteristic of an individual (e.g., Braille); but in some instances, it immortalizes one's failings (e.g., Quisling). Well known are individuals honored in the names of streets, towns, and countries (e.g., America), of machinery (e.g., diesel engine), and even of clothing (e.g., mackintosh raincoat). When an eponym is not capitalized it indicates that the term has become completely absorbed in everyday language, i.e., it has become generic.[3]

Medical Eponyms

Eponyms are found in the sciences as well as in the vernacular. Thus, the ampere is named after André Amperé, Archimede's Principle after the Greek mathematician, and Bunsen Burner after a German scientist.[4] Medicine is not exempt from the eponymic syndrome (the mania to apply names of individuals to medical conditions, structures, or processes). The majority of medical eponyms are derived from names of those who first described a disease, such as Alzheimer's Disease and Bright's Disease. Eponyms are even derived from patients, as for example Lou Gehrig's disease and Christmas disease.[5] Not neglected are the names of mythical, biblical or, fictional characters—Oedipus Complex, Job's Syndrome, and Pickwickian Syndrome among several hundred others.

Although eponyms have become a significant feature of medical terminology, their use is not without controversy. Burchell has listed several advantages and disadvantages of eponyms in medicine.[6] Positive influences are economy of words in communications (medical shorthand), creating interest in medical history, adding spice to dialogue, and immortalization of greats of the profession. Negative aspects are absence of agreed upon definitions, improperly conferred eponyms (Meckel's instead of Hunter's diverticulum), and jargon which limits dissemination of knowledge, and lends itself to parochialism and chauvinism. Confusion may also arise when one person's name is affixed to more than one condition (i.e., von Recklinghausen, Charcot).[7]

More basic problems exist in the use of medical eponyms. They are not descriptive, and often outgrow their utility.[3] One example is the name Tay-Sach's disease, which was originally given to a syndrome of dementia and blindness in infants that is now known to be only one of a group of diseases caused by different biochemical deficiencies. In order to acknowledge the contribution of several coworkers, cumbersome eponyms are sometimes used, such as Hand-Schüller-Christian syndrome or Weaver-Boeck-Schaumann syndrome.[8] Applying a specific name to a condition gives it an aura of being a fully understood entity, and thereby may inhibit further study. An additional concern is that the indiscriminate use of proper names for eponyms creates a nosological nightmare, especially when applied to trivial symptoms or appearances. These advantages and disadvantages of medical eponyms apply as well to those derived from literary sources.

Literature and Medicine

The use of names of fictional characters for medical eponyms falls into the category of Literature and Medicine, a rapidly developing major discipline in the humanities. It is related to the enlarged and humane outlook that results when there is a merger of C.P. Snow's two cultures—literature and science.[9] Both disciplines become enriched, that of the nonscientist by an appreciation of the natural wonder of the world, and that of the scientist by a wider world view. Increasing interest in the hybrid of literature/medicine has resulted in a proliferation of related publications. There are collections of pithy quotations,[10] of tender and moving excerpts,[11] of dramatic and moral segments,[12] of anthologies of short stories,[13] of comprehensive bibliographies,[14] and in 1982 even a journal of commentaries on this neophyte field.[15]

The phrase literature and medicine can be used with various connotations. Even the word literature is open to several interpretations. Dictionary definitions include all writings of a people, era, or activity; elegant and refined artistic writings (belle-lettres); and writings of universal interest, excluding scientific and technical works.[16] The word literature is widely but inappropriately used for scientific medical writings. The current connotation of literature and medicine is, however, generally restricted to fictional works.

On a pragmatic level, this field concerns itself primarily with fictional works having medical content.[17] The quantity of such content varies. Thus, there is medical fiction in which a physician, patient, or disease constitutes the major plot orientation; for example, Somerset Maugham's *Of Human Bondage*[18] and Sinclair Lewis's *Arrowsmith*.[19] The other category can be defined as medical items in fiction in which the medical elements are not an integral part of the story line. Therefore, literature and medicine as now practiced refers essentially to medical content within fictional works.

There is, however, another relationship between medicine and literature, and that is the converse, literature within medicine. The science and practice of medicine have always been influenced by the environment in which they have flourished. These have received considerable study. Examples are technology, science, economics, politics, ethics, culture, social mores, and law. The permeation of and influence on medicine by literature is extensive and has been neglected to a large extent. It can play a significant role in providing a broader and more humane orientation to medicine. Literature impacts on medicine in two forms, the description of disease in characters, and the use of names of its characters as eponyms for medical nomenclature.

Literary Medical Eponyms

Some proponents of eponyms cite as support for their use the need to humanize or even personalize medicine. "I have long worshiped the eponym as one of the last vestiges of humanism remaining in an increasingly numeralized and computerized society."[20] "In defense of the use of eponyms, [they] play an important role in the 'humanistic aspect' of medicine, . . . it [the eponym] provides a familiarity with the subject and establishes a sort of personal relationship between the physician using it and that particular entity."[21] Such statements are even more applicable to the subcategory of literary medical eponyms, which form a surprisingly significant part of medical nomenclature, both scientific and otherwise. They have been considered to be a "satire or caricature—not a rejection or a distortion of reality but an emphasis on certain of its features through the light touch of humor."[22]

In all, even the most trivial literary eponyms link medicine to the mainstream of the society in which it exists. The analysis of their validity can lead to a greater understanding of the medical condition, the literary source, and the impact on medicine of the milieu in which it exists. Literary eponyms can bring medicine in line with the great wealth of human experience that is represented by literature.

More specifically, such literary-related eponyms can, at their best, highlight or clarify a manifestation of disease as illustrated in literary characters. More fundamental, and potentially more important, is their capability to decrease the gulf between science and humanism, and to increase the appreciation of disease as an intensely human experience, both personal and social. This type of eponym helps both physician and patient to put disease in the broader context of human culture; helps them to conceptualize disease in nontechnological clothing; contributes to the humanization of medicine; and enhances sympathy of the profession and laity alike for those afflicted with illness. Such eponyms can decrease the tendency of physicians to dehumanize patients, can envelope diseases in human rather than technological terms, and can increase appreciation of disease as a human experience.

These needs have been well expressed by Charles Odegaard in discussing "theatre, literature, and the other arts."[23]

Familiarity with the works of Shakespeare, Dostoyevsky, and Flaubert also prepares doctors to recognize peculiarities and complexities in the experience of patients that they could not otherwise apprehend. Without the arts and the human sciences, physicians could use only the typifications of human behavior that they have acquired by participation in the everyday world. Such typifications, because of their generic and vague outlines, cannot possibly capture the complicated and unusual interconnections of human experiences that frequently emerge in medical practice. If physicians are to interpret the evidence correctly, then, they must draw on those disciplines and fields that present them with complex and unusual interconnections: the human sciences and the arts.

Delineation of Medical Eponyms

In this encyclopedia, the designation of an eponym as a literary medical eponym is based on the definition of the word literature as given above.[16] These eponyms are taken from the following categories of literature.

A. Mythology
   1. Classical Greece and Rome
   2. Other Cultures
B. Children's Fables
   1. Anthropomorphic Tales
   2. Adventures
C. Scriptural
   1. Old and New Testaments
   2. Saints
D. Literary Prose
   1. Twelfth to Eighteenth Centuries
   2. Nineteenth and Twentieth Centuries
E. Other Literary Forms
   1. Poetry
   2. Performing Arts
F. Art
   1. Drawings and Paintings
   2. Comic Strips and Cartoons

Myths, although fictitious in nature, differ from other types of narrative fiction by "involving supernatural persons, actions, or events, and embodying some popular idea concerning natural or historical phenomenon."[24] They contain "some kind of universal explanation that gives human life its meaning and ethics. . . ."[25] It is this cosmic view and its cultural acceptance that separates primitive and classical mythology from other works of fiction. The adjective scriptural refers to the Bible and to works based upon, derived from, or dependent upon it.[26] These works also provide a universal view of man and his ethos, but differ from myths, as they are based on written works and are related to historical events.

Fables or fairy tales differ from myths, although also fictitious,[27] in that they do not or did not have a cultural basis of belief; often originate from the pen of a specific author; and present specific human problems and morals rather than a universal explanation of nature and man.[28] The other categories in our classification are self-explanatory. Taken in their entirety, these categories of literature in its broad sense encompass all of the aspirations, fears, beliefs, and imaginations of mankind. And when the nature and names of these characters are applied to medical conditions, processes, or structures the result is a humanization of its scientific concepts and of the practice of medicine.

For the purposes of this encyclopedia, we have developed criteria for acceptance of a literary character as a medical eponym. First, the character must depict a human being, or a humanoid (e.g., robot, puppet), or an anthropomorphized creature (e.g., animal, insect). Second, the eponym must have been used for a specific health-related condition, process, or activity (physical or mental diseases, therapy, research, anatomic structures, chemical or physiologic processes, health care delivery or systems). Third, the eponym must have been so named and described in a publication (book, journal, news periodical).

Some of the eponyms consist of only one word, that of the name of the literary character (e.g., Cyclops, Hymen, Moron) or are modified into a noun (e.g., Aphrodisiac, Bovarism, Icarusism). Commoner are two-word eponyms, often with the name followed by the term complex (e.g., Oedipus Complex), or syndrome (e.g., Lot Syndrome), or disease (e.g., Aguecheek's Disease). The term complex was introduced into psychiatry and psychology in the sense of "a group of repressed ideas interlinked into a complex whole, which besets the individual, impelling him to think, feel and perhaps act after a habitual pattern."[29] The term is so used in medical eponyms for essentially psychological conditions, as, for example, Laius Complex.

A syndrome can be defined as a group of signs and symptoms that characterize a specific disease or abnormal condition, and therefore could be mental (e.g., Cinderella Syndrome), biochemical (e.g., Lot's Wife Syndrome), pharmacological (e.g., Atropine), physiological (e.g., Ondine's Curse), anatomical (e.g., Mons Veneris), or morphological (e.g., Leprechaunism) in nature.[30] Syndrome is often used interchangeably with disease—although a syndrome tends to be used more often for a disease with a more obscure etiology and pathogenesis.[31] There are many other words which are used to modify the name of literary characters, examples being Lunar Effect, Janusian Thinking, and Midas Factor.

Discussions of the eponyms are of variable length owing to several factors. These include the medical importance of the condition, prominence in medical writings, complexity of the subject, and, undoubtedly, interests of the coauthors. The discussion of each eponym has the same general format—synopsis of medical condition or state, biographical abstract of the literary character, concordance between the two, other literary references to the condition or state, and related literary, psychosocial, cultural, and historical material. The literary medical eponyms in the encyclopedia provide, to a varying degree, humanistic, historical, and cultural perspectives to microcosms of medicine. In so doing they counterbalance the heavy emphasis of modern health care on detailed information and technology, and help to free students and practitioners from the constraints of traditional beliefs, arcane knowledge, and myopic attitudes.

1. Stein.

2. Frazer, J. G.: *The Golden Bough. A Study in Magic and Religion:* Vol. 1, abridged ed., N.Y., Macmillan, 1951, pp. 284–289.

3. What's in a name? The eponymic route to immortality: *Essays of an Informed Scientist,* 6:384–395, 1983.

4. Espy.

5. Hendrickson.

6. Burchell, H. B.: Thoughts on eponyms: *Int. J. Cardiol.,* 8:229–234, 1985.

7. Gall, E. A.: The medical eponym: *Am. Sci.,* 48:51–57, 1960.

8. Willis, R. A. & Willis, A. T.: *Principles of Pathology and Bacteriology:* 3rd ed., New York, Appleton-Century-Crofts, 1972, p. 676.

9. Snow, C. P.: *Two Cultures and a Second Look:* Cambridge, Massachusetts, Cambridge University Press, 1964.

10. Coope, R.: *The Quiet Art. A Doctor's Anthology*: Edinburgh, E. & S. Livingstone, 1962.

11. Corcran, A. C.: *A Mirror Up to Medicine*: Philadelphia, J. B. Lippincott, 1961.

12. Davenport, W. H. Ed.: *The Good Physician. A Treasury of Medicine*: New York, Macmillan, 1962.

13. Ceccio, J.: *Medicine in Literature*: New York, Longman, 1978.

14. Trautmann, J. & Pollard, C.: *Literature and Medicine. Topics, Titles and Notes*: Philadelphia, Society Health and Human Values, 1976.

15. Rabuzzi, K. A.: Editor's column: *Lit. Med.*, 1:vii–viii, 1982.

16. Stein, pp. 836–837.

17. Rousseau, G. S.: Literature and medicine: The State of the field: *ISIS*, 72:406–424, 1981.

18. Maugham, S.: *Of Human Bondage*: London, W. Heineman, 1915.

20. Lewis, S.: *Arrowsmith*: New York, Harcourt, 1925.

20. Robertson, M. G.: Fame is the spur the clear eponym doth raise: *J.A.M.A.*, 221:1278, 1972.

21. Magalini, S. I. & Scracia, E: *Dictionary of Medical Syndromes*: 2nd ed., Philadelphia, J. B. Lippincott, 1981, p. viii.

22. London, S. J.: The whimsy syndromes. The fine art of literary nosology: *Arch. Int. Med.*, 122:448–451, 1968.

23. Odegaard, C. E.: *Dear Doctor. A Personal Letter to a Physician*: Menlo Park, California, Henry J. Kaiser Family Foundation, 1986, pp. 150–151.

24. OED: VI:818.

25. Jacob, F.: *The Possible and the Actual*: New York, Pantheon Books, 1982, p. 23.

26. OED: IX:284–285.

27. OED: IV:1–2.

28. Heuscher, J. E.: Cinderella, Eros and Psyche: *Dis. Nerv. Syst.*, 24:296–297, 1963.

29. Campbell, p. 120.

30. Thomas, p. 1677.

31. Durham, p. xiii.

Medical Eponyms Derived from Literary Characters

The eponyms followed by another eponym in parenthesis are not given a major heading in the text, but are discussed under a related eponym. The name of the latter is given in parenthesis or indicated by the abbreviation (inf.) if located in the eponym immediately below, and (sup.) if above.

–A–

Abraham Ward
Abraham's Balm (Agnus Castus)
Abram-Man (sup.)
Achilles Syndrome
Achilles Tendon
Acromegalic Pickwickian
    (Pickwickian Syndrome)
Adam Complex
Adam and Eve Evolution
Adam and Eve Syndrome
Adam's Apple
Adam's Deficiency
Advances in Thanatology (Thanatos)
Aesculapian
Aesculapian Board (sup.)
Aesculapius (sup.)
Agnus Castus
Aguecheek's Disease
Ahasuerus Syndrome
Albatross Procedure (inf.)
Albatross Syndrome
Alice in Wonderland Experience
Alice in Wonderland State (inf.)
Alice in Wonderland Syndrome I, II
Ammonia
Ammon's Horn
Anankastic Syndrome (Thanatos)
Andy Gump Deformity
Andy Gump Fracture (sup.)
Angel Wings Sign
Aphrodine (inf.)
Aphrodisiac
Aphrodite Porne (sup.)
Arachnodactyly
Arachnoid Membrane, Space (sup.)
Argus
Athena (Minerva Medica)
Atlas
Atreus Complex
Atropa belladonna (inf.)
Atropine

–B–

Bane of Hypnos (Hypnosis)
Beetle of Aphrodite (Aphrodisiac)
Bellman's Fallacy
Berserk (Lunacy)
Bovarism
Brain of Pooh
Bugs Bunny Bulimia (Falstaff
    Obesity)

–C–

Cain Complex
Cain Factor (sup.)
Cain Personality
Caput Medusae
Cassandra (inf.)
Cassandra Prophecy
Centaur (inf.)
Centaur Figure (inf.)
Centaurius
Charon Complex (Ophelia Complex)
Cheshire Cat Syndrome
Chimera
Cinderella
Cinderella Complex
Cinderella Dermatosis
Cinderella Effect (Cinderella
    Complex)
Cinderella Syndrome
Clio (inf.)
Clio Medica
ClioPedic (sup.)
Clytemnestra Complex (Electra
    Complex)
Collar of Vulcan
Coma
Cupid's Bow Contour
Cupid's Disease (Syphilis)
Curse of Prometheus (Promethean
    Genes)
Cyclopamine (inf.)
Cyclopia

—D—

Daedalus (Icarus Complex)
Dark Warrior Epilepsy (Pac-Man Epilepsy)
Daughter of a Don Juan (Don Juan Syndrome)
Delilah Syndrome
Delphian Node
Delphian Oracle (sup.)
Dermatitis of Onan (Onanism)
Diana Complex
Disbelieving Cassandras (Cassandra Prophesy)
Don Juan of Achievement (inf.)
Don Juan Syndrome
Don Quixote Enterprise (inf.)
Don Quixote Syndrome
Don Quixotism

—E—

Electra Complex
Elfin Facies Syndrome
Elf-shot (sup.)
Elisha Method
Elpenor Syndrome
Ephebiatics (Hebephrenia)
Eros (inf.)
Eros Principle (inf.)
Erotomania
Erysichthon Syndrome
Esau Lady
Ether
Eye of Horus

—F—

Fallen Angel I, II
Falstaff Obesity
Falstaff Snore
Faun's Beard
Faust Complex
Fiacre
Frankenstein Complex
Frankenstein Factor
Frankenstein Monster (sup.)
Frankenstein Syndrome

—G—

Gargoylism
Griselda Complex
Guild of St. Luke, SS. Cosmas and Damian

—H—

Hamlet-Gertrude Complex
Happy Puppet Syndrome
Harlequin Color change
Harlequin Fetus
Hebephrenia
Heir of the Oedipus Complex (Oedipus Complex)
Hemeralopia
Heracles Complex (Laius Complex)
Hercules Morbus (Saint Paul's Evil)
Hermaphrodite
Hermes
Hermes Syndrome (sup.)
Hippocrates (Aesculapian)
Holmesian Technique
Huckleberry Finn Syndrome
Humpty Dumpty Complex (Humpty Dumpty Phenomenon)
Humpty-Dumpty Etymology
Humpty Dumpty Phenomenon
Humpty Dumpty Syndrome I, II
Hygeia (inf.)
Hygiea (inf.)
Hygiene
Hymen
Hymenitis (sup.)
Hymeno- (sup.)
Hypnosis

—I—

Icarus Complex
Icarusism (sup.)
Infant Esau (Esau Lady)
Insurance Hebephrenia (Hebephrenia)
Inverted Oedipus Complex (Oedipus Complex)
Invisible Man Syndrome (Lilliputian Syndrome)
Iris
Isis

—J—

Janiceps Twins
Janus
Janusian Thinking
Jeckyll-and-Hyde Syndrome
Job's Disease (inf.)
Job's Comforter (inf.)

Job's Syndrome
Job's Ward (sup.)
Jocasta Complex I, II
Joseph Complex
Joseph Fantasy (sup.)
Journal of Thanatology (Thanatos)
Judas Goat

–L–

Lady Godiva Syndrome
Laius Complex
Lasthénie de Ferjol Syndrome
Lazarus Complex
Lazarus Illness
Lear Complex
Leontes Syndrome
Leprechaunism
L'herbe de St. Main (Saint Main's
 Disease)
Lilliputian Eyes
Lilliputian Syndrome
Lolita Complex
Lot Syndrome
Lot's Wife Syndrome
Lues Venerea (Venereal)
Lunacy
Lunar Effect (sup.)
Lupus (inf.)
Lycanthropy

–M–

Mad Hatter Syndrome
Madonna-Harlot Syndrome
Madonna Subconscious (sup.)
Manes Ayoul (Job Syndrome)
Mark of Cain (Cain Complex)
Matthew Effect
Medea Complex
Medical Cassandras (Cassandra
 Prophesy)
Medical Messiahs
Medical Nemesis
Medical Odyssey (Ulysses Complex)
Medical Pickwick
Medical Vampire (Vampirism)
Medusa Lock Sign
Medusa's Head
Mercuroform (inf.)
Mercury
Mermaid Deformity (Sirenomelia)

Messiah Complex
Mickey Mouse Marketing (inf.)
Mickey Mouse Sign I, II
Mickey Mouse Syndrome
Midas Factor
Minerva (Minerva Medica)
Minerva Jacket
Minerva Medica
Minerva Pneumatica (Minerva Jacket)
Miss Havisham Syndrome
Mons Veneris
Moron
Morphine
Morphine Abstinence Syndrome
 (sup.)
Moses Complex
Moses Motive (sup.)
Moses Syndrome
Mother Goose Syndrome
Munchausen by Proxy Syndrome
 (inf.)
Munchausen's Syndrome
Myth of Faust

–N–

Narcissism
Nemesis Feeling
New Messiahs (Medical Messiahs)
Nightmare
Noah Urge
Noah's New Flood (sup.)
Nympha (inf.)
Nymphomania

–O–

Oblomov Syndrome
Oedipus Complex
Oedipus-Jocasta Complex (Jocasta
 Complex)
Old Nemesis (Nemesis Feeling)
Old Sergeant Syndrome
Onanism
Onanist Diseases (sup.)
Ondine's Curse
Operation Venus (Venereal)
Ophelia Complex
Ophelia Syndrome
Orestes Complex
Orphan Annie Eyes
Osiris

Othello Syndrome
Our Lady's Sickness (Saint Mary's Disease)

–P–

Pac-Man Phalanx
Pac-Man Tendenitis
Panacea
Pandora's Box
Pandora's Curse (sup.)
Panglossian Paradigm
Panic Terror
Peeping Tom Syndrome
Persephone Syndrome
Peter Pan Profile (inf.)
Peter Pan and Wendy Syndrome
Peter Pan Syndrome I, II
Phaedra Complex
Pickwickian Syndrome
Pied Piper Phenomenon
Pinocchio Appearance
Pinocchio Syndrome
Playboy Bunny Sign
Polle Syndrome (Munchausen Syndrome)
Pollyanna Hypothesis (inf.)
Pollyanna Phenomenon (inf.)
Pollyanna Posture
Pollyanna Principle (sup.)
Pollyanna Process (sup.)
Pollyannaism (sup.)
Popeye Syndrome
Priapism
Principle of Rumpelstiltskin (Rumpelstiltskin Complex)
Procrustean Perspective
Promethean Genes
Prometheus Experiment (inf.)
Prometheus the Imposter
Proteus
Proteus Syndrome
Psyche
Psychological Achilles Heel (Achilles Syndrome)
Pygmalion Complex
Pygmalionism (sup.)

–Q–

Quasimodo Complex (Quasimodo's Tumor)

Quasimodo Syndrome
Quasimodo's Tumor
Queen of Hell Syndrome
Quixotic Medicine

–R–

Raggedy Ann Syndrome
Rapunzel Syndrome
Red Queen Hypothesis
Rhesus Factor
Rip Van Winkle Experience (inf.)
Rip Van Winkle Syndrome
Robin Hood Legacy (inf.)
Robin Hood Syndrome
Romeo Error
Rumpelstiltskin Complex
Rumpelstiltskin Organization

–S–

Saccharum Saturni (Saturnism)
Saint Anthony's Fire
Saint Job's Disease (Job's Syndrome)
Saint Job's Illness (Lazarus Complex)
Saint John's Disease (Saint Vitus Dance)
Saint Main's Disease
Saint Mary's Sickness (Saint Anthony's Fire)
Saint Paul's Evil
Saint Vitus Dance
Santa Claus M.D. (Moses Syndrome)
Sapphism
Satanic Subconscious (Madonna-Harlot Syndrome)
Saturnine Curse (inf.)
Saturnine Gout (inf.)
Saturnism
Satyr Ears (inf.)
Satyriasis
Serendipity
Shandy Syndrome
Sherlock Holmes Method
Sherlock Holmes Test
Sherlockian Ability (inf.)
Sherlockitis
Sick Santa Syndrome
Sirenomelia
Sisyphean Task (inf.)
Sisyphus Pattern (inf.)
Sisyphus Reaction

Sleeping Beauty Syndrome
Snowman Heart
Snow White–Cinderella Theme
Snow White Syndrome (sup.)
Social Frankenstein (Frankenstein Monster)
Somnipherous
Space Invader's Wrist (Pac-Man Phalanx)
Sphincter
Star Fighter Epilepsy (Saint Paul's Evil)
Stentorial Breathing
Straw Peter Syndrome
Svengali (Hypnosis)
Syphilis
Syringe
Syringoadenoma (sup.)
Syringomyelocele (sup.)
Syringotomy (sup.)

–T–
Thanatophoric Dwarf
Thanatopsy (inf.)
Thanatos
Thanatos Syndrome (sup.)
Tom Sawyer Syndrome (Werther Effect)
Traviata Beauty
Tweedledum and Tweedledee Feeling (Alice in Wonderland Syndrome)
Tweedledum and Tweedledee Syndrome

–U–
Ulysses Complex
Ulysses Contract (inf.)
Ulysses Syndrome
Uraniscus

–V–
Vampirism
Venereal
Venus's Grove (sup.)

–W–
Walter Mitty Syndrome
War Nymphomania (Nymphomania)
Wendy Dilemma (Peter Pan and Wendy Syndrome)

Werther Effect
Wizard-of-Oz Phenomenon (Medical Messiahs)

A

Abraham Ward

The Abraham Ward at Bethlem Royal Hospital (Bedlam) had as its inmates lunatics who were indigent beggars, often dressed in colored ribbons and streamers.[1] The eponym is derived from the parable of Abraham receiving in heaven the beggar, Lazarus, who had been turned away by the rich man and was then carried to Abraham's bosom after death by angels.[2] Related is the designation Tom o'Bedlam, which was given to madmen who were discharged from Bedlam and allowed to beg.[3] The term Abra(ha)m-man was used somewhat similarly in the seventeenth to nineteenth centuries for beggars who wandered around England and pretended to be maniacs—an early example of the Munchausen Syndrome.

The name Bethlem is a corruption of Bethlehem, as is the more colloquial Bedlam, which is now used in general to indicate a noisy confusion of excitement and frenzy.[4] The Bethlem Royal Hospital is one of five Royal Hospitals of London.[5] It was founded in 1247 and became a hospital for the mentally ill in the fifteenth century. In the late nineteenth century, the hospital was moved to its present location in Beckenham, Kent.

Another hospital ward named after a biblical figure is Job's Ward of St. Bartholomew's Hospital (see Job's Syndrome).

1. Hinsie, L. E. & Campbell, R. J.: *Psychiatric Dictionary*: 4th ed., New York, London, Oxford University Press, 1970, p. 4.
2. NT: Luke 16:19–31.

3. Partridge, p. 1245.
4. Skinner, p. 64.
5. Allderidge, P. H.: Historical notes on the Bethlem Royal Hospital and the Maudsley Hospital: Bull. N.Y. Acad. Med. 47:1537–1546, 1971.

Achilles Syndrome

(Achilles heel[1])

Designated as the Achilles Syndrome is a psychological vulnerability or insecurity that regularly leads to the downfall of an individual.[2] If the vulnerability is ignored, suppressed, or denied, it has a tendency to reappear when least expected. Examples are fears and insecurities about losing one's temper, being criticized, getting "hurt," and regaining lost weight. Another is the fear of being financially unsuccessful no matter how much money one is making.

Achilles was the son of the goddess Thetis, the beautiful sea-nymph, and a mortal, Peleus, the son of King Aeacus.[3] Thetis made Achilles invulnerable by plunging him into the river Styx. One heel was not immortal, being the anatomical structure by which she held him. Achilles became the hero of Troy, but was finally slain by Paris, who shot a poisoned arrow into his one vulnerable site. Thus, the eponym Achilles Heel is used commonly to refer to any weak point, including the psychological Achilles heel.[4]

Such godlike heroic figures of Greek mythology as Achilles were considered by Jung to be "symbolic representatives of the whole psyche, the larger and more comprehensive identity that supplies the strength that the personal ego lacks."[5] Heroes, symbolic or otherwise, are especially needed when the ego needs strengthening.

1. Espy, p. 39.
2. Bloomfield, H. H.: *The Achilles Syndrome. Transforming Your Weaknesses into Strengths*: New York, Random House, 1985.
3. Gayley, pp. 269. 307–308.
4. Burns, D. D.: *Feeling Good. The New Mood Therapy*: New York, New American *Library*, 1981, p. 234.
5. Henderson, J. L.: Ancient myths and modern man: in Jung, C., pp. 101, 114–115.

Achilles Tendon

(calcaneal tendon, tendo calcaneus)

The Achilles tendon is a broad tendinous structure which has its origin from the two fleshy bellies of the gastrocnemius muscle in the back of the leg. The tendon is inserted into the posterior surface of the calcaneus bone of the heel.[1] It functions as an extensor of the ankle which enhances forward propulsion, a vital function for a soldier such as Achilles. The derivation of the eponym is the same as for Achilles Syndrome.

1. Anson, pp. 591–592.

Adam Complex

The Adam Complex is similar to the Adam and Eve Syndrome in that it relates to guilt, but only occurring after finding out that one has broken a parental law when previously not aware that it existed.[1] It also differs from the syndrome in that it has been applied more specifically to guilt feelings associated with the Oedipus Complex. The Adam story, however, does not appear to be related to the Oedipus Complex in that he did not have a mother, although he had a father, God, at least in the symbolic sense.[2]

The eponym Adam Complex may be more applicable if the original sin is considered as one of "original sex." Levin has suggested that the forbidden fruit may have been pomegranates, which have a high content of estrogen, presumably aphrodisiac in action.[3]

The phrase not to know from Adam is used to indicate naivete,[4] as exhibited by Adam in following Eve's action of eating the forbidden fruit. ADAM Complex is an acronym for a syndrome of congenital anomalies which includes Amniotic Deformity, Adhesions, and Mutilations.[5] Adam's ale is water.[4]

1. Leguay, D.: Le complexe d'Adam: *Evol. Psychiatri.*, 43:761–779, 1978.
2. OT: Genesis 2.
3. Levin, p. 14.
4. Espy, p. 65.
5. Keller, H. et al.: "Adam complex" (amniotic deformity, adhesions, mutilations)—A pattern of craniofacial and limb defects: *Am. J. Med. Genet.*, 2:81–98, 1978.

Adam and Eve Evolution

(monophylectic evolution)

The names of Adam and Eve are used as an eponym for what is labeled more scientifically as monophylectic evolution. It states that a species arises only once and only in one place.[1] This eponym uses the biblical Adam and Eve as representatives of *Homo sapiens*,[2] and thus embraces the evolutionary theory with a universal concept. Although their origin did occur at one location, the garden of Eden, Adam predated Eve. There is a sect, called preadamites, that believes that men existed on earth before Adam.[3]

1. Shaw, A. B.: Adam and Eve, paleontology, and the non-objective arts: *J. Paleontol.*, 43:1085–1098, 1969.
2. OT: Genesis 2.
3. Espy, p. 66.

Adam and Eve Syndrome

Adam and Eve have been invoked for a syndrome of overwhelming guilt and related depression which arises from a belief that one has disobeyed God.[1] This type of self-judgment can lead to self-punishment in order to circumvent the punishment of God, which would be much more severe. Examples of disobedience are sexual misconduct and negative relationships with parents. The eponym has the virtue of placing this psychiatric state in the context of a universally understood concept, linking it to both cultural and religious sources of guilt feelings.

The punishment of the biblical Adam and Eve for eating the forbidden fruit was not only expulsion from Eden, but also the knowledge of good and evil and the need to cover their nakedness.[2] In a more colloquial sense, the phrase Adam and Eve togs is used in the same sense as "birthday suit," and adamatical as synonymous with naked.[3] An adamite is not only a descendent of Adam, but also one who goes naked.[4] The phrase, Adam and Eve, has been used for various other purposes: a comparison of male and female life expectancy,[5] discussion of sex hormonal balances in both sexes,[6] and a consideration of sex differences in the deoxyribonucleic acid (DNA) of the cell nucleus.[7]

1. Sexton, R. O., & Maddock, R. C.: The Adam and Eve syndrome: *J. Religion Health*, 17:163-168, 1978.
2. OT: Genesis 3.
3. Partridge, p. 5.
4. Espy, p. 66.
5. Starkie, C.: Must Adam die before Eve?: *R. Soc. Promotion Health*, 89:286–288, 1969.

6. Federman, D. D.: Adam and Eve: *Calif. Med.*, 114:32–33, 1971.
7. Jones, K. W.: Snake's eye view of Adam and Eve: *Nature*, 268:107–108, 1977.

Adam's Apple

(pomum adami, thyroid cartilage)

Adam's apple is a colloquial designation for the anterior protrusion in the neck at the level of the glottis. It is caused by the anterior portion of thyroid cartilage.[1] The derivation is from a medieval superstition that a piece of the forbidden fruit stuck in Adam's throat.[2] The eponym Adam's Apple is stated to be a literal translation of the Hebrew *tappuah haadam*.[3] The biblical account, however, does not specify an apple. " . . . she took of the fruit thereof, and did eat; and she gave also unto her husband with her, and he did eat."[4] The fruit became an apple in postbiblical legend.

1. Ferner, p. 201.
2. OED: I:100.
3. Safire, W.: I'm Adam. Want an apple, madam?: *Minneapolis Star & Tribune*, Sept. 22, 1986.
4. OT: Genesis 3:6.
5. Chappell, G. S.: *Through the Alimentary Canal with Gun and Camera*: New York, Dover, 1958., p. 36.

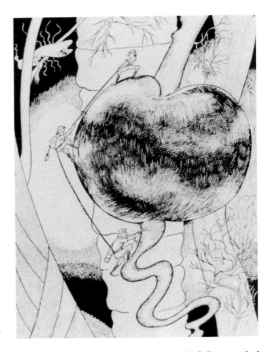

Adam's Apple   Rounding Adam's Apple.[5] (by permission, Dover Pubns., Inc.)

Adam's Deficiency

(congenital lactase deficiency)

A failure of infants to thrive owing to an inability to absorb lactose from the diet was first described in 1959.[1] Lactose is normally hydrolyzed by the enzyme lactase into the absorbable sugars, glucose and galactose. In this condition, lactase is absent from the intestinal mucosa. The result is diarrhea shortly after the newborn begins milk feeding, whether from breast or bottle, and failure to gain weight.[2] This defect is serious because lactose is the only carbohydrate present in any significant amount in milk and represents about 40% of the total caloric value.

The inability to digest lactose to glucose is manifested by a flat blood glucose curve after its ingestion. The basic defect is demonstrated by the absence of lactase activity in an intestinal biopsy.[3] Less than 30 cases have been reported, including several in siblings. Another cause of lactase deficiency is diffuse mucosal damage from various diseases.[4] Whatever the cause, symptoms can be relieved by removal of milk

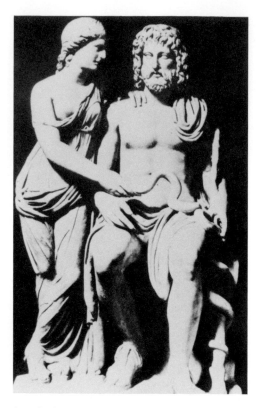

Aesculapian Aesculapius, the god of medicine, with his daughter Hygeia.[13]

from the diet or ingestion of a lactase preparation.

The eponym Adam's Deficiency has been applied to congenital lactase deficiency on the basis that Adam, being the first human, had never been breast fed, and thus had no need for enzymes to digest milk lactose.[5] This rather fanciful eponym is more clever than meaningful. In a similar lighthearted vein is the controversy as to whether or not Adam had a navel, not having been born of a female.

1. Holzel, A. et al.: Defective lactose absorption causing malnutrition in infancy: *Lancet*, 1:1126–1128, 1959.
2. Levin, B. et al.: Congenital lactose malabsorption: *Arch. Dis. Child.*, 45:173–177, 1970.
3. Gardner, L. I. Ed.: *Endocrine and Genetic Diseases of Childhood and Adolescence*: 2nd ed., Philadelphia, W. B. Saunders, 1975, pp. 980–982.
4. Behrman, R. E. & Vaughn, V. C. III: *Nelson Textbook of Pediatrics*: 12th ed., Philadelphia, W. B. Saunders, 1983, p. 938.
5. Levin, p. 19.

Aesculapian

Aesculapian is the name of the journal which was superseded by the *Medical Library and Historical Journal*.[1] The latter in turn was superseded by the present *Bulletin of the Medical Library Association*. Volume 1 of the *Aesculapian* was published in 1908-1909, in Brooklyn, New York.

Aesculapius (Greek Asklepios), the god of medicine, was the son of Apollo and the Thessalian princess, Coronis.[2] When his mother died, the infant was placed in the trust of Chiron, a famous and wise centaur (see Centaurius). He became a great physician: He not only cured the sick, but also restored Hippolytus to life after he had been dashed to death in a chariot accident.

Zeus (Jupiter) killed Aesculapius with a thunderbolt because of the fear that men would escape death altogether through his healing skill. At Apollo's request, Aesculapius was placed in heaven. Machaon, the son of Aesculapius, was a brave warrior as well as a skilled surgeon. He was killed by Eurypylus in the Trojan War;[3] and his ashes were placed in the sanctuary of Gerenia where the sick went for cures. Other members of Aesculapius's family were also involved in healing.[4] His other son,

Telesphorus, represented rehabilitation. His daughters Hygeia and Panacea were goddesses of health and treatment. Even his wife, Epione, soothed pain.

According to René Dubos, Hygeia represented health which "is the natural order of things," and Aesculapius the treatment of disease "to restore health by correcting any imperfections caused by accidents of birth or life."[5] The French psychologist, Diel, proposes that Aesculapius in the broader sense is "a representation of the hope that man may be freed from all evils (even physical disease) by gradual spiritualization . . . those means that are applicable to man as a unity of 'body and psyche.' "[6]

Because of his extraordinary medical skills, Aesculapius's name is indeed worthy for any medical journal. And in fact, the *Index of NLM Serial Titles* lists at least a dozen such, with spellings of the god's name varying with the language of the country of publication.[7] A more recent journal, *Aesculapius*, is the journal of the Medical Heritage Society, being first published in 1971 and dedicated to medical history as well as art and literature.[8] Also of Greek origin, but not mythological, is *Hippocrates*, a medical magazine named after the "father of medicine."[9]

Fictional medical journals are found in literary works. Sinclair Lewis's doctor, Martin Arrowsmith, worked in a research institute that published the *American Journal of Geographic Pathology*.[10] Actual medical journals are also mentioned in fictional works, as for example, the *British Medical Journal*, the *Journal of Psychology*, and the *Lancet* in the Sherlock Holmes stories.[11]

The eponym Aesculapian Board was coined by Joseph Wilde, a thespian, in a long poem entitled *The Hospital*, which was published in 1809.[12] It is based on his admission to a hospital for a "concussion" of the knee caused by a fall on stage. The Aesculapian Board was his term for the medical staff of the hospital. His perception of their rounds provides an excellent insight into the physician/doctor relationship at the beginning of the nineteenth century.

"The daily visit of the prime physicians,
"And still more awful presence of the surgeons."

At the fix'd hour, each cripple ready lays
His wounds all bare; those who are able haste,
And stand before their own peculiar beds, . . .
And each appears a marble momument [sic];
The lame recumbent, and sick erect:
Thus wait they all, in solemn silence hush'd.

1. *Mayo Clinic Library List of Serials*: Rochester, Minnesota, 1971.
2. Gayley, pp. 38, 104, 260, 296.
3. Schmidt, p. 167.
4. Achterberg, J.: *Imagery in Healing*: Boston, New Science Library, 1985, p. 5.
5. Dubos, R.: *Mirage of Health, Utopias, Progress and Biological Change*: New York, Harper & Bros., 1959, pp. 110–111.
6. Diel, p. 199.
7. *Index of NLM Serial Titles*.
8. From the staff of Aesculapius: *Aesculapius*, 1:2, 1971.
9. New magazine set to offer "main course" in health news: *Am. Med. News*, Dec. 6, p. 15.
10. Lewis, S.: *Arrowsmith*: New York, New American Library, 1961, p. 271.
11. Rodin, A. E. & Key, J. D.: *Medical Casebook of Doctor Arthur Conan Doyle*: Malabar, Florida, Robert E. Krieger, 1984.
12. Wilde, J.: *The Hospital, A Poem, Written in the Devon & Exeter Hospital, 1809*: Norwich, England, Stevenson, Matchett & Stevenson, 1809, pp. 7, 38.
13. Bulfinch, p. 226.

Agnus Castus

Medication from the chaste tree (*Vitex agnes castus*) native to the Mediterranean "hath a singular property to procure chastity, for which physicians have named it Agnus castus."[1] Castus is the Latin word for chastity. St. Agnes was a Roman Christian virgin who was stripped naked before a crowd when she refused to offer incense to the alter of Minerva.[2] When her hair fell down and covered her nakedness she was stabbed in the throat (see Lady Godiva Syndrome). Abraham's Balm is another eponym for this ancient medication with the supposed property of reducing sexual desire.[3]

Other substances alleged as having anaphrodisiac action are salicylic acid, quinine, camphor, menthol, and bromides.[4] More ancient is the belief by Pliny that there would be an antiaphrodisiac action on a male if a lizard were dropped into his urine.

1. OED: I:32.
2. Williams, C.: *Saints: Their Cults and Origins*: New

York, St. Martin's Press, 1980, pp. 38–39.
3. OED: I:32.
4. Walker, pp. 9–10.

Aguecheek's Disease

(chronic portal-systemic encephalopathy)

Aguecheek's Disease is an eponym that has been applied to the chronic dementia that occurs in liver disease owing to intolerance of nitrogenous substances.[1] It is characterized by fluctuating personality changes and neurological deterioration.[2] The disease may occur with the ingestion of large amounts of dietary protein, urea, or ammonia salts in patients with cirrhosis,[3] and in those who have had a portocaval shunt operation.[4] The mental changes are due to nitrogenous substances passing through a diseased liver or portosystemic collateral vessels without the usual chemical alteration.[5]

Sir Andrew Aguecheek is a silly, old but immature fop of a knight who exhibits vacillations of his mind in Shakespeare's *Twelfth Night*.[6] He admits that "I am a great eater of beef, and I believe that does harm to my wit." He is considered by Sir Todby Belch to have liver disease. "For Andrew, if he were opened, and you find so much blood in his liver as will clog the foot of a flea, I'll eat the rest of the anatomy." This is a very astute and graphic, albeit satiric, reference to the ischemia that occurs in cirrhosis of the liver.

1. Summerskill, W. H. J.: Aguecheek's disease: *Lancet*, 2:288, 1955.
2. Sherlock, S. et al.: Portal-Systemic encephalopathy. Neurological complications of liver disease: *Lancet*, 2:453-457, 1954.
3. Philips, G. B. et al.: The syndrome of impending hepatic coma in patients with cirrhosis of the liver given certain nitrogenous substances: *N. Engl. J. Med.*, 247:239–246, 1952.
4. McDermott, W. V., Jr. & Adams, R. D.: Episodic stupor associated with an Eck fistula in the human with particular reference to the metabolism of ammonia: *J. Clin. Invest.*, 33:1–9, 1954.
5. White, L. P. et al.: Ammonium tolerance in liver disease: Observations based on catheterization of the hepatic veins: *J. Clin. Invest.*, 34:158–168, 1955.
6. Shakespeare, *Twelfth Night*: I, ii, iii.

Ahasuerus Syndrome

Drug addicts who wander from hospital to hospital simulating disease in order to obtain drugs have been designated as having the Ahasuerus Syndrome.[1] They are considered to

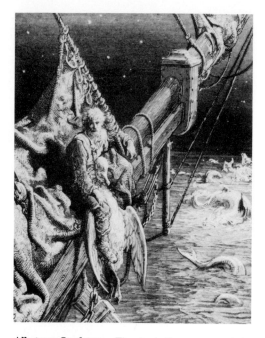

Albatross Syndrome The dead albatross around the neck of the ancient mariner.[3, p. 41] (by Gustave Doré) (by permission of Dover Pubns. Inc.)

have psychopathic personalities. The syndrome is named after the biblical story of Ahasuerus, the "wandering Jew."[2] He was condemned to restless and profitless wandering from place to place ill the Day of Judgement as punishment for insulting Christ on the way to the cross.[3] He is not to be confused with the Ahasuerus who was the king of Persia.[4]

In nineteenth century Europe, the wandering Jew was considered to be afflicted with a traveling neurosis, one manifestation of which was the Diaspora.[5] Charcot, the great French neurologist, considered Jews as a race with a strong propensity for nervous illness, a statement taken by some to be a reflection of the European antisemitism of the time.

The Ahasuerus Syndrome is a variant of the Munchausen Syndrome, used specifically for someone with an addictive need for drugs, narcotics, and/or alcohol.[1] The designation was suggested originally by Wingate as a more suitable name for the generic condition than the Munchausen Syndrome.[6]

1. Wermut, W.: Literary geneologies of some pathologic syndromes: *Psychiatr. Pol.*, 14:69–76, 1980.
2. Anderson, G. K.: *The Wandering Jew*: Providence, Rhode Island, Brown University, 1965.
3. OED: XII:65.
4. OT: Ezra 4:6.
5. Goldstein, J.: The wandering Jew and the problem of psychiatric anti-semitism in Fin-de-Siécle France: *J. Contemp. Hist.*, 20:521–552, 1985.
6. Wingate, P.: Letter to editor: *Lancet*, 1:412–413, 1951.

Albatross Syndrome

(postgastrectomy syndrome with personality defect)

The Albatross Syndrome occurs in postgastrectomy patients who have no demonstrable cause for their symptoms but do have personality defects and neurotic complaints.[1] It is composed of a constellation of complaints, including abdominal pain, nausea, vomiting, drug dependency, and nutritional deficiencies, all without demonstrable cause. The Albatross Syndrome differs from the dumping syndrome in which there is a rapid dumping of food from the postoperative stomach into the jejunum, as demonstrated by x-ray.[2]

The albatross is a large, web-footed seabird

with a wing spread of about 12 feet. It is one of the central characters in the narrative poem *The Rime of the Ancient Mariner* by Coleridge.[3] The killing of an albatross by the mariner was blamed as the cause of the calamity which befell the ship and crew. The dead bird was then hung around his neck to haunt him thereafter.

God save thee, ancient Mariner!
From the fiends, that plague thee thus!—
Why look'st thou so?—With my cross-bow
I shot the Albatross [p. 16].
Ah wel-a-day! what evil looks
Had I from old and young!
Instead of the cross, the Albatross
About my neck was hung [p. 24].

The rash act of killing the albatross is equated with that of the surgeon who is haunted by some postgastrectomy patients who demand that something be done about their symptoms. Postgastrectomy surgery on such patients has been called the Albatross Procedure.[1]

In general, the term an albatross is used to denote a weight around one's neck, or an onerous penalty. In the play *Who's Afraid of Virginia Woolf*, Martha objects that "I wasn't the Albatross . . . you didn't have to take me to get the prize . . . ."[4]

To kill sea birds is considered to be unlucky and to kill an albatross fatal.[5] A literary example is found in Conrad's *Under Western Eyes*,[6] in which Razumov betrays his friend Haldin through fear of his own life. It has been likened to "the Ancient Mariner's killing of the albatross, an abandonment of the ties that bind man and nature."[7] Seagulls have been called ancient mariners because of a superstition that they possess the souls of dead sailors.[8] In fact, the overall theme of *The Rime of the Ancient Mariner* has been equated with life-in-death.[9]

1. Johnstone, F. R. C. et al.: Post-gastrectomy problems in patients with personality defects: The "Albatross" syndrome: *Can. Med. Assoc. J.*, 96: 1559–1564, 1967.
2. Durham, pp. 441–442.
3. Coleridge, S. T.: *The Rime of the Ancient Mariner* (1798): illustrated by G. Doré, New York, Dover, 1970.
4. Albee, E.: *Who's Afraid of Virginia Woolfe?*: New York, Atheneum House, 1962.
5. Partridge, p. 19.

6. Conrad, J.: *Under Western Eyes, A Novel*: London, Methuen, 1911.
7. Cox, C. B.: *Joseph Conrad: The Modern Imagination*: London, J. M. Dent & Sons, 1974, p. 112.
8. Boase, p. 160.
9. Sewell, E.: Poetry and madness, connected or not?—and the case of Hölderlin: *Lit. Med.*, 4:41–69, 1985.

Alice in Wonderland Experience

Contraction and expansion of a prolactin-secreting pituitary tumor has been observed on x-ray films when the patient is treated with an ergot alkaloid which has dopamine-antagonist activity.[1] The exact mechanism is not understood. *Alice's Adventures in Wonderland*[2] is the best known of Lewis Carroll's literary works. Like this syndrome, some episodes of Alice's enlarging and shrinking in size were caused by ingestion of material, in her case, cookies and a mushroom. The changes in size of the pituitary is unlike the Alice in Wonderland Syndrome I in which the distortion in size is psychological. Dreaming of an alteration in body size, either infinitely small or infinitely big, was considered by Jung to be an infantile motif.[3] On a more pragmatic basis, Alice's eating of a specific substance to change her size has been suggested as influencing children toward drug abuse.[4]

1. Williams, R. C. et al.: The "Alice in Wonderland" experience: *West J. Med.*, 138:391–397, 1983.
2. Carroll.
3. Jung, p. 38.
4. Siegel, R. K.: Seduction of the innocent: A clinical note on the effects of cartoons and comics on drug abuse: *J. Psychoactive Drugs*, 17:201–204, 1985.

Alice in Wonderland Syndrome I, II

(hyper- and hyposchematia, metamorphopsia) I The syndrome of bizarre distortions of one's own body image was linked to Alice in Wonderland by Todd,[1] although the condition was described originally by Lippman.[2] It occurs in certain patients with migraine or epilepsy and sometimes in their blood relatives. As described by one such child, "I felt like my hands were made out of tiny twigs with a little mushy flesh on the outside."[3] Another patient who felt short and wide called this a "Tweedledum or Tweedledee feeling," referring to characters from Carroll's other book about Alice, *Through*

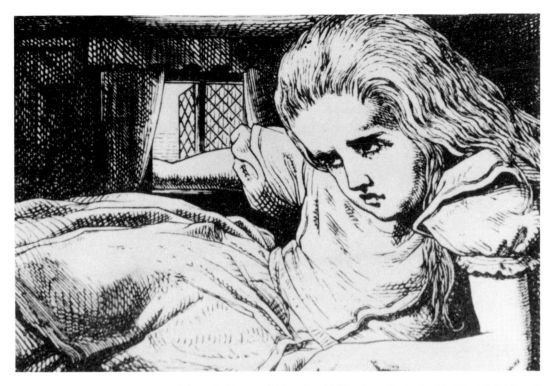

Alice in Wonderland Syndrome   Alice's marked increase in size after drinking from a bottle. (by John Tenniel) (Dodgson)

the Looking Glass. The syndrome can also be caused by psychodelic drugs.[4] Unlike the Alice in Wonderland Experience, there is a perception of change in shape as well as size. Carroll's Alice changed only in her overall size.[5] Another instance is found in the folklore of the Isle of Wight.[6] A man decreased greatly in size when he inhaled some brown powder given to him by fairies.

II The Alice in Wonderland Syndrome has also been applied to children with infectious mononucleosis who may see distortions in sizes, shapes, and spatial relationships of objects rather than of their own body.[7] The syndrome differs from the depersonalization syndrome in which one's body seems changed and no longer one's own.[8]

The phrase Alice in Wonderland has been used for aspects of medical education that are considered to be fantasy or unbelievable, such as some letters of recommendation for residency positions,[9] and the relative neglect of genetics in medical school curriculums.[10] *Through the Looking Glass* has been used as a label for the unreality of physician disinterest in and lack of knowledge of malpractice as a major problem, particularly as it relates to plastic surgery.[11] This may be appropriate because the phrase an Alice is used colloquially for someone who has arrived in strange and fantastic surroundings.[12] Lewis Carroll's are the most often quoted books after Shakespeare's works and the Bible.[13] This is evidenced in part by other syndromes based upon his characters—Cheshire Cat, Humpty Dumpty, Mad Hatter, Red Queen and Tweedledum and Tweedledee.

Comparison with various aspects of Lewis Carroll's *Alice in Wonderland* has been used to highlight conceptual problems in non-Hodgkin's lymphoma, some of which "assume the qualities of surrealistic fantasy."[14] The profusion in staging systems for lymphomas is equated with the caucus race in Carroll's book because neither seems to have a clear start or a clear finish. The extremely complicated approaches to treatment and the unclear degree of success are as difficult to understand as jabberwocky. And when current, conventional treatment of lymphoma is replaced by future research, they will disappear in importance as did the Cheshire cat.

The Alice in Wonderland state has been used to psychoanalyze its author.[15] However, the descriptions of unreality in the book can not be related to Carroll's own migraine headaches because it was written over 25 years before he developed migraine.[16]

There have also been various psychological interpretations of *Alice in Wonderland*: an adult psychological drama with disturbing undertones, a Victorian fantasy about the pains and perils of growing up, and what a young girl thinks of the adult world. Lewis Carroll most likely wrote the story only to entertain his child friends.[17] "The story starts with Alice falling asleep in the sun—does this mean that Carroll intends us to think that Alice dreamt all of this because she developed a sun stroke? No, falling asleep was purely a literary device to give credibility to the make believe."

1. Todd, J.: The syndrome of Alice in Wonderland: *Can. Med. Assoc. J.*, 73:701–704, 1955.

2. Lippman C. W.: Certain hallucinations peculiar to migraine: *J. Nerv. Ment. Dis.*, 116:346–351, 1952.
3. Golden, G. S.: The Alice in Wonderland syndrome in juvenile migraine: *Pediatrics*, 63:517–519, 1979.
4. Vaisrub, p. 22.
5. Carroll, p. 37.
6. Boase, p. 116.
7. Copperman, S. M.: "Alice in Wonderland" syndrome as a presenting symptom of infectious mononucleosis in children: *Clin. Pediatr.*, 16:143–146, 1977.
8. Stockings, G. T.: The depersonalization syndrome: *J. Ment. Sci.*, 93:62–67, 1947.
9. B. M. W.: Is Alice leaving Wonderland?: *Human Pathol.*, 15:401, 1984.
10. Hecht, F.: Teaching medical genetics and Alice in Wonderland: *Am. J. Human Genet.*, 33:138–139, 1981.
11. Rosenthal, S. A. E.: Malpractice—Through the looking glass: *Ann. Plastic Surg.*, 9:326–329, 1982.
12. Hendrickson, p. 10.
13. Clark, A.: *Lewis Carroll. A Biography*: New York, Schocken Books, 1979, p. 139.
14. Glatstein, E.: Lymphomania: Non-Hodgkin's lymphoma as possibly viewed through the eyes of Lewis Carroll: *J. R. Soc. Med.*, 80:70–73, 1987.
15. Schilder, P.: Psychoanalytic remarks on *Alice in Wonderland* and Lewis Carroll: *J. Nerv. Ment. Dis.*, 87:159–168, 1938.
16. Murray, T. J.: The neurology of Alice in Wonderland: *Can. J. Neurol. Sci.*, 9:453–457, 1982.
17. Dunlop, J. M.: The Mother Goose syndrome— A lighthearted look at paediatric literature: *Public Health Lond.*, 88:89–96, 1974.

Ammonia

Ammonia is a colorless gas which has a pungent smell and strong alkaline reaction. It has several pharmacological uses, including correction of metabolic acidosis, an expectorant action, and stimulation of the medullary respiratory and vasomotor centers when inhaled.[1] The name was derived from sal ammonica which is found near the Libyan region of Ammonia, so named for its shrine of Jupiter Ammon, a similar diety to the Egyptian god Amun (Amon).[2] The pungent gas was first observed in the dung of camels left outside of the shrine by supplicants.[3]

1. Gilman, pp. 865–866.
2. Espy, p. 20.
3. Dirckx, p. 73.

Ammon's Horn

(hippocampus)

Ammon's horn is another, albeit infrequently used, name for the hippocampus of the brain.[1] The name is derived from Egyptian mythology, Ammon being a god who is depicted with a ram's head and large curved horns.[2] The basis for the association is the curved nature of the hippocampus. The term hippocampus itself is derived from the shape of a mythical sea monster that the structure is thought to resemble.[3]

1. Anson, p. 986.
2. Ions, V.: *Egyptian Mythology*: New York, Peter Bedrick Books, 1983, p. 90.
3. Dirckx, p. 73.

Andy Gump Deformity

A distinctive appearance is produced by resection of the anterior arch of the mandible and the floor of the mouth, usually for cancer.[1] The appearance resembles that of Andy Gump, the main character in a no longer published comic strip, "The Gumps," begun in 1917 by Sidney Smith.[2] Gump's striking characteristic was absence of the entire lower jaw. The plight of patients with such massive loss of tissue has improved considerably with modern surgical techniques.[3]

The Andy Gump Deformity differs from the congenital anomaly, otocephaly (earhead), which is characterized by severe underdevelopment of the jaw, and is incompatible with extra-uterine existence.[4] It is a very severe variant of the nonliterary Pierre Robin syndrome which has a lesser degree of micrognathia, and is associated with microglossia and palatine fissure.[5]

The Andy Gump Fracture is traumatic, as is the Andy Gump Deformity, but accidental rather than surgical. It is caused by trauma in elderly, edentulous people, with resultant posterior displacement of the chin, prolapse of the tongue, and airway obstruction.[6] This designation is not, however, quite appropriate, as the jaw is still present, although misplaced, and symptomatic unlike that of Andy Gump.

1. Steckler, R. M. et al.: "Andy Gump": *Am. J. Surg.*, 128:545–547, 1974.
2. Daniels, L.: Comix. *A History of Comic Books in America*: New York, Outerbridge & Dienstfrey, 1971, p. 5.
3. Conley, J. & Parke, R. B.: Pectoralis mucocutaneous flap for chin augmentation: *Otolaryngol. Head Neck Surg.*, 89:1045–1050, 1981.

4. Lawrence, D. L. & Bersu, E. T.: An anatomical study of human otocephaly: *Teratology*, 30:155–165, 1984.
5. Durham, p. 489.
6. Seshul, M. B. Sr. et al.: The Andy Gump fracture of the mandible: A cause of respiratory obstruction or distress: *J. Trauma*, 18:611–612, 1978.

Angel Wings Sign

(spinnaker sail sign)

The elevation of the thymus by loculated air in adjacent soft tissues produces an appearance on x-ray film of a curved upper margin and a lower, less curved one resembling an angel's wing.[1] The crescent-shaped density has also been likened to a full-blown spinnaker sail.[2] Angel wings are depicted with various configurations, the commonest being with curved, upper border and a relatively straight lower one.[3] The word angel is derived from the original biblical Hebrew name for attendants and messengers of Jehovah.[4]

1. Eisenberg, p. 279.
2. Moseley, J. E.: Loculated pneumomediastinum in the newborn. A thymic "spinnaker sail" sign: *Radiology*, 75:788–790, 1960.
3. Williams, p. 60.
4. OED: I:323.

Aphrodisiac

An aphrodisiac is a drug or food substance that is alleged to arouse sexual desire or to improve sexual performance.[1] Such a category of drugs is not listed in the Goodman and Gilman authoritative textbook of pharmacology.[2] The effectiveness of some substances, such as psychoactive drugs (cocaine, marijuana, alcohol),[3] may be related to the placebo effect of a strong belief in the aphrodisiac myth.[4] Androgens, however, when given therapeutically have been reported as greatly increasing the sex drive in both females and males.[5] Sigmund Freud, who first promoted cocaine as a therapeutic agent, reported in 1884 that "Among the persons to whom I have given coca, three reported violent sexual excitement which they unhesitatingly attributed to the coca."[6]

Aphrodite (Venus), the Greek goddess of love and beauty, was born out of white foam floating on the surface of waves. She possessed an embroidered girdle (cestus) which had the power of inspiring love.[7] As Aphrodite Urania she became the patron of spiritual love, as Aphrodite Genetrix the patron of marriage, and as Aphrodite Porne the patron of lust and prostitutes (pornography).[8]

Nonscientific approaches to medicine consider many substances as aphrodisiacs, working through analogy, signature, and sympathy.[9] Examples are belladonna, strychnine, garlic, horseradish, leek, hashish, parsnip, chive, and ginseng (extract from an ivy with a penis-shaped root) among many others. In Unani, the Islamic system of medicine, Indragopa (Birbhuti) is a bright-red, eight-legged arachnid. It is taken orally as an aphrodisiac, and applied externally as an ointment to strengthen the penis.[10]

There is one substance which has been considered as an aphrodisiac for many centuries, including the present one. This is Spanish fly, which is obtained from a beetle, *Cantharis vesicatoria*, found in southern France and Spain.[11] The active ingredient in this "Beetle of Aphrodite" is cantharidin, which has an irritant and vesicant action on the skin. As a collodion it is used to remove warts and molluscum contagiosum;[5] but "Despite the lore, it is not an aphrodisiac." There are several possible reasons for the aphrodisiac reputation of Spanish fly.[11] It can cause irritation of the kidneys and bladder with the resultant burning sensation on urination, calling attention to the urethral meatus which is an integral part of the external genitalia; and priapism may occur with toxic doses.

In 1983, a review article on libido stated that the androgen testosterone is the "only true aphrodisiac."[12] Since then several other potential aphrodisiacs have come to the forefront. Yohimbine, a "street" drug (yo-yo), is an alphaZ-adrenergic receptor antagonist derived from the bark of *Pausinystalia yohimbine*, which grows in Africa.[13] It was considered to be the refuge of aging Don Juans in the nineteenth century, but has recently been reactivated as an aphrodisiac in advertisements in a certain pornographic magazine. Its supposed libidinous effect is reflected by its designation as aphrodine, although most researchers in the field consider it to have no such action. In 1986, a report of a study of rat behavior after being given imidazole, an antifungal agent, stated that the results are "interpretable in terms of enhanced sexual arousal and resembling the aphrodisiac effect reported for yohimbine."[14]

Another contender for the libidinous drug of the year is bupropion, an antidepressant similar to amphetamine, which was released by the U.S. F.D.A. in December, 1985. It was distributed under the trade name of Wellbutrin, but it was withdrawn within four months because of a high incidence of seizures in recipients.[15] On April 21, 1987, the national newspaper *USA Today* reported several presentations to be made on Wellbrutin [sic] at the April 30 convention of the American Association of Sex Educators, Counselors and Therapists.[16] Double-blind studies are stated to indicate "boosts in sexual interest and functioning," and noted are efforts by some drug companies for distribution approval for such a use. Not mentioned is that increased sexuality may be the result of a return to a normal libidinous state after relief of depression. The end of the eternal search for Aphrodite, the elusive goddess of love, may not yet be in sight.

A comprehensive list of substances used as aphrodisiacs can be found in a recent book on the subject.[17] Suggested as a biblical aphrodisiac are high doses of estrogen obtained from eating pomegranates (see Adam Complex). More current is a recent report that the addition of an aphrodisiac to flamingo feed at the San Diego Zoo has greatly increased their courting.[18] Its nature is a trade secret. The antithesis of an aphrodisiac is called an anaphrodisiac. One example is the Abraham's Balm (see Agnus castus).

1. OED: I:385.
2. Gilman.
3. Carroll, C. R.: *Drugs in Modern Society*: Dubuque, Iowa, Wm. C. Brown, 1985, pp. 32–33.
4. Rosser, Ms.: The birth of Venus: *Nursing Times*, 80:40–41, 1984.
5. Greenblatt, R. B. et al.: Endocrinology sexual behavior: *Med. Aspects Hum. Sexual.*, 6:119–131, 1972.
6. Shaffer, H.: Uber coca: Cocaine discoveries: *J. Subst. Abuse Treat.*, 1:205–217. 1984.
7. Bulfinch, p. 9.
8. Espy, p. 16.
9. Walker, pp. 13–15.
10. Mahdihassan, S.: Indragopa, a red arachnid, as

an aphrodisiac drug in India, with the significance of the names arya, indra and indragopa.: *Hamdard Natl. Found. Pakistan,* 28:49–59, 1985.

11. Howell, M. & Ford, P.: *The Beetle of Aphrodite and Other Medical Mysteries*: New York, Random House, 1985, pp. 237–267.
12. Greenblatt, R. B. & Karpas, A.: Hormone therapy for sexual dysfunction. The only "true aphrodisiac": *Postgrad. Med.*, 74:78–89, 1883.
13. Linden, C. H. et al.: Yohimbine: A new street drug: *Ann. Emerg. Med.*, 14:1002–1004, 1985.
14. Ferrari, F. et al.: Imidazole has similar behavioural effects to yohimbine: *Psychopharmacology*, 88:58–62, 1986.
15. Bupropion (Wellbutrin by Burroughs Wellcome)—'A Second Generation' Antidepressant: Facts and Comparisons, Dec. 1986 Update: St. Louis, J. B. Lippincott, 1986, p. 760.
16. Elias, M.: Pill to improve sexual interest expected soon: *USA Today*, April 21, 1987, p. 1.
17. Taberner, P. V.: *Aphrodisiacs: The Science and the Myth*: Philadelphia, University of Pennsylvania Press, 1985.
18. Flamingo fertility: *USA Today*, June 11, 1987, p. 1D.

Arachnodactyly

Arachnodactyly refers to long, thin, tapering fingers which are often webbed,[1] and thus have some presumed resemblance to the threads in a spider's cobweb.[2] Its major association is with Marfan's syndrome, a nonliterary eponym which has an X-linked or autosomal recessive inheritance. This entity has many more features than arachnodactyly, including excessive height and thinness, ectopia lentis, and dissecting aneurysms of the ascending aorta due to excessive deposits of mucopolysaccharides.[3]

The word is related to Arachnida, a class of arthropods which includes spiders.[2] In Greek mythology, Arachne was a maiden who was very skillful in weaving and embroidery.[4] She claimed that her skill at weaving was greater than that of Minerva, who, on hearing this boast, challenged her to a contest. Arachne's weaving depicted scenes which showed the failings and errors of the gods. Minerva was so enraged that she made her feel guilt and shame. Arachne then hanged herself, but the goddess brought her back to life and changed her into a spider.

The arachnoid(ea) is one of three membranes which cover the brain and spinal cord. It is located between the outer dura mater and the inner pia mater.[5] The related space is also so named. The derivation of the word is the same as that for arachnodactyly. Its use here categorizes the membrane as being as fine and delicate as a spider web. The pia mater is mentioned three times in the works of Shakespeare.[6] An especially imaginative example is provided by Holofernes, the pedantic schoolmaster in *Love's Labour's Lost*.[7] "This is a gift that I have, simple, simple: a foolish extravagant spirit, full of forms, figures, shapes, objects, ideas, apprehension, motions, revolutions: these are begot in the ventricle of memory, nourished in the womb of *pia mater*, and delivered upon the mellowing of occasion."

1. Thomas, p. 124.
2. OED: I:423–424.
3. Boyd, W.: *Pathology for Physicians*: 7th Ed., Philadelphia, Lea & Febiger, 1965.
4. Bulfinch, p. 132.
5. Anson, p. 1014.
6. Kail, p. 195.
7. Shakespeare, *Love's Labour's Lost*: IV, i.

Argus

Argus is the name of the monthly news bulletin of the American Academy of Ophthalmology. Volume 1 was published in 1977.[1] Headquartered in San Francisco, its circulation reached 14,200 in 1985. Argus was a giant with one hundred eyes. He slept with all except two eyes open.[2] When Jupiter's wife, Juno, suspected that he had been involved in an escapade with Io, Jupiter turned Io into a beautiful heifer in order to protect her. Juno asked her husband for the heifer as a gift, which he could not refuse. She then gave the heifer to Argus to be carefully watched. Jupiter sent Mercury (Hermes) to try to retrieve his mistress in her altered form. Mercury played his pipes and told Argus many stories until all his eyes closed in sleep.[3] Mercury then killed Argus and set Io free. Juno reacted by scattering the hundred eyes of Argus onto the tail of her peacock.

It is hoped that the eyes of patients treated by ophthalmologists have a better fate than those of Argus. The term argus-eyed is in common usage for someone who is sharp-sighted; and one species of pheasant is known as the argus pheasant.[4] A literary example of the argus myth is found in Conan Doyle's short story, "Cyprian Overbeck Wells," in which a frustrated writer has a vision or dream of being visited by several famous writers.[5] Among these was Tobias Smollet, who described Jedediah Anchorstock, a quartermaster. The latter had been subjected in his childhood to an evil-minded person who "had tattooed eyes all over his countenance with such marvelous skill that it was difficult at a short distance to pick out his real ones among so many counterfeits."

Amazon mythology also has a character whose skin was covered with many duplicates of an organ. Atremis of Epheus was a fertility goddess who had many breasts over much of her skin.[6] However, the Atremis Condition has not as yet been proposed as an eponym for polythelia.

1. *Argus*. News of developments that affect eye care: San Francisco, American Academy of Ophthalmology, Vol. 1, 1977.
2. Schmidt, p. 26.
3. Pinsent, J.: *Greek Mythology*: New York, Peter Bedrick Books, 1983, p. 45.
4. Espy, pp. 291–292.
5. Doyle, A. C.: "Cyprian Overbeck Wells." A literary mosaic: in *The Captain of the Polestar and Other Tales*. London, Longman, Green, 1894, pp. 203–229.
6. Guirand, 1968, pp. 121–122.

Atlas

(atlanto-occipital joint)

The first cervical vertebra, which supports the skull by articulating with the occipital bone at the base of the skull, is named after Atlas who was condemned to support the heavens on his shoulders.[1] In Greek mythology, Atlas was a Titan whose bulk surpassed that of any other man.[2] Perseus (the son of Zeus, or Jupiter and Danae, the daughter of King Acrisius of Argos) asked Atlas for food and rest after he had killed the Gorgon, Medusa. Atlas refused because of a prophecy that a son of Zeus would steal his golden apples. In anger, Perseus held up the Medusa's head and Atlas was changed to stone. He increased in bulk until he became a mountain on which the heavens, the stars, and the earth rested, as does the skull on the vertebral column.[3]

This eponym represents the ancient and medieval concept of the centrality of man in the universe. Of a different connotation is the atlas as a book of maps, so named because Mercator's title page contained a picture of the Titan.[4]

1. Ferner, p. 199.
2. Bulfinch, pp. 144–145.
3. Frimmer, S.: *Neverland. Fabled Places and Fabulous Voyages of History and Legend*: New York, Viking Press, 1976, p. 103.
4. Boycott, p. 13.

Atreus Complex

The psychological complex of death wishes of a father against his offspring has been given the name of Atreus of Greek mythology.[1] Atreus, the great-grandson of Jove, wreaked vengeance on his brother, Thyestes, by causing him to eat the flesh of two of his children.[2] Therefore, it would seem more appropriate to call this psychological state the Thyestes Complex. It is related to the Medea Complex in which the mother has such death wishes. Both originate as a desire for revenge against the spouse.

Shakespeare replicated the Atreus legend in *Titus Andronicus*.[3] When Tamora, queen of the Goth, beheaded the two sons of Titus, a Roman general, he retaliated by killing her sons and serving them to her at a banquet. "Why, there they are both, baked in that pie;/Whereof their mother daintily had fed,/Eating the flesh that she herself hath bred."

1. Campbell, p. 122.
2. Gayley, p. 275.
3. Shakespeare, *Titus Andronicus*: V, iii.

Atropine

(belladonna)

Atropine is an anticholinergic drug of the belladonna alkaloid group.[1] It acts on postganglionic effectors innervated by cholinergic nerves, and on smooth muscles which lack cholinergic innervation.

In Greek mythology, Atropos was the oldest of the three fates (also Clotho, Lachesis) who spun the thread of human destiny, which they cut whenever they pleased.[2] Atropos was the one who cut the thread when it was time for someone to die. Atropine occurs in Solanaceae plants, especially the deadly nightshade plant which was used in the middle ages to produce obscure and prolonged poisoning. Therefore, Linné named it *Atropa belladonna* after Atropus who cuts the thread of life.[1]

It has been suggested that the death of

Reverend Dimmesdale in Hawthorne's *The Scarlet Letter*[3] of 1850 may have been due to poisoning with atropine given to him by his physician, Doctor Chillingworth, whose wife the minister had impregnated.[4] There has been disagreement, however, because some statements in the book indicate death due to "the effect of the emotion of guilt on the physical well-being of the patient."[5]

1. Gilman, pp. 130–131.
2. Gayley, p. 38.
3. Hawthorne, N.: *The Scarlet Letter and Selected Tales*: New York, Bantam Books, 1965.
4. Khan, J. A.: Atropine poisoning in Hawthorne's *The Scarlet Letter*: *N. Engl. J. Med.*, 311:414–416, 1984.
5. Kerr, A. J., Jr.: To the Editor: *N. Engl. J. Med.*, 311:1439, 1984.

B

Bellman's Fallacy

(the law of lazy repetition[1])

Some erroneous beliefs in medicine are accepted because of frequent repetition, and perpetuated without question because of lack of reference to original source material on the subject. This reliance on secondary sources, such as statements that Hippocrates described lead poisoning in his writings, has been called the Bellman's fallacy.[2]

The Bellman is the central character in the *Hunting of the Snark* (1876) by Lewis Carroll.[3] He is the leader of an expedition to find the Snark. Bellman is another word for a town crier, and for the "ringer commonly called Le Bellman" at Oxford University, where Carroll matriculated and taught. Le Bellman's duty was to put on the clothes of a deceased person of some rank, and announce their burial by ringing a hand bell.[4] The narrative poem has been interpreted as a satire on such absurd statutes of the university. Carroll does not explain what the Snark is, although the story has been interpreted as the search for the absolute. The eponym, Bellman's Fallacy, is based on several verses.[3]

"Just the place for a Snark!" the Bellman cried,
As he landed his crew with care;
Supporting each man on the top of the tide
By a finger entwined in his hair.

"Just the place for a Snark! I have said it twice:
That alone should encourage the crew.

Just the place for a Snark! I have said it thrice:
What I tell you three times is true."

One example of historical misconception perpetrated by lack of examining primary source material is the almost universal belief that Doctor Arthur Conan Doyle was so unsuccessful a practitioner that he wrote the Sherlock Holmes stories to save himself from starvation.[5] The designation of Bellman's Fallacy, or the rule of three, can be applied to other so-called truths in medicine, both historical and scientific. It appears to be universal.

1. Karlen, A.: *Napoleon's Glands and Other Ventures in History*: Boston, Little, Brown & Co., 1984, p. 45.
2. Waldron, H. A.: Hippocrates and lead: *Lancet*, 2:626, 1973.
3. Carroll, L. (Dodgson, C. L.): The Hunting of the Snark: in *The Annotated Snark*, M. Gardner ed., illustrated by H. Holiday, New York, Bramhall House, 1962.
4. Clark, A.: *Lewis Carroll. A Biography*: New York, Schocken Books, 1979, p. 64.
5. Rodin, A. E. & Key, J. D.: *Medical Casebook of Doctor Arthur Conan Doyle*: Malabar, Florida, Robert E. Krieger, 1984.

Bovarism

Bovarism is defined as the confusion of daydreaming with the facts of the perceptual world, and of the failure to differentiate between fantasy and reality.[1] Fantasy as such is not abnormal unless it becomes uncontrolled owing to insufficient gratification from reality.[2] Thus, fantasies of social prominence and sexual gratification can compensate for the difference between desires and actuality.[3] But they may represent borderline psychotic states with impairment of a person's capacity for normal interrelationships.

The name is derived from the infamous Emma Bovary of Gustave Flaubert's novel of 1857, *Madame Bovary*.[4] She married the sober Doctor Charles Bovary, after which "Domestic mediocrity drove her to lewd fancies, marriage tenderness to adulterous desires." ". . . the lyric legion of these [fictional] adulterous women began to sing in her memory . . . She became herself, as it were, an actual part of these imaginings, and realized the love-dream of her youth as she saw herself in this type of amorous women whom she so envied." Such immersion into fantasy was not cured by two disastrous love affairs. In fact, "She felt herself transported to the reading of her youth, into the midst of Walter Scott." In her agitated depression she felt the reality of an imaginary man "fashioned out of her most ardent memories, of her finest reading, her strongest lusts, and at last he became so real, so tangible. . . ."

Flaubert himself exhibited considerable sexuality in his adolescence and early twenties. Hyposexuality followed the onset of epilepsy at the age of 22.[5] The character of Emma Bovary may have been derived from his own relationships with a doctor's wife and the poetess Loise Colet.[6] Flaubert's writings have also been psychoanalyzed as being influenced by a platonic but very moving love affair at the age of 14.[7] It has been suggested that Flaubert's choice of literature as a career rather than the more bourgeois fields of law or medicine was due to his father's favoritism to an older brother, to his mother's indifference, and to the consequent intensity of love, short of incest, for his younger sister Caroline.[8] He was prosecuted for obscenity, but the case was dismissed after excerpts from the book were read to the approving French judiciary.[6]

Emma Bovary has been psychoanalyzed as having a pathological narcissism, being "indifferent to the qualities of the object except insofar as it enhanced the self or supplied it with gratification."[9] The cause is "a projecting forward of the terror, rage and complete helplessness of the state of infantile separation" from her mother, although at a much older age. When she finally commits suicide it represents "her deepest libidinal wish, fusion with the bad mother." Indeed, Flaubert is on solid psychiatric ground in that fantasies do precede suicidal acts; and sometimes consist of regressive desires for reunion with the mother so as to live again in an ideal state of passivity and infantile gratification.[2]

Madam Bovary's suicide was in desperation after her last lover destroyed the "living out" of her fantasies and ruined her husband financially. She ingested a large amount of arsenic with consequent vomiting of blood, severe epigastric pains, superpurgation (marked diarrhea), brown spots on the skin, faint and irregular pulse, convulsions, and violent breathing.

These are symptoms of an acute gastrointestinal disorder and shock, in themselves suggestive of arsenic poisoning,[10] except possibly for the convulsions. The latter may have been the reason why one commentator cited her death as due to strychnine.[11] Flaubert, however, indicated arsenic by name.[12]

Death due to acute arsenic poisoning is not unknown in other fictional works. In the classic play *Arsenic and Old Lace*,[13] the two Brewster sisters murdered 12 old men with wine containing a poisonous mixture of arsenic, strychnine, and cyanide. Their motive was to bring peace to lonely old men. Not as benevolent is the motive of Jorge, the old medieval monk in Eco's *The Name of the Rose*.[14] He brushed the pages of a blasphemous book on humor with a poisonous substance. When a reader repeatedly moistened his fingers to turn the pages, fingers and tongue turned black, followed by rapid death. The substance is identified as arsenic in the movie of the same name. Death can occur with severe arsenic poisoning within 24 hours.[10]

The eponym, Bovarism, was used by Aldous Huxley in the more generic sense of "the poser granted to man to conceive himself as other than he is."[15]

1. Campbell, p. 88.
2. Kolb, pp. 110–111, 118–119.
3. Chapman, pp. 72–73.
4. Flaubert, G.: *Madame Bovary*: New York, Airmont, 1965.
5. Gastaut, H. et al.: Gaustave Flaubert's illness: A case in evidence against the erroneous notion of psychogenic epilepsy: *Epilepsia*, 25:622–637, 1984.
6. James, B.: Psychiatry, science and the seduction of Emma Bovary: *Aust. N.Z. J. Psychiatry*, 14: 101–107, 1980.
7. Baudry, F. D.: Adolescent love and self-analysis as contributors to Flaubert's creativity: *Psychoanal. Study Child.*, 35:377–416, 1980.
8. Mitzman, A.: The unstrung Orpheus: Flaubert's youth and the psycho-social origins of art for art's sake: *Psychohistory Rev.*, 6:27–42, 1977.
9. Kovel, J.: On reading *Madame Bovary* psychoanalytically: *Sem. Psychiatry*, 5:331–345, 1973.
10. Gilman, p. 1616.
11. Zorn, M.: To the Editor: *N. Engl. J. Med.*, 311:1440, 1984.
12. Vourćh, G.: Madame Bovary died of arsenic poisoning: *N. Engl. J. Med.*, 312:446, 1985.
13. Kesserling, J.: *Arsenic and Old Lace*: New York, Random House, 1941.

14. Eco, U.: *The Name of the Rose*: New York, Harcourt Brace Jovanovich, 1983.
15. Hendrickson, pp. 38–39.

Brain of Pooh

The Brain of Pooh eponym has been used as a designation for the limitations of the human mind, especially in comparison to the complexity of the world about us, including the capabilities of computers.[1] The brain is limited in its degree of preciseness of perception of the outside universe, in the concepts which it can formulate, in the ability of speech to truly express everything we experience, and in the extent of memory. There is considerable evidence that such quantitative limitations of our intellectual capacities are genetically determined. Advances in genetics may lead to the possibility of changing such limitations.

Edward Bear, otherwise known as Winnie-the-Pooh, is the toy bear hero created by A. A. Milne.[2] His mental capacity is indicated in the opening lines of this classic children's story. "Here is Edward Bear, coming downstairs now, bump, bump, bump, on the back of his head, behind Christopher Robin. It is, as far as he knows, the only way of coming downstairs, but sometimes he feels that there really is another way, if only he could stop bumping for a moment and think of it." And yet at times he has the wisdom of the simple-minded. " 'Rabbit's clever,' Said Pooh thoughtfully . . . 'And he has Brain.' . . . There was a long silence. 'I suppose,' Said Pooh, 'that's why he never understands anything.' "

It has been suggested that Pooh had spontaneous functional hypoglycemia as he craved food at about 11A.M., ate a high carbohydrate breakfast of marmalade spread over honeycomb, and became drowsy and unable to concentrate when not given something to eat.[3] Perhaps this might explain his mental confusion, although most humans have no such excuse.

A book designed to please and amuse young patients has been called *The Pooh Get-Well Book*.[4] It contains many references to Pooh and his friends in the forms of puzzles, poems, recipes, and activities with a liberal sprinkling of quotations from the Pooh books.

1. Sinsheimer, R. L.: The brain of Pooh: An essay

on the limits of mind: *Am. Scientist*, 59:20–28, 1971.

2. Milne, A. A.: *The World of Pooh. The Complete Winnie-The-Pooh and The House at Pooh Corner*: New York, E. P. Dutton, 1957.

3. Gault, J. E.: Did Winnie the Pooh have spontaneous functional hypoglycaemia?: *Med. J. Aust.*, 1:942–943, 1965.

4. Ellison, W. H.: *The Pooh Get-Well Book. Recipes and Activities to Help You Recover from Wheezles and Sneezles*: New York, E. P. Dutton, 1973.

C

Cain Complex

A destructive rivalry between brothers has been given the name of Cain, who was the first born son of Adam and Eve.[1] He was a farmer who became enraged when the Lord showed respect for the offering of his brother Abel, a shepherd, but not for his own.[2] Cain then murdered Abel, his brother. The Cain Complex may be related to the Oedipus Complex with the brother instead of the father being the rival.

And the Lord said unto Cain: "Where is Abel thy brother," And he said: "I know not; am I my brother's keeper?" And He said: "What hast thou done? the voice of thy brother crieth unto Me from the ground."

After the murder of Abel, God's retribution was to put a mark upon Cain "lest any finding him should smite him,"[3] a rather surprisingly mild punishment. Legend holds, however, that the mark was actually the curse of Cain in that he was never to die or to reach home again.[4] The Mark of Cain has been interpreted as a patch of eczema on the forehead.[5]

1. Dudzinski.
2. OT: Genesis 4:9–10.
3. OT: Genesis 4:15.
4. Hendrickson, p. 54.
5. Levin, pp. 22–33.

Cain Personality

(Cain factor[1])

Some individuals have a predominantly homicidal personality expressed as rage, anger, vengeance, jealously, and envy.[1] These accumulate to the point of a sudden, explosive attack. It is related to sexual and ego factors. Such human characteristics and consequences have existed since early biblical days when Cain, the first biblical child on record, murdered his brother, Abel, in a jealous rage.[2]

The Cain Personality differs from the Cain Complex in that it does not refer to sibling rivalry, but to the homicidal tendency inherent in all men, and to an excessively overt degree in some. There is a biblical suggestion that Cain's homicidal tendency may have been inherited by later generations, as indicated in the behavior of Lamech, the sixth in the line of descent from Cain: "For I have slain a man for wounding me,/and a young man for bruising me;/If Cain shall be avenged sevenfold,/Truly Lamech seventy and sevenfold."[3]

1. Szondi, L.: Thanatos and Cain: *Am. Imago*, 21:52–63, 1964.
2. OT: Genesis 4:9–10.
3. OT: Genesis 4:23.

Caput Medusae

Portal hypertension can result in distention of superficial periumbilical veins of the skin owing to back pressure of blood from the portal vein which is compressed by cirrhotic liver tissue.[1] The wavy appearance of these distended veins in the skin has been compared to the hair of Medusa. She was one of the three Gorgons of Greek mythology, monstrous females with huge teeth, brazen claws, and snakes for hair.[2]

Medusa was once beautiful, but was deprived of her charms by Minerva (Athena) because she had defiled an Athenian temple by sleeping there with Poseidon (Neptune). Her beautiful ringlets were changed into hissing snakes, and all who looked upon her turned to stone. Her head was cut off by Perseus, who approached her when she was asleep, and only looked at her image reflected in his shield.[3] He gave the head to Minerva and it still retained its power.

The eponym Caput Medusae refers to Medusa's physical appearance rather than her other attributes. Freud suggested that the terror of observing her head was symbolic of the terror of castration, and that her snakes were

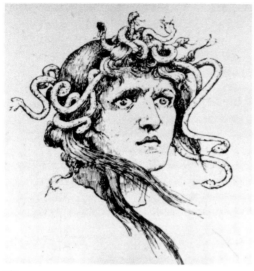

(A)

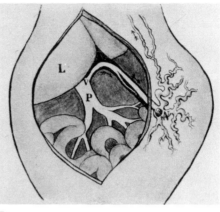

(B)

Caput Medusae   **A.** Head of Medusa with snake's hair.[2, p. 141] **B.** Liver in opened abdomen (left), and distended veins around the umbilicus (right).[1, p. 148]

symbolic of pubic hair.[4] In a different type of literature, but still with psychological overtones, Medusa is variously depicted in comic books as a variety of characters, some evil and some good.[5] All have "snakey" hair. Such an appearance is the reason the name Medusa was given to jellyfish by Linnaeus.[6]

A nonliterary umbilical eponym is the Sister Mary Joseph node named after a surgical assistant at the turn of the century, who noted an umbilical nodule while preparing a patient for surgery at the Mayo Clinic.[7] It is caused by invasion of the umbilicus by an intra-abdominal malignancy, and may be its first sign.

1. Monckeberg, J. G.: *Ribbert's Lehrbuch der Allgemeinen Pathologie und der Pathologischen Anatomie*: 8th Ed., Leipzig, F. C. W. Vogel, 1921, p. 148.
2. Bulfinch, pp. 141–144.
3. Gayley, pp. 209–210.
4. Freud, S.: "Medusa's Head" (1922): in *Sexuality and the Psychology of Love*, P. Rieff, Ed., New York, Collier Books, 1970, pp. 212–213.
5. Adams, K. A.: "Octopoid" genitality and the Medusal Madonna: *J. Psychohistory*, 10:409–462, 1983.
6. Skinner, p. 269.
7. Key, J. D. et al.: Sister Mary Joseph's nodule and its relationship to diagnosis of carcinoma of the umbilicus: *Minn. Med.*, 59:561–566, 1976.

Cassandra Prophecy

Pediatricians working in intensive care may encounter denial and hostility from parents to whom they give (prophetize) a hopeless prognosis for their children.[1] This may result in rejection of the doctor and nurses by parents with counterprophesies of miraculous cures, criticism of health care, or accusations of neglect of their child. The eponym is named after Cassandra of Greek mythology. She was the daughter of Priam, the king of Troy, and Hecuba. Her beauty so affected Apollo that he gave her the gift of prophecy upon her promise to comply with his desires.[2] When she did not comply he ordained that no one should believe her prophecies. Thus, concordance between the goddess and the eponym is excellent.

Idiomatically, a Cassandra is one who always forsees the worst, a compulsive alarmist.[3] Cassandra's name has been used for warnings that were ignored concerning possible carcinogen effects of photodye therapy for herpes simplex.[4] Its relationship to carcinogenesis has, however, been seriously questioned.[5] The phrase disbelieving Cassandra[6] refers to those who consider that a prognosis should not be given in cases of cirrhosis.[7] Medical Cassandras are those whose warnings in the 1950s that syphilis has not been conquered were ignored.[8] Could *Cassandra*, the newsletter of a nurses' group,[9] be so named because some physicians do not listen to their opinions?

1. Waller, D. A., Todres, D., Cassem, N. H. & Anderten, A.: Coping with poor prognosis in the pediatric intensive care unit. The Cassandra prophecy: *Am. J. Dis. Child.*, 133:1121–1125, 1979.
2. Bulfinch, p. 469.
3. Ciardi, p. 62.
4. Berger, R. S. & Papa, C. M.: Photodye herpes therapy—Cassandra confirmed?: *J.A.M.A.*, 238:133–134, 1977.
5. Kaufman, R. H. et al.: Cassandra still a myth: (letter) *J.A.M.A.*, 238:2368, 1977.
6. Atterbury, C. E.: Prognosis in cirrhosis: Disbelieving Cassandra: *J. Clin. Gastroenterol.*, 5:359–360, 1983.
7. Patek, A. J., Jr. & Koff, R. S.: Predicting clinical recovery from alcoholic liver disease: *J. Clin. Gastroenterol.*, 5:303–306, 1983.
8. Rosebury, T.: *Microbes and Morals. The Strange History of Venereal Diseases*: New York, Viking Press, 1971.
9. *Cassandra, Radical Feminist Nurses Newsletter*, vol. 1 1982.

Centaurius

Centaurius, the International Magazine of the History of Science and Medicine, appeared in 1950.[1] It is published in Copenhagen, with the text being in English, French, or German. Another journal named after these hybrid creatures is *Centaur*, first published in 1937 by the Sidney University Veterinary Society (Australia).[1] It seems most appropriate to have a creature that is half man and half beast chosen to designate a veterinary journal.

The centaurs of Greek mythology were born of the union of Ixion, king of the Lapiths, with a cloud that Zeus had shaped to resemble Hera, Zeus's wife whom Ixon had tried to seduce.[2] Centaurus was the father of the centaurs, being the first born. They had a man's bust and a horse's body, and were feared by mortals because of their brutal customs, treachery, and lust for wine and women.[3] One legend is of their attempt to rape Hippodamia at her wedding to Theseus, a demigod ruler of Thebes. The mythical centaurs were probably derived from a real-life ancient race of Thessaly which led a wild and savage life and hunted bulls on horseback.[4] There was one centaur, however, who was an exception: Chiron was the wisest and most just of these hybrids. Apollo and Diana taught him medicine, music, and the art of prophecy. In turn he is stated to have taught the art of healing to Aesculapius (see Aesculapian).[5]

When Shakespeare's *King Lear* was rejected by the two daughters to whom he had given his kingdom, he delivered a diatribe on adultery, comparing them to centaurs.[6] "Let copulation thrive; for Gloucester's bastard son / Was kinder to the father than my daughters / Got 'tween the lawful sheets / . . . Down from the waist they are Centaurs / Though women all above; / But to the girdle do the God's inherit, Beneath is all the fiend's." The imagery of the hybrid centaurs contributes greatly to the effectiveness of Shakespeare's delineation of the dual nature of mankind—the coexistence of both beauty and beast in the same individual.

Doctors in Victorian fiction were depicted as "a kind of 'centaur' figure in whom an idealized partial doctor is merged with the human hero of developing realism."[7] This differs from novels in early nineteenth century fiction, in which the doctor is only sketchily drawn. Such differences in depiction of physicians are a reflection of changing social attitudes. Presumably, the humanistic idealism of physicians is represented by the human bust of the centaur and their scientific pragmatism by its horse's body.

1. *Index of NLM Serial Titles.*
2. Schmidt, p. 60.
3. Guirand, 1964, p. 120.
4. Bulfinch, p. 470.
5. Martí-Ibáñez, R.: *Ariel. Essays on the Art and the History and Philosophy of Medicine*: New York, MD Publications, 1962, p. 47.
6. Shakespeare, *King Lear*: IV,vi.
7. Hill, J.: The doctor as hero in nineteenth-century British fiction: *Pharos*, 50:31–33, 1987.

Cheshire Cat Syndrome

Appropriate medical diagnoses may not be made because all of the accepted criteria are not present in patients with a forme fruste of a disease.[1] In some patients there may be a forme sine, with only one or a few of the criteria evident. Three such cases of polyarteritis nodosa have been described under the label of the Chesire Cat Syndrome, or "innate common sense untrammeled by the rigorous laws of proof."[1] These patients were diagnosed as such during life with considerably less than the usual clinical criteria, and did have one or two focal areas suggestive of polyarteritis at autopsy.[1] However, one is always in danger of finding what one wants to find if one wants to find it badly enough.

When Alice was in Wonderland, she encountered the Cheshire cat, who disappeared so slowly that for a short while only its grin remained—"a grin without a cat."[2] Lewis Carroll may have named the Cheshire cat after John Cathedral of Chester, who bared his teeth in a grin when angry and whose coat of arms included a cat.[3] Another, but less interesting suggestion, is derivation from a strange engraving in the Cranleigh Church in Surrey.[4] The phrase grins like a Cheshire cat was in common use long before Carroll's "Alice," being defined in Grose's *Dictionary of the Vulgar Tongue* (1785)[7] as "said of anyone who shews his teeth and gums in laughing." The Cheshire cat is not a specific breed of cat, but probably derived from an old, lost folktale.[6]

The Cheshire cat may not be quite appropriate for this eponym as the cat (disease manifestations) did appear fully at first and only the grin (forme sine) was left at the end; instead of the reverse with presentation being only a few features of the disease and subsequent investigation revealing the rest of the features. (see Procrustean Perspective).

1. Bywaters, E. G. L.: The Cheshire cat syndrome: *Postgrad. Med. J.*, 44:19–22, 1968.
2. Carroll, p. 88–91.
3. Clark, A.: *Lewis Carroll. A Biography*: New York, Schocken Books, 1979, p. 18.
4. Crocknell, B.: Famous Surrey names: in *Surrey County Guide*, Gloucester, British Publishing Co., n.d.
5. Grose, F.: *1811 Dictionary of the Vulgar Tongue*: London, Bibliophile Books, 1984.
6. Ciardi, p. 69.

Chimera

(Chimaera)

In general, the terms chimera and mosaic have been applied to animals containing the tissues of two or more distinct genetic types.[1] More specifically, in a mosaic the different genetic tissues are derived from the same cell as a genetic mutation in which there is an abnormal division of chromosomes.[2] In a chimera, the cause of the different genetic tissues is the addition of tissues from one individual to another. The classic example of the latter is that of nonidentical twins who share one placenta. This permits the intermingling of blood and blood-forming cells between the twins while in utero, creating the chimera state. A related situation is found in patients who have received blood-forming cells from donors after their own were destroyed by radiation.

In Greek mythology, Chimaera was the offspring of Echinda and Typhon.[3] Echinda was both a woman and a serpent, and had given birth to such monsters as the Sphinx, dragons, and the eagle that gnawed the liver of Prometheus; she was finally killed by the hundred-eyed Argus while she slept. Typhon was a horrible monster covered with scales, and who had a hundred mouths which vomited flames; he was killed by Zeus and buried under Mount Aetna, which is said to still emit his flames. Chimaera herself had the head of a lion, the body of a she-goat, and the tail of a dragon. She terrorized Lycia by vomiting flames and eating all humans who crossed her path. Chimaera was finally killed by Bellerophon mounted on the winged horse Pegasus. He filled her with lead arrows which were melted by the heat of her own flames and burned her to death.

The mythological Chimaera is actually a hybrid, which is the offspring of two distinct species with the resultant creature being a composite of different body areas derived from the two different species.[4] The griffins, who guarded the treasures of Apollo, were also hybrids, having the head of an eagle and the winged body of a lion.[5] These differ from the biological definitions of chimera and mosaic which denote an intermingling of the different tissues not evident to the naked eye. An exception is the phrase interspecific chimerism which has been used for the result of combining embryonic cells of two different species with resultant characteristics of both.[6] An example is the sheep-goat with strongly curved goat horns and wool containing patches of fibers, some of which are characteristic of goats and others of sheep. The three terms are even less clearly distinguished in general usage.

The terms chimera and chimerical have been applied to the skull of Piltown man, first discovered in 1912 and then exposed as a hoax about 40 years later.[7] The head proved to be that of a human about 500 years old, and the carefully altered jaw was that of an orangutan.

1. Stedman, chimera, p. 263.
2. Dixon, B.: Engineering chimeras for Noah's Ark: *Hastings Center Report*, 14:10–12, 1984.
3. Schmidt, pp. 64–65.
4. Thomas, p. 783.
5. Schmidt, p. 114.
6. Fehilly, C. B. et al.: Interspecific chimaerism between sheep and goat: *Nature*, 307:634–636, 1984.
7. Blinderman, C.: *The Piltdown Inquest*: Buffalo, New York, Prometheus Books, 1986.

Cinderella

A popular designation for any area of medicine that is relatively neglected or overlooked is Cinderella. So-called have been an amazing cornucopia of medical items: colorectal surgery,[1] cancer of the uterus,[2] endocrinology,[3] forensic medicine,[4] fractures,[5] general practice,[6] geriatrics,[7] geriatric nursing,[8] health promotion,[9] the history of pharmacy,[10] hyperbaric oxygen therapy,[11] *Listeria monocytogenes*,[12] mental retardation,[13] occupational medicine,[14] postnatal care,[15] postoperative analgesia,[16] preventative medicine,[7] primary health care,[17] rheumatology, [18] the virus of hepatitis A,[19] and the physically handicapped.[20]

Cinderella is the heroine of a world-wide folk story with hundreds of variations, the oldest one known being a ninth century Chinese version.[21] English variants are derived from translations from the French of Charles Perrault's "Cendrillon" in his 1697 collection of *Tales of Mother Goose*.[22] The basic elements include being verbally demeaned by her stepmother and stepsisters, forced to do menial work, and given only rags for clothes. Only through her fairy godmother is she able to meet the prince. The plot is one variant of the universal theme of boy meets girl, boy loses girl, boy finds girl, to live happily every after.

The eponym is not a perfect fit, as Cinderella is purposely neglected and not just ignored. Cinderella as a word has the further connotation of eventually achieving recognition of affluence.[23] Freud psychoanalyzed Cinderella's disappearance and the inability of the prince to find her as an unmistakable symbol of death.[24] The Cinderella story has also been considered as symbolic of patients who use neurotic and psychotic fantasies and dreams to escape conflicts between wish fulfillment and reality,[25] as occurs in Bovarism. It has been used as an example of the significant role of fairy tales in the growth of children, by portraying specific human problems.[26] CINDERELLA is an acronym for a computerized patient data system.[27]

1. Leading Article: Colorectal surgery—The Cinderella specialty: *Br. Med. J.*, 283:169–170, 1981.
2. De Muelenaere, G. F. G., & Fichardt, T.: Carcinoma of the corpus uteri: The Cinderella of cancer therapy: *S. Afr. Med. J.*, 47:245–255, 1973.
3. Greep, R. O.: The Presidential address of the Endocrine Society—Endocrinology: Orphan and Cinderella science: *Endocrinology*, 79:823–827, 1966.
4. Birrell, J. H.: "Where death delights to help the living." Forensic medicine—Cinderella?: *Med. J. Aust.*, 57:253–261, 1970.
5. Allgower, M.: Cinderella of surgery fractures?: *Surg. Clinics North Am.*, 58:1071–1093, 1978.
6. Rhodes, P.: Educating the doctor: Postgradu-

ate, vocational, and continuing education: *Br. Med. J.*, 290:1808–1810, 1985.

7. Shennan, D. W.: The second Cinderella: *Central Afr. J. Med.*, 29:70–72, 1983.
8. We Say: The Cinderella Service: *Nursing Mirror Midwives J.*, 141:33, 1975.
9. Chappell, A.: "Health promotion—Cinderella or challenge for nurses"?: *N.Z. Nurses J.*, 75:6–8, 1982.
10. Crellin, J. K.: Commentary—Cinderella and big sister: A case for closer relationships: *Bull. Hist. Med.*, 7(H. E. Sigerist suppl.):87–90, 1982.
11. Editorial: Hyperbaric oxygen therapy—The Cinderella in the management of anaerobic infection: *J. Infect.*, 6:1–3, 1983.
12. Bottone, E. J. and Sierra, M. F.: Listeria monocytogenes: Another look at the "Cinderella among pathogenic bacteria": *Mt. Sinai J. Med.*, 44:42–59, 1977.
13. Tarjan, G.: Cinderella and the prince: Mental retardation and community psychiatry: *Am. J. Psychiatry*, 122:1057–1059, 1966.
14. Joslin, G.: Occupational health. The 'Cinderella' of medicine: *Australas. Nurses J.*, Dec. 21, 1971, p. 15.
15. Special Correspondent: The Cinderella of the service?. Postnatal care: *Midwife Health Visit Commun. Nurse*, 14:389, 1978.
16. Mather, L. E.: Postoperative analgesia: The Cinderella of surgery: *Curr. Therapeut.*, 21:15–16, 1980.
17. Dowling, T. P.: Primary care—The Cinderella of health care and of nursing too: *J. N.Y. State Nurses Assoc.*, 9:21–24, 1978.
18. Bennett, B. L. et al.: Rheumatology—The 'Cinderella' specialty—An examination of doctors' attitudes to training and careers: *Br. J. Med. Ed.*, 6:232–237, 1972.
19. Thomas, H. C.: Cinderella virus: *Br. Med. J.*, 290: 1977, 1985.
20. Miller, F. H. & Miller, G. A. H.: The painful prescription. A procrustean perspective: *N. Engl. J. Med.*, 314:1383–1386, 1986.
21. *Encyclopaedia Britanica*: II:940.
22. Perrault, C.: *Cinderella or The Little Glass Slipper*: New York, Henry Z. Walck, 1971.
23. Espy, p. 122.
24. Freud, "The Theme of the Three Caskets": S.E., V.12, p. 293.
25. Huckel, H.: One day I'll live in the castle! Cinderella as a case history: *Am. Imago*, 14:303–314, 1957.
26. Heuscher, J. E.: Cinderella, Eros and Psyche: *Dis. Nerv. Syst.*, 24:286–297, 1963.
27. Salomon, J. et al.: Cinderella—A clinical nuclear medicine retrieval and filing on-line stand-alone system for patient data: *Nucl. Med.*, 19:80–84, 1980.

Cinderella Complex

Proposed in a book by Dowling is the concept that women have an unconscious desire to be taken care of by others, based primarily on a fear of being independent.[1] Its thesis is that ". . . the deep wish to be taken care of by others—is the chief force holding women down today . . . largely repressed attitudes and fears that keep women in a kind of half-light, retreating from the full use of their minds and creativity. Like Cinderella, woman today are still waiting for something external to transform their lives." The oppressed Cinderella of Perrault's folktale certainly does have desires (daydreams) and hopes for a miracle which finally arrives in the form of a fairy godmother.[2]

The relationship of the fictional heroine to the Complex is valid only in a general, extrapolated sense, as Cinderella's attitudes are not suppressed. She is seeking not independence, but a much more romantic and ennobling dependence. Other studies have shown a relationship between positive attitudes of women and ego maturity.[3] The Cinderella story has also been used as an example of psychological problems which can be created by family pathology,[4] and of the portrayal in fairy tales of significant psychological factors in the growth of the child.[5] Thus, her ambivalent father may be a phallic symbol, and the dancing at the prince's ball sexual arousal from which Cinderella at first flees.

Another eponym, the Cinderella Effect, relates to the Cinderella Complex (coined five years later) in that both depict females as having an unconscious desire to be looked after by others. The Effect is based on a study that revealed a greater percentage of adolescent girls than boys do not plan to implement their values and self-perceptions.[6] Nearly one-fourth of high school senior girls have no educational or vocational plans, although they have as positive academic values and self-estimated ability to succeed in school as do boys. Such a gender difference in behavior may be the result of females receiving more cues to control self-assertion than do males. The Cinderella of folklore was not assertive, but her three stepsisters certainly were.

1. Dowling, C.: *The Cinderella Complex. Women's Hidden Fear of Independence*: New York, Summit Books, 1981.
2. Perrault, C.: *Cinderella or The Little Glass Slipper*:

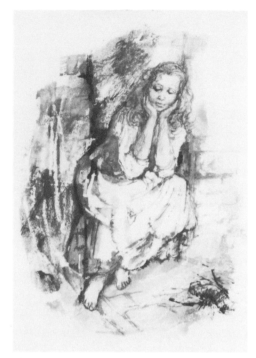

(A)

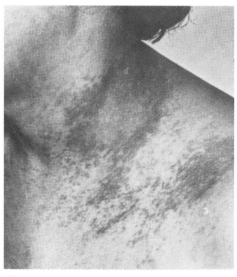

(B)

Cinderella Dermatosis **A.** Cinderella daydreaming at the fireplace.[3] (by permission, Random House) **B.** Ashy Dermatosis.[1] (by permission, copyright, Amer. Med. Assoc.)

New York, Henry Z. Walck, 1971.

3. Erickson, V. L.: Beyond Cinderella: Ego maturity and attitudes toward the rights and roles of women: *Counselling Psychologist*, 7:83–88, 1977.
4. Roseman, S.: Cinderella: Family pathology, identity-sculpting and mate-selection: *Am. Imago*, 35:375–396, 1978.
5. Heyscher, J. E.: Cinderella, Eros and Psyche: *Dis. Nerv. Syst.*, 24:286–292, 1963.
6. Rapoza, R. S. & Blocher, D. H.: The Cinderella effect: Planning avoidance in girls: *Counseling and Values*, 21:12–19, 1976.

Cinderella Dermatosis

(ashy dermatosis, dermatosis cenicienta, erythema chromicum figuratum melanodermicum,[1] erythema dyschromicum perstans)

Ashy dermatosis is characterized by nonspecific, ash-colored macules scattered on the skin, with shadings of grayish pigment, and varying in size from 1 cm to very large plaques. Histological changes consist of follicular hyperkeratosis, decreased melanin, vacuolation of some epidermal cells, degeneration of the basal layer, and a perivascular dermal infiltrate.[1] Ashy dermatosis appears in early adult life, coming in successive outbreaks.[2] It is commoner in South America than in the northern sections of the hemisphere.

The cause is not known, and there has been no response to treatment. The ashlike lesions do not occur on the scalp, palms, and toes, unlike those of Cinderella, whose name is derived from her habit of sitting by the fireplace.[3] "When her work was done, Cinderella would creep to the chimney corner and sit there in the ashes."

1. Knox, J. M. et al.: Erythema dyschromicum perstans: *Arch. Dermatol.*, 97:262–272, 1968.
2. Ramirez, C. O.: The ashy dermatosis (erythema dyschromicum perstans)—Epidemiological study and report of 139 cases: *Cutis*, 3:244–247, 1967.
3. Perrault, C.: Cinderella or The Little Glass Slipper: New York, Henry Z. Walck, 1971.

Cinderella Syndrome

Three adopted girls, 9 and 10 years of age, falsely accused their adoptive mothers of keeping them in rags, making them do all the chores, and favoring their stepsiblings.[1] All three girls were abused in a former placement, had loss of a mothering figure, and received emotional abuse at former adoptive homes.

There was, however, some psychopathology in the adoptive home, such as intense rivalry with stepsiblings and emotionally distant adoptive fathers. The accusations were those of Cinderella, although hers were not false.[2] This could be considered as a variant of the Munchausen Syndrome, with simulation of neglect being used to obtain psychological help.

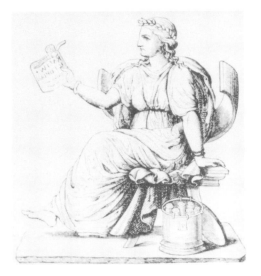

Clio Medica   Clio, the Muse of History. (3, p. 11)

1. Goodwin, J. et al.: Cinderella syndrome: Children who simulate neglect: *Am. J. Psychiatry*, 137:1223–1225, 1980.
2. Perrault, C.: *Cinderella or The Little Glass Slipper*: New York, Henry Z. Walck, 1971.

Clio Medica

Clio Medica is the name used for the published proceedings of the Academiae Internationalis Historiae Medicinae.[1] Volume 1, No. 1 appeared in November 1965. Clio was one of the nine Muses, daughters of Jupiter and Mnemosyne (memory), who presided over song and memory.[2] Each of the muses were assigned patronage to a department of literature, art, or science, with Clio being the Muse of history.[3]

Another journal named after Clio is *Clio, An Interdisciplinary Journal of Literature, History, and the Philosophy of Medicine*.[4] It appeared in 1971. *The ClioPedic* is the name of the Bulletin of the Center for the History of Foot Care and Foot Wear.[5] *Clio Medica* is also the name of a series of books which present in a concise manner specific areas in the history of medicine. It was under the general editorship of E. B. Krumbhaar, who authored one of the books himself.[6] Clio, as the goddess of history, is featured on the seal of the Association for the History of Medicine.[7] She is depicted standing in front of the Temple of Knowledge with a column around which is entwined a snake representing medicine.

1. *Clio Medica*: Vol. 1. No. 1, November, 1965.
2. Bulfinch, pp. 11–12.
3. Gayley, p. 37.
4. *Clio, An Interdisciplinary Journal of Literature, History, and the Philosophy of Medicine*: Vol. 1, 1971.
5. Holloway, L. M.: What's in our name?: *The ClioPedic*, 1:5–6, 1984.
6. Krumbhaar, E. B.: Pathology: Vol. 9 of *Clio Medica. A Series of Primers on the History of Medicine*, E. B. Krumbhaar Ed., New York, Hafner, 1937.
7. Editor: The Association's seal: Newsletter, *Am. Assoc. Hist. Med.*, Oct. 1986, p. 2.

Collar of Vulcan

An irritant dermatitis can be caused by burns around the neck of welders exposed to flying sparks.[1] The distribution of this type of dermatitis in the collar area has been named after Vulcan, the son of Juno and Jupiter. He was the god of fire—volcanic eruptions, incendiary flames, and the glow of the forge or hearth. He was also the blacksmith of the gods, his forge providing shields, spears, brass hoofs, and artistic works.[2] Vulcan was lame, either born as such or because he was hurled out of heaven. In Roman mythology, his assistants were the Cyclopes.[3]

Welders may also develop dermatitis from actinic rays of the arc and from irritant vapors and fumes of the metal or the flux.[4] Another irritant dermatitis has been reported on areas covered by clothing in welders who reline blast furnaces. In this instance, the dermatitis has been attributed to dust containing highly alkaline material from the limestone blast furnace.[5]

1. Dirckx, p. 73.
2. Gayley, pp. 24–25.
3. Croft, P.: *Roman Mythology*: London, Octopus Books, 1974.
4. Schwartz, L. et al.: *Occupational Diseases of the Skin*: Philadelphia, Lea & Febiger, 1947, p. 893.
5. Rycroft, R. J. G. & Calnan, C. D.: Irritant dermatitis during the relining of a blast furnace: *Contact Dermatitis*, 3:745–778, 1977.

Coma

Coma is "A state of profound unconsciousness from which one cannot be aroused."[1] The word is derived from Comus of Greek mythology.[2] He was the guardian of banquets and indulged in nightly orgies which resulted in a state of profound insensibility caused by a drunken stupor.[3] Alcoholic intoxication is, however, only one of many possible causes of coma.

Harrison's Principles of Medicine[4] lists 49 causes, "the pathophysiologic basis being either mechanical destruction of crucial areas of the brain stem or cerebral cortex (anatomic coma), or global disruption of brain metabolic processes (metabolic coma)." Alcoholic stupor resembles the latter category.

The words comic and comical are also derived from the god of festive mirth.[2]

1. Stedman, p. 303.
2. Espy, p. 31.
3. Bulfinch, p. 471.
4. Braunwald, pp. 114–120.

Cupid's Bow Contour

A normal concavity on the inferior aspect of the third, fourth, and fifth lumbar vertebrae resembles the archery bow of Cupid when viewed on frontal x-ray.[1] Cupid (Eros) was the winged and mischievous son of Venus, who became jealous of the great beauty of the mortal Psyche.[2] Venus asked Cupid to give Psyche a passion for some low, mean, and unworthy being. Cupid placed a few drops from a bitter fountain on her lips while she was asleep and touched her side with the point of his arrow. She startled him by awakening and he accidentally wounded himself with his own arrow. Thus, they became destined for each other.

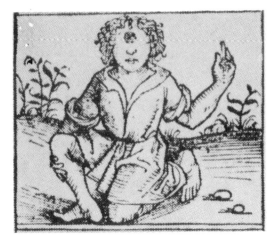

(A)

1 Dietz, G. W. & Christensen, E. E.: Normal Cupid's bow contour of the lower lumbar vertebrae: *Radiology*, 121:577–579, 1976.
2. Bulfinch, pp. 100–103.

Cyclopia

(cyclopism, cyclops, monoculus, monophthalmus, monops[1])

Cyclopia is the designation for the presence of only one palpebral space in the mid-line, below an elongated, tubelike probiscus.[2] Cyclopia may have one or two eye globes within the single orbit; although more strictly speaking, synophthalmos is defined as two fused globes, and cyclopia the much rarer complete fusion.[3] It may be a hereditary condition. One patient and some members of his family had a missing third chromosome and a supplementary C chromosome.[4] These fetuses are stillborn because of related malformations, particularly of the central nervous system.

The name is derived from the Cyclopes of Greek and Roman mythology. They were referred to by Homer as a one-eyed, gigantic, and lawless race of shepherds in Sicily who devoured human beings. The Cyclopes served as assistants to Vulcan, and were killed by Apollo for having furnished Zeus with thunderbolts.[5] The Arimaspians were yet another mythical people who had only one eye each. They lived in Sycthia, north of the Black Sea, and sought

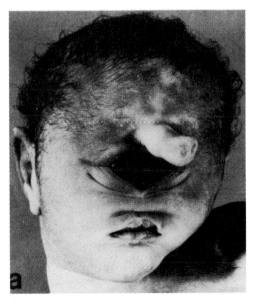

(B)

Cyclopia **A.** A Medieval Cyclops[13] **B.** Stillborn with cyclopia.[2] (by permission, Alan R. Liss, Inc.)

to steal the treasures of the griffins.[6] In African folklore, the wengwa of Gabon is a reanimated corpse which has only one eye in the center of its forehead.[7]

Cyclopia has been reported in many animals: horse, cow, pig, sheep, goat, cat, guinea pig, and rat.[8] In rabbits, it may be inherited. Cyclopia may occur in fetuses of pregnant ewes which feed upon or are given the plant *Veratrum californicum* about the fourteenth day of pregnancy.[9] Such teratogenic activity is due to cyclopamine, a steroidal alkaloid extracted from the plant.[10] Anatomical defects include absence of one optic nerve, of the olfactory nerve, and of various small bones of the cranium and face.[11]

Quevedo y Villegas, in his 1626 book titled *Graces and Disgraces of the Eye of the Ass* likened the anus not only to a eye, but also to the Cyclopes.[12] The justification was that the eye of the "ass" is median and is only one "for so it comes to resemble the Cyclopes, who themselves were one-eyed and descended from the gods of sight."

1. OED: II:1300.
2. Kokich, V. G. et al.: Cyclopia: An anatomic and histologic study of two specimens: *Teratology*, 26:105–113, 1982.
3. Duke, E. S.: Anomalies of fusion: in *System of Ophthalmology*, 2nd ed., V. III, St. Louis, C. V. Mosby, 1964, pp. 429–451.
4. Pfitzer, P. & Muntefering, H.: Cyclopism as a hereditary malformation: *Nature*, 217:1071–1072, 1968.
5. Bulfinch, pp. 471–472.
6. Schmidt, p. 114.
7. Hill, D.: *The History of Ghosts, Vampires, and Werewolves*: Ottenheimer, Memphis, 1973, p. 14.
8. Saunders, L. Z. & Rubin, L. F.: *Ophthalmic Pathology of Animals*: Basel, S. Harger, 1975, p. 202.
9. Bryden, M. M. et al.: Cyclopia in sheep caused by plant teratogens: *J. Anat.*, 110:307, 1971.
10. Keeler, R. F. & Binns, W.: Teratogenic compounds of Veratrum californicum (Durand). II.: *Can. J. Biochem.*, 44:829–838, 1966.
11. Gimeno, M. et al.: Malformáciones Congénitas en La Oveja: Ciclocéfalos: *Anat. Histol. Embryol.*, 9:129–133, 1980.
12. Quevedo [y Villegas], F. G. de: *Graces and Disgraces of the Eye of the Ass*: 1626, as quoted by Gonzales-Crussi in *Three Forms of Sudden Death*, New York, Harper & Row, 1986, p. 130.
13. Schedel, H.: *Woodcuts from Hartman Schedel*: Neurenberg, 1498.

D

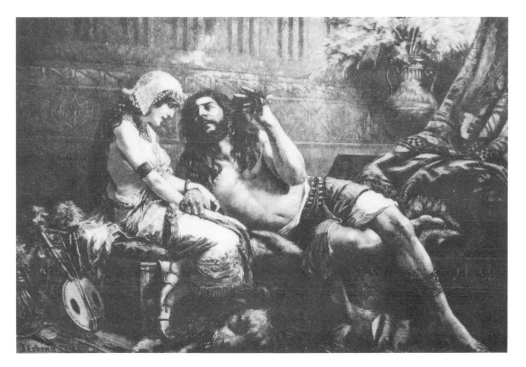

Delilah Syndrome   Delilah seducing Sampson.[4]

Delilah Syndrome

Delilah's name has been given to a syndrome of marked sexual promiscuity arising from the fear and dislike of a strong, dominant, aggressive father.[1] These women unconsciously switch roles with their fathers in seducing and overcoming males. Samson fell in love with Delilah, who had been raised by the Philistines and became their agent.[2] She was offered 1100 pieces of silver by the Philistines to find out the source of Samson's great strength. After considerable pleading he told her, and then she had seven locks of his hair shaven off while he was asleep.

The shearing of Samson's hair is considered as a symbolic castration.[1] "Like Delilah, these women could not break the Philistine's (father's) hold, nor could they successfully challenge it. Instead they approach, seduce, and overcome their Samsons and symbolically (as well as physically) render them weak." The Delilah Syndrome appears to be a form of nymphomania. In the vernacular, "a delilah" is a temptress.[3]

1. Gerson, A.: The Delilah syndrome (or the father's role in female promiscuity): *Perspect. Psychiatr. Care*, 12:74–79, 1974.
2. OT: Judges 16:4–22.
3. Espy, p. 72.
4. Brewer, 4:12.

Delphian Node

The Delphian lymph node is located in the mid-line fascia of the anterior neck, overlying the thyroid isthmus. It is so-called because if abnormal in appearance when exposed at surgery, it is indicative of disease in the underlying thyroid, but not of any one obvious type.[1]

Delphi was a city on the slopes of Parnassus in Phocis, and the supposed center of the earth. Goats feeding at this mountain had convulsions. A goat herder when inhaling a peculiar vapor arising from a deep cleft in the mountainside had convulsions, and his ravings were taken to be divinely inspired and attributed to Apollo. A priestess, named Pythia, was chosen to sit on a tripod over the cleft and her inspired words were interpreted by priests.[2] Delphian came to refer to anything obscure or ambiguous,[3] as were the responses of the Delphic oracle.[4] Pytho was the first name for Delphi, the latter being found in Homer.[5]

Lourie[6] states that delphic nodes are pretracheal nodes, and so named because they were thought to be of uncertain significance (although there are no anterior pretracheal nodes). The term Delphian oracle was used in the seventeenth century for the belief that all diseases could be diagnosed by the observation of urine. "[They] are nothing at all ashamed, by the urine alone to deliver their Delphian oracles concerning all diseases."[4]

The adjective delphian (or delphic) refers, in general, to anything that is ambiguous or obscure,[3] and is derived from the oracle at Delphi.

1. *Dorland's Illustrated Medical Dictionary*: 26th ed., Philadelphia, W. B. Saunders, 1981, p. 897.
2. Bulfinch, pp. 372–373.
3. Espy, p. 23.
4. OED: III:169.
4. Dempsey, T.: *The Delphic Oracle. Its Early History, Influence and Fall*: Oxford, England, B. H. Blackwell, 1918.
6. Lourie, J. A.: *Medical Eponyms: Who Was Coudé*: London, Pitman, 1982, p. 45.

Diana Complex

Psychological masculine tendencies in women have been labeled as the Diana Complex, as demonstrated by engaging in traditional male activities.[1] Diana (Artemis) was a virgin Greek goddess noted for her modesty, grace, and vigor. She despised the weakness of love, and imposed on her nymphs vows of perpetual maidenhood.[2] As the twin sister of Apollo, she took part in most of his adventures. She was both a huntress and a guardian of wild beasts. Diana was not an Amazon, as she had feminine grace and modesty in addition to her love of adventure and hunting. Akin to this goddess is Wonder Woman, a comic book character and later television heroine, whose everyday name is Diana.

Doctor James Barry (1800–1865), a British military physician, is considered to have been a female who impersonated a male.[3] This was based upon the observations by the charwoman who laid out the body after death.[4] Suggested have been hermaphrodism and Kleinfelter's disease, which have secondary sex characteristics which differ somewhat from the normal genotype. He or she did, however, attain the rank of inspector general in the British Army.[5]

More consistent with the Diana Complex is Dr. Mary Edwards Walker (1832–1919), who became a contract surgeon in the United States Army in 1864.[6] She was an undoubted biological female, who adopted aggressive male behavior and attire. Walker has been diagnosed as having a paranoia with "a militant and determined ego that revolted against its sex . . . in . . . open, and complete as possible, switch to the opposite sex,"[6] unlike the goddess Diana (see Don Juan Syndrome). Similar to Dr. Walker is a woman who contravened the rule in classical times that forbad women to study medicine. Hyginus described how Agnodike "cut off her hair, dressed as a man and became the student of Herophilus," who practiced in the fourth and fifth centuries B.C.[7] When she went to help a women in labor, the patient refused until Agnodike lifted up her own clothes to reveal her femininity.

Several nineteenth century authors could be considered as a forme fruste of the Diana Complex. The masculine tendency of Lucie Dupin (1804–1876), the French romantic novelist, was restricted to the adoption of a male pseudonym (George Sand) and a rejection of ties that bind wives to husbands against their will (although she certainly was not a virgin).[8] Other Victorian female writers who hid their gender under an alias were the Brontë sisters (Acton, Currer, and Ellis Bell) and Mary Ann Evans, (George Eliot).[9]

The related syndrome in the male is the Don Juan Syndrome. The acronym DIANA refers to a Fortran program for the analysis of ultracentrifugation patterns.[10]

1. Dudzinski.
2. Gayley. pp. 29–31.
3. Smith, K. M.: Military man—or woman?: *Can. Med. Assoc. J.*, 126:854–857, 1982.
4. Bensusan, A. D.: The medical history of Dr. James Barry: *South Afr. Med. J.*, 39:1074–1075, 1965.
5. Kirby, P. R.: Dr. James Barry, controversial South African medical figure: A recent evaluation of his life and sex: *South Afr. Med. J.*, 44:506–516, 1970.
6. Brussel, J. A.: Pants, politics, postage and physic: *Psychiatr. Q. Suppl.*, 35:332–345, 1961.
7. King, H.: *Agnodike and the Profession of Medicine*: Proceedings of the Cambridge Philological Society, 212:53–77, 1986.
8. Drabble, M., Ed.: *Oxford Companion to English Literature*: 5th ed., Oxford, England, Oxford University Press, 1985, p. 864.
9. Johnson, W. S.: *Living in Sin. The Victorian Sexual Revolution*: Chicago, Nelson-Hall, 1979, p. 83.
10. Trankle, E.: Description of Diana 2: *Comput. Programs Biomed.*, 7:45–55, 1977.

Don Juan Syndrome

(Don Juanism,[1] satyrism)

The Don Juan Syndrome has been applied

to excessive sexual behavior in males. About 50% of cases of hypersexuality represent efforts of impotent males to prove themselves.[2] They feel little emotion in their relationships with women. This syndrome has also been considered as an expression of the Oedipus complex in which the promiscuous male is searching for his mother's love in other women,[3] or as a manifestation of repressed homosexuality.

Don Juan is a popular Spanish legend dating back to the seventeenth century.[4] At the height of his career, he seduced the daughter of a noble family and killed her father when he tried to avenge her. Don Juan refused to repent and was sent to eternal damnation. Thus, he is regarded as the symbol of libertinism and the archetype of the heartless seducer.

The legend of Don Juan was propagated by Mozart's 1787 opera, *Don Giovanni*,[5] which has helped to transform him into a universal character. *Man and Superman*,[6] a play by George Bernard Shaw, contains a long act (Don Juan in Hell) which is based on the Juanian legend. Shaw, in his introduction, provides a generic definition of the prototype. He "is a man who, though gifted enough to be exceptionally capable of distinguishing between good and evil, follows his own instincts without regard to the common, statute or canon law;. . . ." The description is more that of a sociopath than of a psychopath. There have been at least nine other Don Juan plays in the past five centuries, with a varying orientation based on the social attitudes of the time.[7] A Don Juan type is also portrayed in Dostoevsky's novel, *The Eternal Husband*,[8] in the character of Velchaninov.

A related syndrome is the Daughter of a Don Juan, the female child of a father who exhibits the Don Juan Syndrome.[9] She experiences intense feelings of both arousal and rejection with the inability to develop "a viable psycho-sexual identity because of a lack of an adequate ego-ideal, and ultimately might develop a male identity as a last effort to gain her father's love." This could also be a cause of the Diana Complex.

In real life, Pushkin, Byron, Alfred de Musset, Benjamin Constant, and Casanova have been called Don Juans.[10] Casanova, the eighteenth century Italian writer and libertine, resembles the fictional character in particular, lacking any emotional or sentimental feelings toward his conquests. The phrase, Don Juans of achievement, has been applied to people compelled to "pile one success upon another in an attempt to undo previous failures and allay guilt."[11]

The name Don Juan has also been used for a figure known as Kokopelli, depicted in paleolithic drawings on rocks in the southwestern United States.[12] He is a hunchback who is depicted with priapism. The latter suggests spinal irritation related to the vertebral disease, and also the reason for the linkage with the fictional Don Juan. Another Don Juan occurs in a series of four books written by Carlos Castaneda. He is an elderly Mexican Yaqui Indian,[13] and rather than the prowess in sex associated with the legendary Don Juan, it is in mystical knowledge and perception that he excels.[14]

1. Holzbach, E. Von: Don-Juanismus. Sexuelle Stilbildung als Kulturhistorisches Phänomen und Psychiatrisches Problem: *Schwiez. Arch. Neurol. Neurochir. Psychiatr.*, 120:227–241, 1977.
2. Freedman, pp. 1507–1508.
3. Fenichel, O.: *The Psychoanalytical Theory of Neurosis*: New York, W. W. Norton, 1945.
4. *Encyclopaedia Britannica*: III:621–622.
5. Mozart, W. A.: Don Giovanni: in the *New Milton Cross Complete Stories of the Great Operas*, K. Kohrs, ed., Garden City, New York, Doubleday, 1955, pp. 177–186.
6. Shaw, G. B.: *Man and Superman. A Comedy and a Philosophy*: London, A. Constable, 1903.
7. Jones, A. D. et al.: Socialization and themes in popular drama: An analysis of the content of child-rearing manuals and Don Juan plays in sixteenth to twentieth centuries: *Eur. J. Soc. Psychol.*, 4:65–84, 1974.
8. Pratt, B. E. B.: The Role of the unconscious in *The Eternal Husband*: *Lit. Psychol.*, 21:29–39, 1971.
9. Guiora, A. Z.: Daughter of a Don Juan—A syndrome: *Psychiatr. Q.*, 40:71–79, 1966.
10. Martí-Ibáñiez, F.: Casanova, then and now: in *Ariel. Essays on the Arts and the History and Philosophy of Medicine*: New York, MD Publications, 1962, p. 221.
11. Campbell, pp. 185–186.
12. Wellmann, K. F.: Kokopelli of Indian paleology. Hunchbacked rain priest, hunting magician, and Don Juan of the old southwest: *J.A.H.A.*, 212:1678–1682, 1970.
13. Scotton, B. W.: Relating the work of Carlos Castaneda to psychiatry: *Bull. Menninger Clin.*, 42: 223–238, 1978.

14. Smith C. U. M.: Don Juan and the vision of vision: *Perception*, 10:435–453, 1981.

Don Quixote Syndrome

The existence of a sufficient amount of incompetence in dentistry to warrant compulsory continuing education is considered to be an erroneous assumption.[1] This premise has been compared with Cervantes's "Don Quixote," who imagined that evil lurked everywhere. Thus, inappropriateness of mandated education of professionals is equated with Quixote's assumption that windmills are evil dragons.[2]

The Don Quixote Syndrome could apply as well to mandated continuing medical education by many states.[3] The assumption has been that the major cause of the increased number of malpractice suits against physicians is a lack of keeping up to date with medical knowledge. The number of mandated continuing education hours have, however, been less than that actually spent in the past by a good majority of physicians; not to mention the erroneous assumption that cognitive learning in itself guarantees appropriate application. The eponym Quixotic Medicine refers not only to false premises, but also to pre–twentieth century physicians who fought imaginary diseases. Called a Don Quixotic Enterprise was the research by a psychiatrist on the harmful effects of comics on children, the context being that of a futile effort.[4]

1. Kennedy, L. M.: The Pandora's box: Why compulsory continuing education: *Ohio Dent. J.*, 44:317–319, 1970.
2. Cervantes, M. de: *The Adventures of Don Quixote de La Mancha*: New York, Dodd, Mead, 1971.
3. Chouinard, J. L.: Compulsory continuing education: It's just around the corner: *Can. Med. Assoc. J.*, 122:595–600, 1980.
4. Wertham, R.: *Seduction of the Innocent*: New York, Rinehart, 1954, p. 15.

Don Quixotism

Adults have been described who behave in the manner of a young adolescent boy whose unfulfilled love and eternal fidelity for a female help to repress sexuality.[1] This has been compared to the behavior of Cervantes's "Don Quixote," who adopted the lifestyle of knight errantry.[2] At about the age of 50, he became enamored of Aldonza Lorenzo, whom he called Dulcinea and ascetically idolized. Quixote saw her only rarely, and when he did he became apprehensive and embarrassed. Such a reaction, more abnormal in the adult than the adolescent, may be a narcissistic overcompensation for the severe frustration of one's repressed sexuality.[1] The Arthurian ideal of knighthood, which Quixote emulated, had similar implications.

It has been suggested that Cervantes had a significant influence through his book, *The Adventures of Don Quixote de la Mancha*[2] on Freud's creation of psychoanalysis.[3] In letters written in 1883, when Freud was reading this book, he referred to the conflict between reading Don Quixote and his study of the anatomy of the brain. Freud stated that "we were all noble knights passing through the world caught in a dream." Suggested as particularly influential on Freud are Cervantes's presentation of madness as a complex but intelligible phenomenon; his major theme of what is reality and what is truth; and the impact of an individual's convictions on his environment.

1. Deutsch, H.: Don Quixote and Don Quixotism: *Psychoanal. Q.*, 6:215–222, 1937.
2. Cervantes, M. de: *The Adventure of Don Quixote de La Mancha*: New York, Dodd, Mead, 1971.
3. Grinberg, L. & Rodríguez, J. F.: The Influence of Cervantes on the future creator of psychoanalysis: *Int. J. Psychoanal.*, 65:155–168, 1984.

E

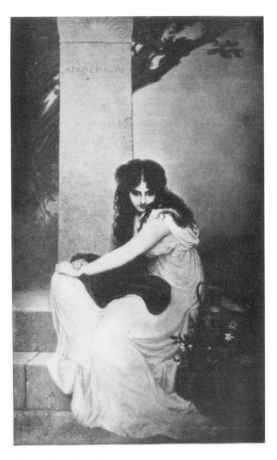

Electra Complex   Electra lamenting.[8]

Electra Complex

The Electra Complex is the female counterpart of the Oedipus situation (see Oedipus Complex), occurring in girls who see their mother as the most powerful member of the family, and their father as their chief source of nurturence.[1] Electra of Greek mythology was the daughter of Agamemnon and Clytemnestra. She and her brother, Orestes, killed their mother and their mother's lover, Aegisthus, in retaliation for murdering their father.[2] Tragedies based on Electra have been written by Sophocles, Aeschylus, Euripides, and, more recently, Eugene O'Neill (*Mourning Becomes Electra*). In Euripides' tragedy, Orestes bewails, "Take it! shroud my mother's dead flesh/in my cloak, clean and close the/sucking wounds./You carried your own death in your womb." Electra replies, "Behold! I wrap her close in the robe,/the one I loved and could not love."[3]

The existence of an exact female equivalent to the Oedipus Complex has been rejected by some on the basis that "the feminine and masculine minds are fundamentally different in their mechanisms and methods of approaching a situation."[4] The explanation given is that women are said to be more intuitive, more superstitious, and narrower in their outlook; whereas men are more rational, more logically oriented, and broader in outlook. The premise of the Electra Complex would, however, be acceptable to Freud, who was convinced that girls as well as boys experience the Oedipus Complex.[5]

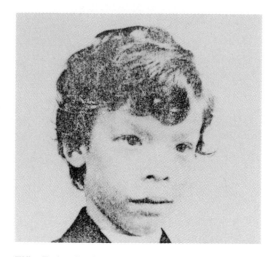

Elfin Facies Syndrome A boy with the Elfin Facies Syndrome.[3] (by permission, Annales Génétique)

Closely related to the Electra Complex is the Clytemnestra Complex in which a wife kills her husband so that she may possess one of his male relatives.[6] It is named after Clytemnestra whose lover Aegisthus was the nephew of her husband, Agamemnon, whom they killed.[2] A similar circumstance is the essence of Shakespeare's *Hamlet*, in which the King of Denmark is killed by his brother, who then marries the widowed queen.[7]

1. Garai, J. E. & Frohock, J. A.: Revelations of the Electra complex and sibling rivalry in the kinetic family drawings of seven-year-old identical twin girls: *Prog. Clin. Biol. Res.*, 24A:33–41, 1978.
2. Bulfinch, p. 291.
3. Euripides: *Electra*: E. T. Vermule translator, in *The Complete Greek Tragedies*, Vol. 4, Chicago, University of Chicago Press, 1959, pp. 397–454.
4. Coleman, S. M.: Misidentification and non-recognition: *J. Ment. Sci.*, 79:42–51, 1933.
5. Wilner, D.: The Oedipus complex, Antigone, and Electra. The woman as hero and victim: *Am. Anthropol.*, 84:58–78, 1982.
6. Campbell, p. 121.
7. Shakespeare, *Hamlet*.
8. Brewer, 1:366.

Elfin Facies Syndrome

(Williams elfin facies syndrome)

The typical Elfin Facies Syndrome is that of infantile hypercalcemia associated with peculiar coarse facies, supravalvular aortic stenosis, mental retardation, and retarded growth. Other more variable anomalies may be present.[1] The abnormal facies is characterized by short palpebral fissures, stellate pattern in the iris, medial eyebrow flare, depressed nasal bridge, anteverted nares, and thick lips. A study of 19 patients with such a facial appearance revealed 32% with cardiac anomalies and none with hypercalcemia.[2] Occurrence of the syndrome is sporadic and it is of unknown etiology. One patient has, however, been described with a 12p/15p chromosomal translocation.[3]

In early Teutonic mythology, elves were supernatural beings of dwarfish form with magical powers and given to capricious interference in human affairs.[4] They were believed to cause various diseases and nightmares, and to steal children, replacing them with changelings. The modern concept of an elf is that of a more playful, mischievous creature, equivalent to a fairy or sprite.[5]

The choice of an elf as representative of this syndrome appears to be related to retarded growth and a supposed resemblance of the abnormal facies to elves, although the latter are not usually so depicted. The medical designation depends on the author's image of an elf, which appears to be more that of a sprite or pixie (see Leprechaunism). In northern Europe, elves were depicted as graceful winged creatures that looked after flowers.[6] In Scotland, they were ugly and evil. The term elf-shot in Scottish dialect indicates disease produced by evil elves by means of an elfin arrow that makes an invisible wound.

1. Williams, J. C. P. et al.: Supravalvular aortic stenosis: *Circulation*, 24:1311–1318, 1961.
2. Jones, K. L. & Smith D. W.: The Williams elfin facies syndrome. A new perspective: *J. Pediatr.*, 86:718–723, 1975.
3. Fryns, J. P. et al.: The Elfin face syndrome and the short arm of chromosome 15: *Ann. Genet.*, 25:181–182, 1982.
4. OED: III:88–89.
5. Stein, p. 463.
6. Cohen, D.: *The Magic of the Little People*: New York, Julian Messner, 1974, pp. 26–28.

Elisha's Method

(expired-air artificial respiration, mouth-to-mouth respiration)

Mouth-to-mouth resuscitation has become accepted as suitable for use by laymen and taught as part of first aid.[1] Its eponymic name is derived from Elisha, a Hebrew prophet who succeeded Elijah in the struggle to maintain the worship of their God, Yahweh, against the cult of the Phoenician god Baal.[2] Described in the Second Book of Kings is the following.

And when Elisha was come into the house, behold, the child was dead, and laid upon his bed . . . And he went up, and lay upon the child, and put his mouth upon his mouth, and his eyes upon his eyes, and his hands upon his hands; and he stretched himself upon him; and the flesh of the child waxed warm . . . and the child sneezed seven times, and the child opened his eyes.[3]

The revival of the boy by Elisha has been interpreted differently by Wislicki.[4] He considers the initial diagnosis not as death, but as heatstroke leading to central depression with consequent imperceptible respiration and hypothermia. Elisha's therapy, then, could be that of resuscitation of a case of hypothermia by rewarming with his own body. In the First Book of Kings, Elisha's predecessor, Elijah, also brought a boy back to life by stretching himself upon the child three times and praying, "O Lord my God, I pray Thee, let this child's soul come back into him."[5] In this instance there is no mention of mouth-to-mouth application. The respiratory difficulty may have been due to laryngeal obstruction caused by infection or a foreign body.[6]

There is yet another death of a child in the First Book of Kings. King Solomon was presented with the dilemma of two women claiming the same newborn, as they had each delivered a baby three days before. Each accused the other of having killed her own "because she overlay it" and switched the infant with the live one during the night.[7] This is the earliest reference for the sudden infant death syndrome, which was previously thought to be due to suffocation by bed clothes or the mother rolling on top of the baby.[8]

There are more recent examples of historic resuscitations. In 1865, army surgeon Charles Leale used mouth-to-mouth breathing and cardiac massage in an attempt to resuscitate Abraham Lincoln after he had been shot by Booth.[9] In 1910, Dr. J. B. Johnston of Sherbrooke, Quebec, used prolonged mouth-to-mouth breathing to resuscitate a seven-week-old infant who had been given tincture of opium by mistake.[10] Such an "intimate" resuscitative method was not widely adopted, however, until 1960.[11] Similar to the mouth-to-mouth method is forced breathing into a tracheostomy tube. This was described in an appendage to an eighteenth century account of resuscitation after hanging.[12]

A more primitive use of oral contact for instilling life is the dancing corpse (rolang) of Tibetan lore.[13] It is animated by a sorcerer, lying mouth-to-mouth on the corpse. As a result the corpse rises and threshes about. The sorcerer then bites off its tongue, the corpse collapses, and its tongue used as a potent magical object.

Elisha's medical activities were not restricted to resuscitation. Naaman, captain of the king of Aram's army, came to Elisha's door requesting a cure for his leprosy. Elisha did not come out to see him, but sent a messenger to tell him to bathe in the river Jordan seven times.[14] Naaman was upset at Elisha's nonappearance and his simple remedy, but rejoiced when it resulted in a cure. Gordis[15] considers this an example of the primacy of the quality and effectiveness of care over a warm bedside manner. A letter to the editor has stressed the equal need for both.[16]

The bones of Elisha have been credited with at least one miraculous cure.[17] When a man was about to be buried a band of enemy Moabites appeared and he was thrown into Elisha's grave: "and as soon as the man touched the bones of Elisha, he revived and stood up on his feet." The Bible contains several instances of revival of the dead by prayer (see Lazarus Complex). Today, there is the additional emphasis on cardiopulmonary resuscitation, although concern has been expressed that there is insufficient training being done for this technique.[18]

1. Editorial: New methods of resuscitation: *Br. Med. J.*, 2:1592–1593, 1962.
2. *Encyclopaedia Britannica*: III:853–854.
3. OT: 2 Kings 4:32–37.
4. Wislicki, L.: A biblical case of hypothermia—Resuscitation by rewarming (Elisha's method): *Clio Med.*, 9:213–214, 1974.
5. OT: 1 Kings, 17:17–24.
6. Levin, p. 44.
7. OT: 1 Kings, 3:19.
8. Russell-Jones, D. L.: Sudden infant death in history and literature: *Arch. Dis. Child.*, 60:278–281, 1985.
9. Brooks, S. H.: *Our Assassinated Presidents. The True Medical Stories*: New York, Bell, 1966, pp. 30–31.
10. Quintin, T. J.: The "Elisha" maneuver . . . Sherbrooke, 1845: *Can. Med. Assoc. J.*, 115:731, 1976.
11. Wright-St. Clair, R. E.: The development of resuscitation: *N.Z. Med. J.*, 98:339–341, 1985.
12. *The Wonderful Monitor or Memorable Repository*: Boston, E. Russell, 1788, pp. 17–18 (privately reprinted by H. G. Huston, 1986.
13. Hill, D.: *The History of Ghosts, Vampires and Werewolves:* Memphis, Ottenheimer, 1973, p. 15.
14. OT: 2 Kings 5:1–14.
15. Gordis, L.: An early commentary on medical care: *N. Engl. J. Med.*, 292:44–45, 1975.
16. Dynes, T. F.: Elisha's bedside manner: *N. Engl. J. Med.*, 292:929, 1975.
17. OT: II Kings 13:20–21.

18. Johnson, R. W. G.: Resuscitating resuscitation: *Br. Med. J.*, 295:71, 1987.

Elpenor Syndrome

(postsleep fugue, sleep intoxication)

A disturbance of consciousness may occur when awakening after overindulgence in alcohol or drugs in a strange place. The resultant abnormal behavior may be antisocial and criminal,[1] such as jumping out of windows, theft, or murder.[2] The eponym for this mental state is named after Elpenor, who was one of the companions of Odysseus during his wanderings.[3] On suddenly awakening from a drunken sleep on a roof, he sprang up, fell from the roof, and died of a fractured cervical vertebra; "and his soul went down to the house of Hades." Elpenor returned as a ghost, pleading with Odysseus to bury his body.

Elpenor's behavior on awakening was not antisocial or criminal as is that of the patients to whom the eponym is applied.

1. Wermut, W.: Literary geneologies of some pathologic syndromes: *Psychiatr. Pol.*, 14:69–76, 1980.
2. Dudzinski.
3. Homer.

Erotomania

The definition of erotomania is insanity arising from passionate love.[1] In Greek mythology, sexual love is personified by Eros.[2] Eros (Cupid), the son of Venus and the god of love, shot darts of desire from his bow into both gods and men.[3] He is sometimes represented with his eyes covered because of the blindness of his actions.[4]

Some restrict the use of the term erotomania to involvement in imagination only, and others include nymphomania, satyriasis, and sexual deviations.[5] An example of erotomania is found in Chaucer's "The Knight's Tale"[6] in which Arcite's love sickness results in loss of judgment, palor, sighing, pulse variation, insomnia, and anorexia.[7] Shakespeare, who used many medical allusions,[8] provided another literary example of erotomania in *Troilus and Cressida*.[9]

I tell thee I am mad
in Cressid's love; thou answer'st, she is fair;
Pour'st in the open ulcer of my heart
Her eyes, her hair, her cheek, her gait, her voice.

The novels of nineteenth century authors, such as Balzac, Sand and Zola, were condemned as being erotic.[10] Erotic as an adjective also has the connotation of the passionate rather than the pornographic.[11] The term erotogenic (erogenous) zones has, however, a definite sexual meaning.[12] The term erotica refers to any collection of sexually stimulating books or objects.[13] The journal *Eros* has as its motto Plato's aphroism: "Love-Eros-makes his name in men's hearts /, but not in every heart . . . and he whom love touches not walks in darkness."[14] The contents have an emphasis on the sexual aspects of love. Jung used the eponym Eros Principle to denote the capacity of women for relationship, for seeing how things and people can be brought together.[15]

1. OED: III:274.
2. Jaeger, p. 53.
3. Weekley, p. 522.
4. Gayley, p. 35.
5. Walker, pp. 92–94.
6. Chaucer, G.: The Knight's Tale: in *The Canterbury Tales*, A. C. Spearing, ed., Cambridge, England, Cambridge University Press, 1966, pp. 98–99.
7. Ciavolella, M.: Medieval medicine and "Arcite's love sickness": *Florioegium*, 1:222–241, 1979.
8. Gandevia, B.: Shakespeare and Chaucer: Their use of medical allusion in the story of Troilus and Criseyde: *Melbourne Hosp. Clin. Rep.*, 23:8–12, 1953.
9. Shakespeare, *Troilus and Cressida*: I,ii.
10. Johnson, W. S.: *Living in Sin. The Victorian Sexual Revolution*: Chicago, Nelson-Hall, 1979, p. 7.
11. Espy, p. 224.
12. Kern, S.: *Anatomy and Destiny. A Cultural History of the Human Body*: New York, Bobbs-Merrill Co., 1975, pp. 180–187.
13. Cicardi, p. 121.
14. Ginzburg, R., Ed.: *Eros*: Vol. 1, 1962.
15. Martin, P. W.: *Experiment in Depth. A Study of the Work of Jung, Eliot and Toynbee*: London, Routledge & Kegan Paul, 1955, p. 31.

Erysichthon Syndrome

A syndrome has been described of dietary hyperlipidemia and progression of coronary atherosclerosis in obese individuals who continue overeating in spite of warnings.[1] It is named after Erysichthon of Greek mythology, who despised the gods. He cut down a venerated oak in a grove sacred to the goddess Ceres (Demeter). She ordered Famine to instill Erysichthon with insatiable hunger. The more

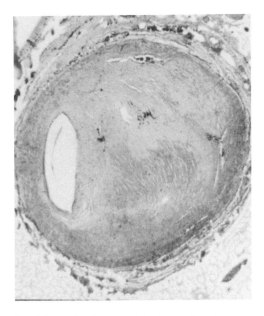

Erysichthon Syndrome   Marked narrowing of a coronary artery by atherosclerosis.[6] (by permission, J.B. Lippincott Co.)

he ate the more he craved. He repeatedly sold his daughter for money to buy more food, and finally devoured himself.[2]

There is no indication that Erysichthon was obese or had atherosclerosis or any of its manifestations. Thus Falstaff Obesity, or bulimia, would be a better designation for individuals with an insatiable appetite.[3] The word bulimia itself has been altered from its ancient Greek derivation. Originally it designated exhaustion, exposure, and hunger, and now is used for a mental state of insatiable desire for eating.[4] Examples are Samuel Johnson and the fictional Sir John Falstaff.

The association between elevated cholesterol levels and diet became a national concern in the 1980s because of its relationship to heart disease. This has resulted in a National Education Program geared toward low fat diets. The success of such a program has been called "A nation of Jack Sprats," referring to the nursery rhyme character who would eat no fat.[5]

1. Nash, D. T. et al.: The Erysichthon syndrome. Progression of coronary atherosclerosis and dietary hyperlipidemia: *Circulation*, 56:363–365, 1977.
2. Gayley, pp. 191–192.
3. Williams, J. F. et al.: Hand lesions characteristic of bulimia: *Am. J. Dis. Child.*, 140:28–29, 1986.
4. Tobe, B. A. & Wolinsky, J.: From exhaustion, exposure, and hunger to extreme voraciousness: Bulimia: *Br. Med. J.*, 293:1647–1648, 1986.
5. Marwick, C.: A nation of Jack Sprats?: *J.A.M.A.*, 256:2775, 2779, 1986.
6. *U.S. Naval Medical School: Color Atlas of Pathology*: Vol. I, Philadelphia, J. B. Lippincott, 1954, p. 236.

Esau Lady

(bearded woman[1])

The occurrence of a considerable amount of hair on the chin and upper lip of women is well known because of bearded females in circus side shows.[1] The designation of Esau Lady was, however, given to one individual in particular, Annie Jones-Elliot, who was born in Marion, Virginia, in 1865.[2] She had a moustache at birth and a fully developed beard by the age of two. Her hirsutism is stated to have occurred only on her upper lip and chin. The biblical Esau was the twin brother of Jacob.[3] He was born with a mantle of hair over his entire body.

"And Jacob said to Rebekah his mother: 'Behold, Esau my brother is a hairy man, and I am a smooth man.'" Annie, unlike Esau, was a female.

Another bearded lady, Julia Pastrana, had a generalized hypertrichosis and not a full beard.[4] This is similar to Ambroise Paré's description and drawing in the sixteenth century of a girl born "as furry as a bear" because her mother had "looked too intensely at the image of Saint John [the Baptist] dressed in skins . . . which picture was attached to the foot of her bed while she was conceiving."[5]

Generalized hirsutism in females may be caused by various conditions which result in increased androgenic secretion and menstrual abnormalities. It may also be the result of medicinal or surreptitious use of synthetic androgens.[6] About one-third of women aged 15 to 45 have some upper lip hair increase, and a few of these also have hair on the chin. Abnormally increased hair due to increased androgen concentrations appears most commonly along the mid-line of the abdomen and the nasal or auricular vibrissae, or as a beard or moustache.[7] This type of hair is the so-called terminal hair which is coarse, corkscrew curled, and strongly pigmented.

In a young male child, excessive hirsutism may develop as a feature of adrenocortical hyperplasia. This has been offered as the cause of Esau's excessive hair.[8] Esau may have had another manifestation of adrenocortical hyperplasia—low blood sugar (hypoglycemia) on the basis of his request for food (red pottage) when he felt faint.[9]

Hirsutism without virilization is designated as idiopathic or familial hirsutism and begins after puberty.[10] Occurring in either sex is the Cornelia de Lange syndrome, which consists of growth and mental retardation, a peculiar facies, congenital anomalies, bushy eyebrows, and generalized hirsutism.[11] None of these variations appear to apply to the Esau Lady. There is the possibility of an inherited hirsute trait. The son of a side show bearded lady was called the Infant Esau because he had a beard by the age of four.[12]

A different cause of hirsutism resulted in the beard of St. Wilgefortis. She was the daughter of a Portuguese King who had arranged for her marriage to the King of Spain, not knowing that she had taken a vow of chastity. Her prayers were answered by the growth overnight of a beard which repelled her fiance.[13] A literary example of the Esau Lady is found in Shakespeare's *Macbeth*. When confronted by the three witches he observed that "you should be women, / And yet your beards forbid me to interpret / that you are so."[14] Another fictional example is found in Vonnegut's novel *Galápagos*[15] in which Hisako gave birth to Akiko whose skin was "covered with a fine, silky pelt like a fur seal's. . . ." The mother had been exposed to radiation at Hiroshima and the daughter in turn gave birth to furry babies.

A reverse condition to the Esau Lady was called the disease of the Scythians by Hammond in 1882, in which there is disappearance of the beard in men as well as other physical and "moral attributes" of males.[16] Recently, idiopathic hirsutism has been treated by the aldosterone antagonist spironolactone with significant improvement.[17]

1. Gould, G. M. & Pyle, W. L.: *Anomalies and Curiosities of Medicine*: New York, Julian Press, 1956, pp. 229–232.
2. Mould, R. F.: *Mould's Medical Anecdotes*: Bristol, England, Adam Hilger, 1984, pp. 24–25.
3. OT: Genesis 27:11.
4. Miles, A. E. W.: Julia Pastrana: The bearded lady: *Proc. R. Soc. Med.*, 67:160–164, 1974.
5. Paré, p. 38.
6. Liddle, G. W.: *Hirsutism*:, R. H. Williams, ed., *Textbook of Endocrinology*, 6th ed., Philadelphia, W. B. Saunders, 1981, pp. 280–281.
7. Cittandini, E. et al.: Diagnosis of virilizing syndromes: Gynecological parameters: in *Androgenization of Women. Pathophysiology and Clinical Aspects*, Molinatti, G. M. et al., eds., New York, Raven Press, 1983, pp. 115–119.
8. Taub, J.: Endocrinology in the Bible: *Horafé Haivri*, 2:164–156, 1955.
9. Greenblatt, R. B.: *Search the Scriptures. A Physician Examines Medicine in the Bible*: Philadelphia, J. P. Lippincott, 1963, pp. 11–15.
10. Braunwald, pp. 648–650.
11. Ptacek, L. J. et al.: The Cornelia de Lange syndrome: *J. Pediatr.*, 63:1000–1020, 1963.
12. Durand, A. & J.: *Pictorial History of the American Circus*: New York, A. S. Barnes, 1957, p. 104.
13. Williams, p. 39.
14. Shakespeare, *Macbeth*: 1,ii.
15. Vonnegut, K.: *Galápagos*: New York, Dell, 1986.
16. Hammond W. A.: The disease of the Scythians (morbus feminarium) and certain analogous

conditions: *Am. J. Neurol. Psychiatry*, 1:339–355, 1882.

17. Evans, D. J. & Burke, C. W.: Spironolactone in the treatment of idiopathic hirsutism and the polycystic ovary syndrome: *J. R. Soc. Med.*, 79: 451–453, 1986.

Ether

The word ether is used to designate diethyl ether, an anesthetic agent, although many other ethers also have anesthetic properties.[1] In the beginnings of Greek mythology there was a vast and dark space, called Chaos. Chaos gave birth to Erebus and Nox (night) to whom were born Aether (light) and Hemera (day).[2] Aether gradually organized the cosmic matter in the sky.[3] This assumed the shape of an egg, around which Nox formed a shell.

Ether was first discovered in the thirteenth century by Lullius as a white fluid called sweet vitriol. In 1730, Frobenius of Germany named it ether,[4] after the subtle fluid that supposedly permeates the clear sky formed originally by Aether.[5] It was not until the nineteenth century that ether came into general use as an anesthetic. In occultism, ethcrosis is the term used for disorders of the "second body" (non-material) of man, such as emotional and psychosomatic disorders.[6]

1. Stedman, p. 490.
2. Espy, p. 16.
3. Guirand 1964, pp. 11, 13.
4. Keys, T. E.: *The History of Surgical Anesthesia*: New York, Dover, 1963, p. 9.
5. Weekley, p. 526.
6. Walker, pp. 94–98.

Eye of Horus

The eye of Horus (Utchat) was a very common amulet used throughout early Egyptian history to protect the health of the bearer.[1] The sun was the center of Egyptian worship, being Horus in the morning, Ra at noonday, and setting as Tum.[2] Osiris was Horus's father and Isis his mother. He later became identified with the latter. In a fight with the demon Set Horus lost his eye. Thoth, the god of wisdom, spat on the wound and thus returned the eye to Horus, the sun.[1] This eye, drawn within a modified R, became a symbol of a miracle and a talisman to ward off evil. In the Middle Ages, the eye was used by artists to denote God as well as satanism.[3]

The Egyptian symbol was an ℞ with an eye painted in the top circle. At the time of Nero, the ℞ sign was introduced as a graphic that indicated that physicians were subject to the power of the church.[3] In medieval Latin, it was a symbol for a recipe, a form of the verb recipere, "to take, receive."[4] It gradually turned into the sign for prescriptions—its early use being to ward off any harmful effects of medication. It is used at present to indicate "take thou."[5] Horus is also still with us in the form of his other symbol, the sharp-eyed falcon which is carved on the so-called Cleopatra Needle on the London embankment.[6]

1. Krause, A. C.: Ancient Egyptian ophthalmology: *Bull. Inst. Hist. Med.*, 1:258–276, 1933.
2. Bulfinch, p. 365.
3. Marti-Ibáñez, F.: Symbols and Medicine: in *Ariel. Essays on the Arts and the History and Philosophy of Medicine*: New York, MD Publications, 1962, pp. 40–49.
4. Editors of the American Heritage Dictionaries.
5. Guthrie, D.: *A History of Medicine*: London, Thomas Nelson & Sons, 1945, p. 20.
6. Hayward, R. A.: *Cleopatra's Needles*: Buxton, Derbyshire, Moorland, England, 1978, p. 124.

F

Fallen Angel I, II

I   The Fallen Angel eponym derives from the Victorian concept of a women being pure (angelic).[1] When she discards her purity for sexual indiscretion there can be no return to her original virtuous state, thus comparing her with Lucifer who fell from God's grace. In contrast is the male who can retain his state of grace even if he is the seducer. The eponym and its implicit double standard relates in part to the biblical depiction of the first woman, Eve, who committed the first sin by plucking the forbidden fruit from the tree of knowledge.[2] The original purity of the first and all subsequent women is reflected in much of the literature of the nineteenth century. On a more modern, psychological basis this all-or-none attitude toward women has been called the Madonna-Harlot Complex.

II   Inept, careless, and poorly trained parachute jumpers can sustain injuries to their lower extremities on landing, such as a torn Achilles tendon, a malleolar fracture, and fractured long bones.[3] Such individuals who make jumps to raise money for hospital-sponsored charities have been called Fallen Angels. The eponym is more a "cute" pun than appropriate, as it is used to denote someone doing a good (although foolhardy) deed (and Lucifer was certainly not so inclined).

The eponym Fallen Angel was originally applied to the devil, Lucifer, an angel who fell (descended) into hell when he tried to usurp the position of the monotheistic god of Western

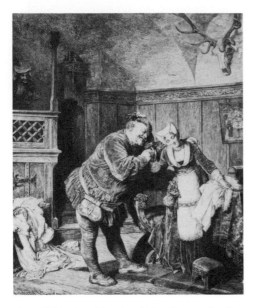

Falstaff Obesity   The obese Falstaff romancing.[12]

religions.[4] The phrase is now used literally for one who has fallen out of previous good graces, such as a defaulter.[5]

1. Mitchell, S.: *The Fallen Angel. Chastity, Class and Women's Reading*, 1835–1880: Bowling Green, Ohio, Bowling Green University Popular Press, 1981.
2. OT: Genesis.
3. Jessop, J. H.: Fallen angel: How not to raise money for charity: *Br. Med. J.*, 291:1282, 1985.
4. *Encyclopaedia Britannica*: III:502–503.
5. Partridge, p. 377.

Falstaff Obesity

An eponym denoting obesity due to the excessive consumption of food[1] has been derived from Shakespeare's comic knight in the *Merry Wives of Windsor, Henry IV*, I & II, and *Henry V*.[2] Falstaff is depicted as being addicted to food and drink, with consequent marked obesity. The eponym is related to the Erysichthon Syndrome, but without the direct connotation of atherosclerosis. Falstaff is, in general, considered as the embodiment of self-indulgence, good humor, and bulimia (excessive and insatiable appetite).[3]

In his dying moments in *Henry V* Falstaff's nose was described by Mistress Pistol as "sharp as a pen, and a' babbled of greene fields."[4] The former could be indicative of a Hippocratic facies, which results from emaciation due to disease; and the latter possibly to jaundice caused by cirrhosis consequent to the fatty liver of obesity and alcoholism.[5] There is, however, considerable controversy over the cause of his death, the most popular reason offered being a type of anemia with green skin (chlorosis), although it occurred in females, or a "broken heart" (febris amatoria).[6] Another interpretation is a great fever such as typhoid or peritonitis.[7]

There is considerably more concern with obesity and diets today than in Falstaff's day. This is due in part to a change in esthetic preference from the pleasantly plump, nubile females of renaissance paintings to the more suave, slender females seen in today's advertisements and television commercials. The concern is also based on the knowledge of the relationship between obesity and atherosclerosis, cirrhosis, hypertension, and diabetes. It has been estimated that about 20% of United States teenagers are overweight and that "at any one time about half of all Americans are on a diet."[8]

Excessive ingestion of only one kind of food differs from the eating habits of bulimic individuals such as Falstaff who will eat almost anything. Some nutritional faddists ingest excessive amounts of carrots which contain a significant amount of carotene, a vitamin A precursor, with resultant carotenemia.[9] The large amount of this pigment in the blood results in yellowing of the serum and the skin, most marked in the palms and soles. Carotenemia has been labeled as Bugs Bunny Bulimia, named after a cartoon rabbit who was continually eating and protecting his hoard of carrots (although his skin is not depicted as yellow).[10] This anthropomorphized rabbit, the product of Leon Schlesinger Productions, became the most popular animated animal of the 1940s.[11] Bugs Bunny's wisecracking confidence and spirited defense of his home have been credited with contributing to morale during World War II.

1. Dudzinski.
2. Shakespeare.
3. Espy, p. 128.
4. Shakespeare, *King Henry*: V, II, iii.
5. Fleissner, R.: Putting Falstaff to rest: "Tabulating" the facts: *Shakespeare Studies Res. Crit. Rev.*, 14:57–74, 1983.
6. Fleissner, R. F.: Falstaff's green sickness unto death: *Shakespeare Q. (Wash.)*, 12:47–55, 1961.
7. Simpson, R. R.: *Shakespeare and Medicine*: Edinburgh, E. & S. Livingstone, 1962, pp. 52–57.
8. Dunea, G.: Sweet tooth maketh a sour disposition: *Br. Med. J.*, 293:120–121, 1986.
9. Wilson, J. D.: Vitamin excess: in Braunwald, E. et al., eds., *Harrison's Principles of Internal Medicine*, 11th ed. New York, McGraw-Hill, 1987, p. 417.
10. Chase, M.: Solace for us slobs: Being fit and pretty can be bad for you: *Wall Street J.*, July 14, 1986, pp. 1, 8.
11. Daniels, L.: *Comix. A History of Comic Books in America*: New York, Outerbridge & Dienstfrey, 1971, p. 52.
12. Brewer, 2:2.

Falstaff Snore

Falstaff's name has been used for the heavy snoring which may occur in obese people.[1] In Shakespeare's *Henry IV*, Part II, Falstaff is caricatured as being fast asleep and breathing noisily.[2] "Sheriff: 'A gross fat man.' Carrier 'As

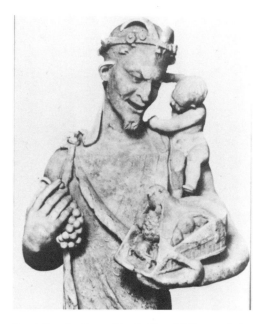

Faun's Beard Faun with tufted beard.[2] (by permission, Giraudon)

fat as butter . . ..' Peto: 'Falstaff! Fast asleep behind the arras, and snorting like a horse.' Prince: 'Hark, how hard he fetches his breath.' " Falstaff's snoring, however, may have been due more to alcoholic intoxication than to obesity.[3] One study has suggested an association between habitual and frequent snorers and ischemic heart disease and strokes.[4] In these instances, the snoring is likely related to obstructive sleep apnea which results in hypoxia and increased packed red cell volume, the latter being in itself a cause of ischemic heart disease.[5]

1. Adler, J. J.: Did Falstaff have the sleep-apnea syndrome?: *N. Engl. J. Med.*, 308:404, 1983.
2. Shakespeare, *Henry IV*: Part 1, II,iv.
3. Junghans, R. P.: Falstaff was drunker than he was fat: *N. Engl. J. Med.*, 308:1483, 1983.
4. Koskenvuo, M. M. et al.: Snoring as a risk factor for ischaemic heart disease and stroke in men: *Br. Med. J.*, 294:16–19, 1987.
5. Yates, P.: Letter to Editor: *Br. Med. J.*, 294:371, 1987.

Faun's Beard

The tuft of hair which may be associated with spina bifida occulta[1] is considered to have some resemblance to the beard of the faun of Roman mythology.[2] Fauns were playful, rural Latin deities with horns, pointed ears, beards, goats' hooves, and tails. Their name is derived from Faunus, the grandson of Saturn, who was the god of fields, shepherds, and prophecy.[2] It is the tufted beards of fauns which have a commonality with patients afflicted with spina bifida, rather than their playful behavior.

1. Dirckx, p. 73.
2. Guirand 1968, p. 215.

Faust Complex

The Faust Complex has been defined as "a distorted and maladaptive hypertrophy of the strivings for omnipotence, omniscience and boundless sexual gratification."[1] There is also an overwhelming desire for wish fulfillment which results in an almost magical mode of thinking.

The historical Faustus, a German magician and charlatan, was Doctor Johannes Faustus, who died in 1540. Thereafter arose the legendary, literary Faust who sold his immortal soul to the devil, Mephistopheles, in exchange for knowledge and power.[2] He used his magical power to journey all over the world and to evoke Helen of Troy. After many years he suffered remorse and wanted to repent; but it was too late and he was seized by Mephistopheles. According to Jungian psychology, Faust had not lived out an important part of his early life.[3] Therefore, he was an incomplete person who took on a quest for metaphysical goals that proved to be useless. Faust's behavior has been analyzed as the striving for a form of superiority that occurs in individuals with a continuous overwhelming inferiority feeling.[4]

The universal nature of the Faust theme is evidenced in a play by Christopher Marlowe in the sixteenth century,[5] a dramatic poem by Goethe in the nineteenth century,[6] and an opera by Gounod (1859).[7] In a more recent version, Thomas Mann's *Doctor Faustus*, Faust is represented by a composer, Adrian Leverkuhn, who developed neurosyphilis. He made a contract with the devil for 24 years of musical creativity in return for the eternal damnation of his soul.[8] There have been suggestions that illnesses may enhance creativity,[9] as, for example, the tuberculosis of Keats, Dostoevsky's epilepsy, Poe's alcoholism, De Quincy's opium addiction, and Beethoven's headaches and deafness.[10]

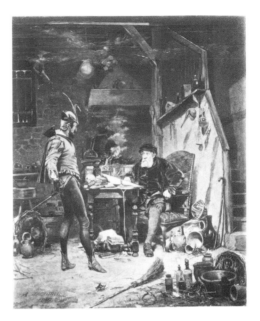

Faust Complex   Faust and Mephistopheles.[11]

1. Werman, D. S. & Rhoads, J. M.: The Faust legend seen in the light of an analytic case: *J. Am. Psychoanal. Assoc.*, 24:101-121, 1976.
2. Butler, E. M.: *The Fortunes of Faust*: Cambridge, England, Cambridge University Press, 1952.
3. Henderson, J. L.: Ancient myths and modern man: in Jung, C., p. 112.
4. Osherson, S.: An Alderian approach to Goethe's Faust: *J. Individ., Psychol*, 21:194-198, 1965.
5. Marlowe, C.: *The Tragical History of Doctor Faustus*: London, Golden Hours Press, 1932.
6. Goethe, J. W. von: *Faust. A Tragedy*: A. Raphael translator, New York, Jonathan Cape & Harrison Smith, 1930.
7. Gounod, C. F.: *Faust* (1859): New York, Crown, 1939.
8. Mann, T.: *Doctor Faustus. The Life of the German Composer, Adrian Leverkuhn, as Told by a Friend*: H. T. Lowe-Porter translator, New York, Alfred A. Knopf, 1948.
9. Forschbach, G.: Tuberculosis and creative man: *Bull. Int. Union Tuberc.*, 59:107-110, 1984.
10. Meehan, M. C.: A medical version of the Faust legend: *J.A.M.A.*, 196:156-160, 1966.
11. Brewer, 3:41.

Fiacre

Fiacre is a medieval name for hemorrhoids, fistula-in-ano, and all diseases of the rectum.[1] It is an eponym derived from St. Fiacre, an Irish hermit of the seventh century.[2] He moved to France where he built a hospice for travelers, and became widely known for his healing powers. In particular he was noted as a healer of all intestinal afflictions.[3] Fiacre was summoned by Bishop Faron for an inquest, but then was made to wait sitting on a large stone for several days. The stone miraculously became softer and retained the print of the Saint's buttocks. The stone was then granted the power of curing diseases of the anus of anyone sitting on it. Cardinal Richelieu's hemorrhoids were not, however, cured in 1632 by the saint's relics.

St. Fiacre is known as the patron saint of proctology,[3] and was also invoked for the cure of venereal disease.[4] Early Parisian cabs were named fiacres after the Hotel Saint-Fiacre rather than after the Saint directly. They may well have aggravated hemorrhoids rather than cured them. Perhaps riding in cabs contributed to the fistula of the King of France in Shakespeare's *All's Well That Ends Well*.[5] St. Fiacre's skills in gardening and growing medical herbs has resulted in yet another patronage, that of gardeners.[1]

1. Murphy.
2. Delaney, J. J.: *Dictionary of Saints*: Garden City, New York, Doubleday, 1980, p. 225.
3. Racouchot, J. E. et al.: Saint Fiacre: The healer of hemorrhoids and patron saint of proctology: *Am. J. Proctol.*, 22:175-179, 1971.
4. Dewhurst, J.: Saint who's?: *Br. Med. J.*, 293: 1618-1621, 1986.
5. Shakespeare, *All's Well That Ends Well*: 1,i.

Frankenstein Complex

There exists for some the fear that machines and robots will supplant humanity.[1] An example is the potentiality of artificial intelligence technology to create robots that may replace physicians in the future.[2] Such fears have been labeled as the Frankenstein Complex, derived from Mary Shelley's novel of 1818, *Frankenstein*.[3] The association is a bit stretched because the recreated monster was only one individual, unlike those in Capek's *Rossum's Universal Robots*.[4] Frankenstein was not the first artificial being in literature, although, unlike others, he was created by Baron Victor Frankenstein by the effect of electricity on the dead.[5]

The name Frankenstein is generally used for anything that destroys its creator,[6] although the Baron died of infirmities rather than at the hands of his monster. His wife, however, was killed on their wedding day.

A relationship between Mary Shelly and the character of her monster has not been neglected.[7] She suffered considerable parental neglect, her mother having died of sepsis from a retained placenta shortly after Mary's birth. Her father was unable to provide any warmth or love. Thus, it has been proposed that such deprivation is expressed by Frankenstein's crying out for love and acceptance.

No father had watched my infant days, no mother had blessed me with smiles and caresses. I ought to be thy [Victor's] Adam; but I am rather the fallen angel, whom thou drivest from joy for no misdeed. Everywhere I see bliss from which I am irrevocably excluded.

This Gothic novel has been considered as "the first work of science fiction . . . a symbol of the discoveries in science . . . a classic example of man's playing god."[8]

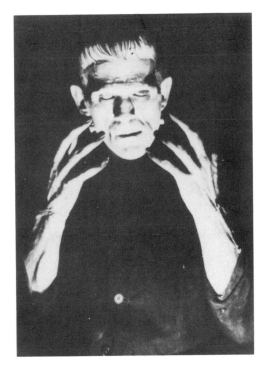

Frankenstein Factor   Boris Karloff as Frankenstein.[12]

1. Asimov, A.: *Asimov on Science Fiction*: Garden City, New York, Doubleday & Co., 1981, pp. 153-154.
2. Bloom, K. J. & Weinstein, R. S.: Expert systems: Robot physicians of the future?: *Human Pathol.*, 16:1083-1084, 1985.
3. Shelley.
4. Capek, K.: *R.U.R. (Rossum's Universal Robots)*: Garden City, New York, Doubleday, Page & Co., 1923.
5. Cohen, J.: *Human Robots in Myth and Science*: London, George Allen & Unwin, 1966.
6. Espy, p. 133.
7. Myers, W. A.: Mary Shelley's *Frankenstein*: Creativity and the psychology of the exception: *J. Psychoanal. Psychother.*, 9:625-645, 1982-83.
8. Wygant, A.: Shelley, Hawthorne, and Wells: Images of medicine in early science fiction: Bookman, 8:3-8, 1981.

Frankenstein Factor

The Frankenstein Factor refers to an antitechnology bias due to concern for possible mistakes or unknown horrors of genetic research with recombinant deoxyribonucleic acid (DNA).[1] Ethical concerns have also been raised in respect to genetic construction.[2] The more esoteric and intricate a scientific technique, the more mysterious and feared it is by the lay person, as represented by Shelly's Frankenstein monster.[3] Frankenstein was created by Mary Shelley as an innocent and naive being. He was thwarted by people who responded negatively to his physical appearance to such a degree that he became transformed to hatred and despair.[4]

Sophisticated and detailed genetic control of man is no longer entirely in the realm of science fiction.[5] The birth of hundreds of babies after in vitro fertilization of human embryos could be the first step.[6] The Asilomar conference of 1985 recommended that research with recombinant DNA should be postponed until safety guidelines could be developed.[5]

Related to the Frankenstein Factor is the Frankenstein Monster, an experiment or enterprise that has gone awry or amok.[7] Also related to the Frankenstein Monster is the Social Frankenstein which states that "human endeavors even though initiated through the best of intentions, often come to grief through misdirected applications of noble intentions."[8] Events compared with a Frankenstein monster out of control are the American medical education system which is not meeting its objectives[9] and health-related expenditures in the United States[10] and in Britain (see Icarus Complex).[11]

1. Gaylin, W.: The Frankenstein factor: *N. Engl. J. Med.*, 297:665-667, 1977.
2. Lynch, A.: Brave new world in reproductive techniques and genetic construction — A dream or a nightmare? 1984: The pre-ethical agenda.: *Ann. R. Coll. Phys. Surg. Can.*, 17:505–508, 1984.
3. Shelley.
4. Morowitz, H. J.: Frankenstein and recombinant DNA: *Hosp. Pract.*, 14:175–176, 1979.
5. Redaksie, V. D.: Die 'Frankenstein Faktor': *South Afr. Med. J.*, 53:154–155, 1978.
6. Smith, T., Ed.: Experiments on embryos: Do they have rights?: *J. R. Soc. Med.*, 78:503–504, 1985.
7. Dirckx, p. 74.
8. Thorne, F. C.: Social science-created Frankensteins: *J. Clin. Psychol.*, 29:112, 1973.
9. Iberti, T. J.: American medical education. Has it created a Frankenstein?: *Am. J. Med.*, 78:179–181, 1985.
10. Prior, J. T.: Dr. Frankenstein, I presume?: *N.Y. State J. Med.*, 81:1266–1268, 1981.
11. Nazer, G.: Who can control this son of Frankenstein?: *Nursing Mirror*, 148:7, 1979.

12. Glut, D. F.: *The Frankenstein Catalog*: Jefferson, North Carolina, McFarland & Co., 1984, frontispiece.

Frankenstein Syndrome

The Frankenstein Syndrome has been used to represent man's ambivalent attitude toward knowledge and power. It is exemplified by the contrast between Aristotle's praise of knowledge of any kind and God's punishment of Adam and Eve for eating from the fruit of the tree of knowledge.[1] This Janus-faced attitude toward knowledge is evident in the reverence given to scientists such as Pasteur, Curie, Reed, and Sinclair Lewis's fictional Doctor Arrowsmith on the one hand, and to the fear of genetic manipulation and the fictional Frankenstein on the other hand. Baron Victor Frankenstein was filled with the hope of creating life, but terrified that he was mocking the Creator of the universe.[2]

The four eponyms named after Frankenstein relate in different ways to the possible results of unrestricted scientific and social experimentation upon humanity, and to whether the means justifies the ends.[3] It is a fear of our own godlike creations.[4] The Frankenstein monster was created by the Baron with the best of intentions, the subtitle of the book being *A Modern Prometheus*—the Greek Titan who stole fire from the sun for the benefit of mankind;[5] and the fire has now reached its ultimate form, the hydrogen bomb.

1. Graubard, M.: The Frankenstein syndrome: Man's ambivalent attitude to knowledge and power: *Perspect. Biol. Med.*, Spring, 1967, pp. 419–443.
2. Shelley.
3. Comroe, J. H., Jr.: Frankenstein, Pickwick, and Ondine: *Am. Rev. Respir. Dis.*, 111:689–692, 1975.
4. Roth, N.: Early electromedicine and the Frankenstein myth: *Med. Instrument.*, 12:248, 1978.
5. Bulfinch, pp. 19–28.

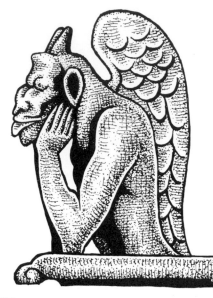

(A)

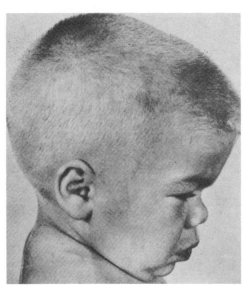

(B)

Gargoylism **A.** A gargoyle on the Cathedral of Notre Dame, Paris.[8] (by permission, Dover Pubns. Inc.) **B.** A patient with Hunger-Hurler's Disease.[7] (by permission, J.B. Lippincott Co.)

G

Gargoylism

(dysostosis multiplex,[1] Hunter's syndrome, Hunter-Hurler disease, Hurler's syndrome, lipochondrodystrophy, Thompson's syndrome)

Gargoylism is a mucopolysaccharide disorder of metabolism. Heparin sulfate and dermatan sulfate accumulate in cellular lysozymes of connective tissue, liver, spleen, kidney, and brain owing to deficiency of the enzyme, alpha-L-iduronidase.[2] This results in hepatosplenomegaly, dwarfism, and very coarse facial features (large face, puffy eyes, saddle nose, large thick nostrils and lips, large tongue).[3] Sex-linked inheritance is associated with gargoylism.[4]

A gargoyle is a rain spout found in Gothic architecture representing a grotesque animal or human figure which projects from a gutter and carries rain water clear of the walls.[5] The word gargoyle was derived from the French word for throat (gargouille). The commonality between the figure and the condition is the grotesque appearance of affected patients and dwarfism.[6] Thus, this eponym is derived from an art form. More humane is the labeling of these unfortunates with the names of those who have delineated this disorder—Hunter, Hurler, and Thompson.

The snorter dwarfism occurring in cattle has similar metabolic defects and morphological abnormalities to that found in Hunter-Hurler's disease, including a short nose with labored breathing (snorter), large tongue and head, and short neck and stature.[7]

1. Durham, p. 262.
2. Scarpelli, D. G.: Cell injury and errors of metabolism: in *Anderson's Pathology*, 7th ed., J. M. Kissane, Ed., St. Louis, C. V. Mosby, 1985, pp. 101–102.
3. Beebe, R. T.: Hunter's syndrome. Gargoyles–Washington Irving–"Rip Van Winkle": *Bull. Hist. Med.*, 44:582–585, 1970.
4. Beebe, R. T.: Gargoylism: Sex-linked transmission in nine males: *Trans. Am. Clin. Climatol. Soc.*, 66:199–205, 1954.
5. OED: IV:57.
6. Shipley, J. T.: *Dictionary of Word Origins*: New York, Philosophical Library, 1945, p. 166.
7. Lorincz, A. E.: Hurler's syndrome in man and snorter dwarfism in cattle: *Clin. Orthop. Related Res.*, 33:104–118, 1964.
8. Huber, R.: *Treasury of Fantastic and Mythological Creatures*: New York, Dover, 1981, p. 30, fig 2.

Griselda Complex

In the Griselda Complex, the father subconsciously resents but grudgingly gives up his daughter to another man as a wife and future mother. This represents a reactivation of his Oedipal yearning for his own mother.[1] The father usually assumes an altruistic concern for his daughter's welfare.

Griselda appears in the tenth story of Boccaccio's *Decameron*[2] as the daughter of a poor peasant, Giannucole. Gultieri, the Marquis of Sanluzzo, married Griselda, who was so obedient and submissive that she did not openly object to his insults on her low origin of birth, to his pretense of killing their two children, or to driving her out in only a shift on the pretense of taking another wife. "My lord, do with me whatever you think best for your honor and happiness, and no matter what, I shall be happy for I realize that I am of lower birth than they and am not worthy of honor which your courtesy has bestowed upon me."

Griselda's patient endurance finally changed her husband's attitude toward her and she became highly honored.[2] It is not evident from Decameron's "Tenth Day, Tenth Story" that Griselda's father had any of the psychological processes compatible with the Griselda Complex.

More in accord with the tenth story is the vernacular use of the name Griselda for a woman who is a paragon of purity, virtue, and endless patience, carried to the ultimate ex-

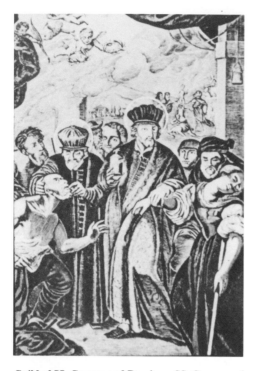

Guild of SS. Cosmas and Damian SS. Cosmas and Damian in the process of healing the ailing.[8] (by Franz Ambros Dietel, 1730)

treme.[1] Boccaccio used Griselda as an example of highly religious Christian women who, to obtain eternal glory, forced themselves to tolerate adversities beyond all reason.[3] Related is the eponym Dorcas, which was applied to a Christian disciple named Tabitha who was "full of good deed and acts of charity."[4] It is used for an ideal housewife.[5]

1. Campbell, pp. 121–122.
2. Boccaccio, G.: Tenth day, tenth story: in *The Decameron*, M. Musa & P. Bondanella translators, New York, W. W. Norton, 1982, pp. 672–689.
3. Jordan, C.: Feminism and the Humanists.: The Case of Sir Thomas Elyot's Defence of Good Women: *Renaissance Q.* 36:182–201, 1983.
4. NT: Acts 9:36–39.
5. Hendrickson, p. 333.

Guild of St. Luke, SS. Cosmas and Damian

St. Luke, SS. Cosmas and Damian is the name of the guild of the Catholic Association of Doctors of Medicine in Great Britain.[1] The alternate name of the *Catholic Medical Quarterly* journal is the same as that of the guild.[2] These saints are depicted in the crest of the Royal Society of Medicine.

Saint Luke was the author of one of the Gospels and probably of Acts of the Apostles of the New Testament.[3] He was called "the beloved physician" by the Apostle, Paul.[4] St. Luke lived during the first century, but little is known of his life.[2] Some modern biblical scholars consider him to have been a practicing physician in Malta before he became an evangelist[5] because the Gospel and Acts contain 23 technical terms not used elsewhere in the Bible, as, for example, diagnosis, dysentery, thrombi, and syndrome.[6]

Little more is known of the other two patron saints of the Guild. SS. Cosmas and Damian (c. third century) were twin brothers who were born in Arabia, studied in Syria, and became renowned for their medical skill, which was provided without fees.[7] They lived in Aegea in Cilicia, but were beheaded during the persecutions of Christians. Legends ascribe miraculous cures to them, such as replacing an amputated leg with one from a corpse, and after their death, to healing the ill that slept in a church in Constantinople.[8] The former legend has been depicted in many paintings.[9]

Saints Luke, Cosmas, and Damian are considered as the patron saints of physicians and surgeons in general, unlike other medically related saints who have been assigned to specific diseases. Luke is also claimed as a patron saint of painters,[7] and Cosmas and Damian as that of a variety of other groups, such as barbers, bandagers, hernia healers, apothecaries, druggists, wet-nurses, physicists, and shopkeepers.[8]

1. Matthews, L. G.: SS. Cosmas and Damian—Patron saints of medicine and pharmacy. Their cult in England: *Med. Hist.*, 12:281–288, 1968.
2. *Index of NLM Serial Titles.*
3. Thurston, IV:142–143.
4. NT: Col. 4:14.
5. Walsh, J. J.: St. Luke the physician: *N.Y. Med. J.*, 91:159–164, 1910.
6. Short, A. H.: A doctor investigates: *Sphincter*, 20:23–27, 1957.
7. Thurston, III:659–661.
8. Gerlitt, J.: Cosmas and Damian, the patron saints of physicians: in *Saints in Medicine*, G. Rosen, Ed., *Ciba Symp.*, 1:118–121, 1939.
9. Zimmerman, L. M.: Cosmas and Damian. Patron saints of surgery: *Bull. Soc. Med. Hist. Chicago*, 5:69–87, 1937.

H

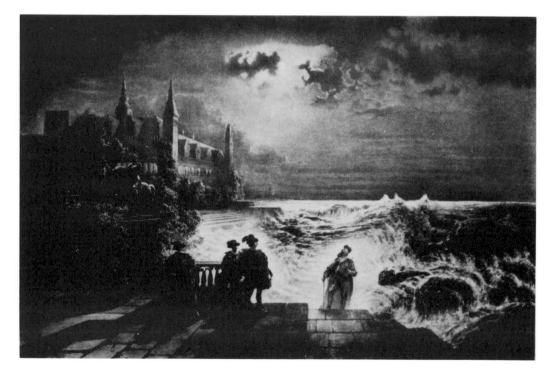

Hamlet-Gertrude Complex   Hamlet and his father's ghost.[7]

Hamlet-Gertrude Complex

A repressed Oedipus Complex that originates in infancy can result in inhibition of actions because of feelings of guilt.[1] The results are self-reproach, scruples of conscience, and the affected person's feeling that "he himself is literally no better than the sinner whom he is to punish." The complex is demonstrated by Shakespeare's *Hamlet*[2] who hesitated and was reluctant to seek revenge against the man who murdered his father; that is, Hamlet's father's brother, who then married his brother's widow, Hamlet's mother, Queen Gertrude.[3]

According to Freud, "Hamlet is able to do anything—except take vengeance on the man who did away with his father and took that father's place with his mother, the man who shows him the repressed wishes of his own childhood realized."[4] Another view is that the text of *Hamlet* is indicative not of a patricidal drive but of a consuming hostility against his mother and a struggle against feelings of matricide.[5] It has been suggested that Hamlet's reactions may be a reflection of Shakespeare's own state of mind.[4] The Hamlet-Gertrude Complex may also apply to D. H. Lawrence.[6]

1. Macy, J.: Introduction: in *Sons and Lovers* by D. H. Lawrence, New York, Modern Library, 1922, pp. viii, 82, 211, 238, 427.
2. Shakespeare, *Hamlet*: 1,ii.
3. Edgar, I. I.: The psychoanalytic approach to Shakespeare's Hamlet: *Can. Psychiatr. Assoc. J.,* 6:353–355, 1961.
4. Freud, S.: "Material Sources and Dreams": *S.E.,* Vol. IV, 1953, pp. 264–265.
5. Wertham, F.: The matricidal impulse. Critique of Freud's interpretation of Hamlet: *J. Crim. Psychopathol.,* 2:455–464, 1940.
6. Ober, pp. 104–105.
7. Brewer, 2:142.

Happy Puppet Syndrome

(Angelman syndrome, puppet children[1])

In the Happy Puppet Syndrome, the affected children have flat heads, their movements are jerky, and they are easily provoked to prolonged paroxysms of laughter.[1] The characteristic facies consists of protruding jaw and tongue and a smiling but otherwise expressionless face.[2] The syndrome also includes horizontal occipital depression, microcephaly, some cerebral atrophy, ventricular dilatation, optic atrophy, profound mental retardation, and ataxia. The electrocardiograms reveals spikes and slow waves.[3] Unilateral cerebellar atrophy has been demonstrated by computerized axial tomographs.[4] The disease is nonprogressive[5] and the etiology is unknown.[6]

These children do have superficial similarities to jointed puppets, which are animated with strings or wires to produce jerky movements and laughter is a frequent part of puppet shows.[7] Justification for the eponym by its originator is that it is "an unscientific name but one which may provide for easy identification."[1] Disorders of laughter have been classified as (1) genuine laughter but excessive for the stimulus, (2) laughter that continues long after the stimulus, and (3) laughter as part of an epileptic seizure with no appropriate stimulus.[8] Lesions in the cortex of the brain result in lack of inhibition of the hypothalamus, which is the center for release of emotional responses.[9] Kuru has been called the laughing death[10] because foolish laughter is part of the marked emotionalism, general tremors, and ataxia. The disease is one of the subacute spongiform viral encephalopathies caused by a slow virus.[11] It occurred exclusively in the Fore tribe of New Guinea, being spread by cannibalistic eating of the brain of those who had recently died.

Another laughter eponym is related to a Greek epic author—the Homeric Laughter syndrome, in which there are recurrent violent fits of uncontrollable, mirthless laughter.[12] The source of this eponym is Homer's *Odyssey*, in which the following line appears: "An unextinguishable laughter shakes the sky."[13] Presumably, the laughter was that of Momus, the god of laughter, and was caused by Vulcan's snaring of Cytherea (Venus) and Mars with a net during their amorous encounter.

The ability to laugh has been cited by William Osler as a valuable quality for a physician.[14] "The comedy, too, of life will spread before you, and nobody laughs more often than the doctor at the pranks Pluck plays upon the Titanias and the Bottoms among his patients." Laughter has also been recommended as a nonspecific but effective therapeutic agent.[15] Norman Cousins attributes his own recovery from ankylosing spondylitis to have been due in good part to laughter—inducing jokes, literature, and films.[16]

1. Angelman, H.: 'Puppet' children. A report on three cases: *Develop. Med. Child. Neurol.*, 7:681–688, 1965.
2. Elian, M.: Fourteen happy puppets. Two new cases and a review: Clin. Pediatr., 14:902–908, 1975.
3. Bower, B. D. & Jeavons, P. M.: The 'happy puppet' syndrome: *Arch. Dis. Child.*, 42:298–302, 1967.

4. Williams, C. A. & Frias, J. L.: The Angelman ("happy puppet") syndrome: *Am. J. Med. Genet.*, 11:453–460, 1982.
5. Moore, J. R. & Jeavons, P. M.: The "happy puppet" syndrome: Two new cases and a review of five previous cases: *Neuropediatrie*, 4:172–179, 1973.
6. Bjerre, I. et al.: The Angelman syndrome or "happy puppet" children: *Acta Pediatr. Scand.*, 74:398–402, 1984.
7. Collodi, C.: *The Adventures of Pinocchio*: C. C. Chiesa translator, ill. A. Mussino, London, Collier Macmillan, 1969.
8. Martin, J. P.: Fits of laughter (sham mirth) in organic cerebral disease: *Brain*, 73:453–464, 1950.
9. Davison, C. & Kelman, H.: Pathologic laughing and crying: *Arch. Neurol. Psychiatry*, 42:595–643, 1939.
10. Howell, M. & Ford, P.: The ghost disease: in *The Beetle of Aphrodite and Other Medical Mysteries*, New York, Random House, 1985, p. 130.
11. Gajdusek, D. C.: Unconventional viruses and the origin and disappearance of kuru: *Science*, 197:943–960, 1977.
12. London, S. J.: The whimsy syndromes. The fine art of literary nosology: *Arch. Int. Med.*, 122:448–452, 1968.
13. Homer, VIII:116.
14. Anon.: On staying sane despite being a headache doctor: *Headache*, 25:375, 1985.
15. Gonzalez-Crussi, F.: *Three Forms of Sudden Death*: New York, Harper & Row, 1986, pp. 140–142.
16. Cousins, N.: *Anatomy of an Illness*: N. Engl. J. Med., 295:1459–1463, 1976.

Harlequin Color Change

(harlequin syndrome)

A difference in color between the two sides of the body has been described in 22 neonates.[1] One-half of the body becomes much paler than the other half, which remains the usual pink, with a sharp line of demarcation running vertically through forehead, nose, chin, neck, and trunk, involving upper and lower extremities on the same side. The lips and tongue are not involved. It begins in the first few days of life as attacks lasting for only a few minutes; the syndrome passes off in a few days. First proposed was that the color difference between the two halves of the body is determined by gravity, the paler part always being uppermost. The description of another patient considers the lighter side to be normal and the darker an abnormal diffuse redness.[2] Suggested has been a temporary instability of the vasomotor

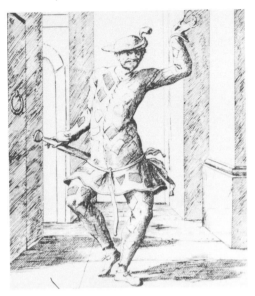

(A)

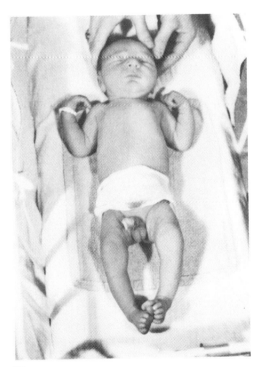

(B)

Harlequin Color Change **A.** A Harlequin clown.[6, p. 26] **B.** Unilateral skin color change in a newborn.[2] (Reprinted with permission from the American College of Obstetrics & Gynecology)

control of skin arterioles related to hypothalamic dysfunction.[3] Discrepancy remains as to which side is abnormal.

Harlequin is a clown who originated in sixteenth century Italian plays as one of the comic servants of principal characters. His costume consists of many colors,[4] as did that of the biblical Joseph. There is no unilateral color difference, but many patches of different colors, unlike the syndrome for which the name has been usurped. More appropriately, the term Harlequin has been applied as a descriptor for many specific species of flora and fauna that are multicolored: bat, beetle, brant, cabbage-bug, deer, duck, garrot, moth, pigeon, rose, and snake.[5]

Clowns have not been neglected by psychoanalysts. They have been labeled as having manifestations of female identification (make-up); as showing exhibitionistic-fetishistic-transvestic denials of castration,[6] and as being a father figure assuming the sexual and aggressive Oedipal guilt of the son.[7]

1. Neligan, G. A. & Strang, L. B.: A "harlequin" color change in the newborn: *Lancet*, 2:1005–1007, 1952.
2. Birdsong, M. & Edmunds, J. E.: Harlequin color change of the newborn. Report of a case: *Obstet. Gynecol.*, 7:518–521, 1956.
3. London, S. J.: The whimsy syndromes. The fine art of literary nosology: *Arch. Int. Med.*, 122:448–452, 1968.
4. Glennon, W.: *The Adventures of Harlequin*: Pittsburgh, Pittsburgh Playhouse Press, 1968.
5. OED: V:93–94.
6. Beaumont, C. W.: *The History of Harlequin*: New York, Arno Press, 1976.
7. Simons, R. C.: The clown as a father figure: *Psychoanal. Rev.*, 52:75–91, 1965.

Harlequin Fetus

(collodion baby, congenital icthyosis)

The collodion baby is covered at birth by gray, dry, scaly, parchmentlike, cracked skin with deep fissures.[1] Microscopically, hyperkeratosis, atrophy of rete pegs, and absence of the stratum granulosum are apparent. Additionally, there are ectropionized eyelids, a fish-shaped mouth, deformed earlobes, and plump extremities.[2] If severe, these infants die of infection in the first few days of life. This rare keratinizing disorder has an autosomal recessive inheritance.[3]

The so-called Harlequin Fetus has only one color, resembling collodion, unlike the multi-colored patches of the medieval Italian clown after whom the condition is named (see Harlequin Color Change).[4] A more appropriate name for this syndrome is congenital icthyosis, so-called because the dry, scaly skin resembles that of fish.[5] A milder icthyosis with roughness and dryness of the skin may occur in older individuals.

1. U.S. Naval Medical School: *Color Atlas of Pathology*: Vol. 2, Philadelphia, J. B. Lippincott, 1954, p. 372.
2. Moll, H.: *Atlas of Pediatric Diseases*: W. Kleindienst translator, Philadelphia, W. B. Saunders, 1976, pp. 190–191.
3. Solomon, L. M. & Esterly, N.: The skin and the eye: in *Genetic & Metabolic Disease*, M. F. Goldberg, Ed., Boston, Little, Brown, 1974, pp. 515–516.
4. Glennon, W.: *The Adventures of Harlequin*: Pittsburgh, Pittsburgh Playhouse Press, 1968.
5. Behrman, R. E. & Vaughan, V. C., III: *Nelson Textbook of Pediatrics*, 12th ed., Philadelphia, W. B. Saunders, 1983, pp. 1896–1897.

Hebephrenia

Hebephrenia is a somewhat outdated designation for a chronic form of schizophrenia that has a gradual onset in adolescence. There is profound emotional withdrawal, grimaces, giggling, and inappropriate smiling, hallucinations, bizarre delusions, and disregard for conventions.[1] It may at times resemble manic-depressive psychosis.[2] The prognosis is poor. Adolescent dementia was first described in 1863, and named after Hebe in 1871.[3] In Greek mythology, Hebe was the daughter of Zeus and Hera (Juno). She was the goddess of youth and spring, and cupbearer of the gods, but lost this position when she was given in marriage to Hercules.[4]

The term Hebe has been used in general to refer to an involuntarily alluring waitress, barmaid, or young woman.[5] The suffix phrenia (Gr., the mind) denotes a mental disorder.[6] Ephebiatrics, also derived from Hebe, is a Greek word used for Athenian youth of military age; and for adolescent medicine in general.[7] The bizarre and inappropriate behavior of Shakespeare's Ophelia after the murder of her father by Hamlet has been considered as

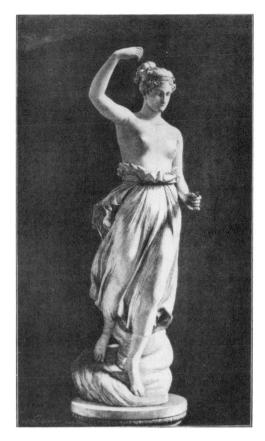

Hebephrenia   Hebe, the Goddess of Youth and Spring.[9]

The figure of Hermaphrodite twinnes cleaving together with their backes.

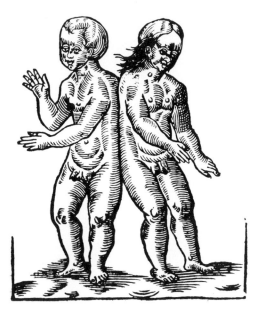

Hermaphrodite   Medieval "Twinnes, both Hermaphrodites."[17]

an example of hebephrenia (see Ophelia Complex).[8]

The phrase insurance hebephrenia has been applied to schizophrenic patients who present initially as a compensation neurosis. The patients' complaints then become increasingly absurd, illogical, and bizarre.[2] The derivation of the name is in part inappropriate as this neurosis is not identified with adolescence.

1. Chapman, p. 271.
2. Campbell, pp. 276–278.
3. Skinner, p. 205.
4. Gayley, p. 36.
5. OED: V:182.
6. Jaeger, pp. 105–106.
7. Stedman, p. 473.
8. Stone, A. A. & Stone, S. S.: *The Abnormal Personality Through Literature*: Englewood Cliffs, New Jersey, Prentice-Hall, 1966, pp. 64–65.
9. Brewer, 2:155.

Hemeralopia

(day blindness)

Hemeralopia refers to decreased vision in sunlight and other bright lights.[1] Hemera is the Greek word for day, aloas for blind, and ops for eye. It has been noted in albinism, retinitis with central scotoma, toxic amblyopia, coloboma of the iris and choroid, lens opacity, and conjunctivitis with photophobia.

At the beginning of the world of Greek mythology, it was from Chaos that two children issued, Erebus and Nox (night).[2] They wedded with the resultant birth of two daughters, Aether (light) and Hemera (day). Mother and daughter were never together, Nox leaving the palace in a chariot when Hemera returned. Hemera is also the name of a geological time period in which any species was most abundant; i.e., "had its day."[3]

1. Thomas, p. 741.
2. Gayley, p. 4.
3. Espy, p. 16.

Hermaphrodite

(hermaphroditism[1])

Of rare occurrence is an individual with a mixture of both male and female gonads, external genitalia, and sexual characteristics. When this occurs the affected individual is known as a hermaphrodite.[1] Either or both ovarian and testicular tissue may be functional. Most have a

46 XX chromosomal karyotype, but 46 XY and mosaics have occurred.[2] A pseudohermaphrodite has a normal karyotype, gonads of one sex, and external genitalia of the other. This occurs in the testicular feminization syndrome due to failure of an androgen-sensitive receptor to use testosterone during fetal development.[3] Related to hermaphroditism is the freemartin of cattle.[4] Occasionally when cows have twins of different sex, the female one may have marked male characteristics, probably caused by stimulation of the female embryo by testosterone from the male embryo.

In Greek and Latin mythology, Hermaphroditus was the son of Hermes (Mercury) and Aphrodite (Venus), the goddess of love. While Hermaphroditus was bathing in a lake, the nymph Salmacis, who ruled the lake, saw him and fell in love. When the shy youth resisted her advances, she pleaded with the gods that nothing would ever separate them. Immediately they were united as one, neither man nor woman, and yet both.[5] In another version, the name Hermaphroditos originated from roadmarkers called herms in honor of Hermes, the god of travelers.[6] These markers were at first topped by representations of Hermes, but later by other dieties such as Aphrodite. Although this etymological version is probably more accurate, the former is humanistically appealing and more compatible with psychological and morphological conditions which relate to a blending of the two sexes.

The original man was considered to be hermaphroditic by the earliest races.[7] In the biblical story of Adam and Eve, both male and female existed in the male before the miraculous excision and transformation of the rib. Adam rejoiced that "This at last is bone of my bones, and flesh of my flesh: she shall be called Woman, because she was taken out of man."[8] It has been postulated that Eve arose from the adrenal gland underlying Adam's lower rib, a gland which secretes female as well as male hormones.[9] In fact, the human embryo is undifferentiated as to sex until the sixth or seventh week of life, and can therefore be considered as hermaphroditic. In medieval times, hermaphrodites were also called androgynes and hommes et femmes.[10] The cause was considered to be an equal amount of "seed" furnished by both the male and female, with each competing to make its likeness.

Another Greek character with hermaphroditic qualities was the soothsayer Tiresias, who was stricken blind by Minerva after he saw her bathing.[11] By one account, he was changed into a woman when he killed two serpents that were mating.[12] When he again met two entwined snakes seven years later he recovered his original male form. T. S. Eliot used Tiresias in his poem *The Waste Land* as symbolic of the melding of the two sexes.[13] "I Tiresias, although blind, throbbing between two lives, / Old man with wrinkled female breasts. . . ." In some ancient myths, Hermaphrodite was depicted as a young man with female breasts and long hair.[14] In some cultures, hermaphrodites were killed, as were other morphological deviants from the normal.

In Jungian psychological terms, the unconscious of each individual has both a female element, the anima, and a male element, the animus.[15] In medieval times, this inner dual nature was symbolized as a hermaphroditic figure with the right and left sides being of different sexes.

On a more mundane level, ambiguous external genitalia of hermaphrodites or pseudohermaphrodites may result in serious social problems.[16] Anne Grandjean, born in 1732, was a typical psychological and physiological girl until the time of puberty when she developed male characteristics and was attracted to girls rather than boys. It was determined by her religious confessor that she must live as a boy henceforth. She assumed the male name Jean-Baptiste and married. Jean-Baptiste's wife rejected him because of gossip by his prior lover that he was neither male or female. He was imprisoned on the basis of purposeful indulgence in sexual aberration, but then released on the condition that he never marry again. This differs from the Diana Complex in which masculine behavior of a female is of psychological origin rather than of indeterminate genitalia origin.

1. OED: V:243.
2. Kraus, F. T.: Female genitalia: in *Anderson's Pa-*

thology, J. M. Kissane, Ed., 8th ed., St. Louis, C. V. Mosby, 1985, pp. 1455–1457.

3. Strickland, A. L.: Picture of the month: Testicular feminization syndrome: *Am. J. Dis. Child.*, 140:565–566, 1986.

4. Keller, R.: Hermaphroditism in the animal kingdom: in *Ciba Symposium*, Vol. 2, No. 3, 1940, pp. 478–485.

5. Guirand 1964, p. 132.

6. Keller, R.: Historical and cultural aspects of hermaphroditism: *Ciba Symposium*, Vol. 2, No. 3, 1940, pp. 466–470.

7. Taub, J.: Endocrinology in the Bible: *Harofé Haivri*, 2:164–156, 1955.

8. OT: Genesis 2:23.

9. Levin, p. 17.

10. Paré, pp. 26–33.

11. Bulfinch, p. 231.

12. Schmidt, p. 270.

13. Eliot, T. S.: *The Waste Land* 1922: in *Collected Works*, New York, Harcourt, Brace & World, 1963, pp. 51–76.

14. Bartsocas, C. S.: Goiters, dwarfs, giants and hermaphrodites: *Prog. Clin. Biol. Res.*, 200:1–18, 1985.

15. Jung, Chap. 3.

16. Gonzalez-Crussi, F.: *Three Forms of Sudden Death*: New York, Harper & Row, 1986, pp. 40–64.

17. *The Workes of Ambrose Parey*: London, Cotes & Young, 1634.

Hermes

Hermes was an early but short-lived medical journal, also titled the *Journal du Magnétisme Animal*, which had only four volumes, 1826 to 1829.[1] Hermes is the Roman name for Mercury, the messenger of the gods, who also presided over commerce and everything which requires skill and dexterity, including science.[2] He carried a rod entwined with two serpents, called the caduceus, which is used extensively as a symbol of medicine.[3] It is, however, considered inappropriate by some to have the god of commerce used as the motif of medicine, especially as Aesculapius is represented with only one serpent.[4]

The two entwined serpents of Hermes staff can be considered as representing the act of sexual union and thus a symbol of fertility.[5] In a symbolic sense, Jungian psychology relates this union to Hermes' erect phallus. As a messenger, Hermes led souls to and from the underworld. "His phallus therefore penetrates from the known into the unknown world, seeking a spiritual message of deliverance and healing."[5] Hermes was also the Greek patron god of alchemy "which prepared medicines enhancing reproductivity to best assume longevity" (see Mercury).[6]

Hermes is also the origin of another bibliophilic eponym, the Hermes Syndrome,[7] applied to the greatly increasing number of thefts of books from medical libraries, in other words, bibliokleptomania.[8] The rationale is that Hermes was also the god of thieves because on the day of his birth he stole fifty divine heifers from Apollo.[9] Some bibliophiles do consider books to be divine; as, for example, devotees of Conan Doyle's Sherlock Holmes, who call the collected stories the canonical or sacred writings.[10]

1. *Hermes. Journal du Magnétisme Animal*: Union List of Serials in Libraries of the United States and Canada, 2nd ed., W. Gregory, Ed., New York, H. W. Wilson Co., 1943, p. 1203.
2. Bulfinch, p. 11.
3. Bunn, J. T.: Origin of the caduceus motif: *J.A.M.A.*, 202:163–167, 1967.
4. Rakel, R. E.: One snake or two?: *J.A.M.A.*, 253:2369, 1985.
5. Henderson, J. L.: Ancient myths and modern man: in C. Jung, p. 155.
6. Mahdinassan, S.: Systems of alchemy and their associated dieties: Hermes, Shiva and Tso-Chun: *Hamdard*, 28:27–44, 1985.
7. What's in a name? The eponymic route to immortality: in *Current Comments, Essays from an Information Scientist*, 47:384–395, 1983.
8. V. (Vaisrub) S.: Mythologic eponyms Updated: *J.A.M.A.*, 220:724, 1972.
9. Guirand 1964, p. 51.
10. Key, J. D.: Keeping the Holmes fires burning: *Mayo Alumnus*, 17:42–43, 1981.

Holmesian Technique

(argument by exclusion)

The term Holmesian Technique has been used to designate the determination of causes of changes in population mortality rates by first eliminating some possible influences, and then proposing that the remainder are the probable causes.[1] The term was applied in a criticism of studies by McKeown[2] on the reasons for overall decline in mortality in Victorian England. Woods and Woodward objected that McKeown had "played down if not completely eliminated . . . the positive influence of medicine, health care and hospitals."[1] Sir Arthur Conan Doyle created a universal character, Sherlock Holmes, who was endowed with acute deductive abilities.[3] Several of his adages relating to ratiocination are widely quoted by aficionados. The one referred to as the Holmesian Technique is found in "The Adventure of the Beryl Coronet." "It is an old maxim of mine that when you have excluded the impossible, whatever remains, however improbable, must be the truth."[4] Its application as the Holmesian Technique is not fully justified, as the example rules out several possible influences on a decline in mortality rates rather than impossible ones.

This Holmesian adage can be criticized on the basis that even when the impossible is eliminated several possibilities may be left, all of which may not necessarily be true.[5] Butterfield, a prominent historian, has compared his approach to the study of history with the logical methods of Sherlock Holmes—the refusal to force facts, the suspension of judgment until they offer their own answer, and the ability not to prejudge anything.[6] He gives Holmes more than his due, however. A less serious reference to the sleuth is the name of a short play, *Sherlock Chromosomes, Scientific Detective*. It is an educational demonstration that "solves" the mystery of the structure of deoxyribonucleic acid (DNA), produced by Science Museums of Charlotte, North Carolina.

The application of Holmesian reasoning to medicine has not been neglected, as, for example, another of his adages: "It is a capital mistake to theorize before you have all the evidence."[7] However, this method of reasoning is contrary to the early hypothesis generation so necessary for clinical diagnosis.[5] It is the characterization of Holmes as both an acute observer and astute reasoner that is fundamental to clinical medicine. For example, an unusual and complex case of factitious pheochromocytoma has been labeled as "a case for Sherlock Holmes."[8] More general is the following reminiscence by a physician. "When I taught clinical haematology I used to show my students a picture of Sherlock Holmes to impress on them that all diagnostic work is detective work: 'The baffling case of the enlarged spleen,' and 'the lady with the mysterious anaemia' are true mysteries of everyday medicine."[9]

The basis for the seemingly impossible conclusions made by Sherlock Holmes has been compared with the methods used for the attribution of paintings by Morelli to rightful artists and for the psychological interpretations of Freud.[10] "In all three cases tiny details provide the key to a deeper reality, inaccessible by other methods. These details may be symptoms, for Freud, or clues, for Holmes, or features of paintings, for Morelli."

1. Woods, R. & Woodward, J.: Mortality, poverty and the environment: in *Urban Disease and Mortality in Nineteenth-Century England*, R. Woods & J. Woodward, Eds., New York, St. Martin's Press, 1984, pp. 29–33.
2. McKeown, T. & Record, R. G.: Reasons for the decline of mortality in England and Wales during the nineteenth century: *Population Studies*, 16:94–122, 1962.
3. Baring-Gould, W. S., Ed.: *The Annotated Sherlock Holmes. The Four Novels and the Fifty-Six Short Stories Complete by Sir Arthur Conan Doyle*: 2nd ed., 2 Vols., New York, Clarkson N. Parker, 1967.
4. Doyle, A. C.: "The Adventure of the Beryl Coronet": *Strand Mag.*, 3:511–525, 1892.
5. Rodin, A. E. & Key, J. D.: The scientific Holmes. A survey of science, medicine and deduction: *Sherlock Holmes Rev.*, 1:81–86, 116–122, 1987.
6. Watson, A.: Introduction: in *The Origins of History*, H. Butterfield, New York, Basic Books, 1981, pp. 7–9.
7. Doyle, A. C.: "A Study in Scarlet": *Beeton's Christmas Annual*, No. 29, 1887.
8. Portioli, I. & Valcavi, R.: Factitious pheochromocytoma: A case for Sherlock Holmes: *Br. Med. J.*, 283:1660–1661, 1981.
9. Bottiger, L. E.: The head that wore a crown and other stories: *Br. Med. J.*, 292:1060, 1986.
10. Ginzburg, C.: Morelli, Freud and Sherlock Holmes: Clues and scientific method: A. Davin translator, *Hist. Workshop J.*, 9:5–36, 1980.

Huckleberry Finn Syndrome

(persistent truancy[1])

The Huckleberry Finn syndrome is one of frequent truancy arising from severe parental rejection, strong feelings of inadequacy, worthlessness, and depression in an individual with superior intelligence.[2] A study of truants has revealed a high incidence of defense mechanisms such as withdrawal, isolation, and aggression.[3] This truancy syndrome may extend into adulthood in the form of repeated absenteeism from work and frequent job changes.[2]

Mark Twain's Huckleberry Finn[4] ran away not only from school, but also from the mores of society, being a liar, irreligious and unwashed.[5]

His truancy, however, was not overriding and suggests masochism or relief of guilt by incurring punishment. "At first I hated the school, but by-and-by I got so I could stand it. Whenever I got uncommon tired I played hookey, and the hiding I got next day done me good and cheered me up."[4]

Huckleberry Finn's passivity, lack of anger and concern with death have been subjected to a detailed psychoanalytical study. Conclusions include a death wish so that he could be reunited with his dead mother, and a subconscious rage against her due to abandonment through death.[6] This analysis was done in spite of Mark Twain's warning at the beginning of the novel that "Persons attempting to find a motive in this narrative will be prosecuted; persons attempting to find a moral in it will be banished; persons attempting to find a plot will be shot."[4] Mark Twain has been labeled as a Skinnerian behaviorist[7] on the basis of another book, *What Is Man?*[8]

The behavior of Huckleberry Finn's bosom friend, Tom Sawyer, has also been psychoanalyzed as due to the death of his mother. In Tom's case the result was a feeling of helplessness and sadness with resultant "repression, omnipotence, denial and identification with the victim and aggressor."[9] In most instances of truant children, the cause may be child abuse and neglect rather than the desire to just play hooky.[10]

1. Roe, P. F.: Eponymous disorders: *Lancet*, 2:794, 1978.
2. Andriola, J.: Truancy syndrome: *Am. J. Orthopsychiatry*, 12:174–176, 1946.
3. Pandey, R. S. & Nagar, S.: Personality dynamics of early truants: Indian J. Clin. Psychol., 7:71–72, 1980.
4. Clemens, S. L. (Mark Twain): *The Adventures of Huckleberry Finn*: New York, W. W. Norton Co., 1977, p. 18.
5. Brauer, A.: Life is still perilous for Huck Finn: *MD*, June, 1984, pp. 117–133.
6. Barchilon, J. & Kovel, J. S.: Huckleberry Finn. A psychoanalytic study: *J. Am. Psychoanal. Assoc.*, 14:775–814, 1966.
7. Morgan, W. G.: Mark Twain: Behaviorist: *J. Behav. Exp. Psychiatry*, 15:99, 1984.
8. Twain, M.: *What Is Man?*: New York, De Vinne Press, 1906.
9. Palmer, A. J.: Tom Sawyer: Early parent loss: *Bull. Menninger Clin.*, 48:155–169, 1984.

10. Diven, B.: Playing hooky? Forget Huck Finn; Absences may mean problems at home: *Albuquerque J.*, Sept. 16, 1984, Sec. D, p. 1.

Humpty-Dumpty Etymology

The use of some prefixes in coining medical terms can be confusing and inappropriate.[1] Examples are platy- and ortho-[2] for such words as platypnea and orthodeoxia.[3] Analagous is the dismay of Alice, of looking glass fame, when confronted by the linguistic creativity of Humpty Dumpty.[4]

"When *I* use a word," Humpty Dumpty said, in a rather scornful tone, "it means just what I choose it to mean—neither more nor less."

"The question is," said Alice, "whether you can make words mean so many different things."

"The questions is," said Humpty Dumpty, "which is to be master—that's all."

Inappropriate etymology (derivation of words) is not limited to prefixes in medicine. Humpty Dumpty's confusion of words has also been invoked against the designation of an up to 70% rate of occurrence of capsular contracture after breast implants as a complication rate.[5] The objection is that this phrase is imprecise and has many different connotations, some of which are much more onerous than an increase in firmness. William Bean has provided a more general and satirical indictment of what he calls logomania, or word madness in medical papers. "The medical profession [is] overwhelmed by misuse of words, obscurity of style, the puffery of redundancy, and the compulsive lapse into those foot-and-a-half long sesquipedalian words that scarify and cicatrize our medical journals. . . ."[6]

Humpty Dumpty has also been used as the main character in a coloring book, which is given to children as a means of becoming familiar with hospital routine and thereby being less anxious.[7] Other fictional characters from children's stories have been used to decorate x-ray suites in order to allay fear.[8] Examples include Dr. Seuss characters, Batman and Robin, the Flintstone family, and clowns.

On a hudibrastic level is the "Dumpty Dictionary of Techno-talk" which is used by sales people for personal computer customers.[9] Thus, a beginner is "a person who believes more than one-sixteenth of a salesperson's spiel," and an advanced user "a person who has managed to remove a computer from its packing materials."

1. Robin, E. D.: To the Editor: *N. Engl. J. Med.*, 295:345, 1976.
2. Cormier, Y. & Newball, H. H.: Humpty-Dumpty etymology.: *N. Engl. J. Med.*, 295:344, 1976.
3. Robin, E. D. et al.: Platypnea related to orthodeoxia caused by true vascular lung shunts: *N. Engl. J. Med.*, 294:941–943, 1976.
4. Carroll, p. 269.
5. Brody, G. S.: Humpty Dumpty on capsular contracture and complications: *Plast. Reconst. Surg.*, 73:658–659, 1983.
6. Bean, W.: Logomania, or word madness: *Postgrad. Med.*, 77:233–236, 1985.
7. Sparks, L.: Humpty Dumpty goes to the hospital: *Can. Nurse*, 64:34–36, 1968.
8. Anonymous: Batman joins the fight against frightening children in the x-ray suite: *Mod. Hosp.*, 113:94–95, 1969.
9. Manes, S.: "The Dumpty Dictionary," Version 2.0: *PC Mag.*, Oct. 28, 1968, pp. 111–112.

Humpty Dumpty Phenomenon

The eponym Humpty Dumpty Phenomenon has been applied to picturesque but befuddling names used in relationship to disturbances in cerebral blood flow. Examples are intracerebral steal, inverse cerebral steal (Robin Hood Syndrome), luxury perfusion, and hypercarbia.[1] Like Lewis Carroll's anthropomorphized egg inside Alice's looking glass,[2] these terms may obscure rather than provide enlightenment on the relationship between regional cerebral blood flow and the type of anesthetic needed.[1]

Like the Humpty Dumpty Etymology, the Phenomenon can result in difficulties in communication. There is also a danger that the careless use of eponyms may obscure ignorance of basic medical phenomena.

1. Wollman, H.: The Humpty Dumpty phenomenon: *J. Anesthesiol.*, 33:379–381, 1970.
2. Carroll, chap. 4.

Humpty Dumpty Syndrome I, II

(disability neurosis)

I Protracted disability may develop in a patient following apparent recovery from a so-

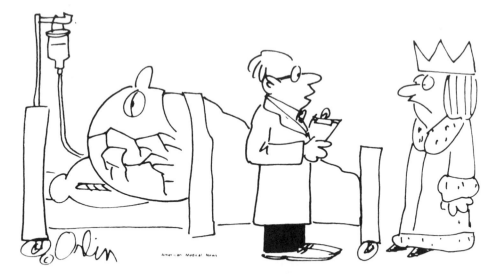

Humpty Dumpty Syndrome "The cracks will heal, but I'm worried about his cholesterol level."[8] (Copyright 1984, American Medical News. Reprinted by permission)

matic disease or injury.[1] This can occur in previously conscientious employees who have childhood histories of marked, severe deprivation, abuse, and abandonment by parents (often by death). Affected individuals frequently belong to a racial minority. There is anger at their employers and physicians, who become authority figures, taking the place of their parents. Treatment is often no more curative than the attempts to resurrect Humpty Dumpty: "All the King's horses and all the King's men couldn't put Humpty Dumpty back together again."[2] This failure has been contrasted with the 75% success rate of microsurgery in reestablishing the lumen of the vas deferens after vasectomy.[3]

II   The Humpty Dumpty Syndrome has also been used allegorically, equating the shattering of his shell after a fall with that of the fragmentation of general surgery into many subspecialties.[4] These syndromes could be considered symbolically as the king being the physician, his men as other health workers, and the horses as his diagnostic and therapeutic armamentarium.[5] The designation of a Humpty

Dumpty Syndrome would be more appropriate for the accident-prone syndrome.

The imagery of Humpty Dumpty's traumatic fall has been used in Wilson's play *Talley's Folly*,[6] as symbolic of the fear of leaving oneself open emotionally and psychologically to others. "All people. He said all people are eggs. Said we had to be careful not to bang up against each other. Crack our shells, never be any use again. . . . So we never can really communicate. . . . We all have a Humpty Dumpty Complex." Humpty Dumpty is also invoked for a more sophisticated psychiatric condition, the borderline personality disorder. One variant is represented by "the egg shell fragility of a Humpty Dumpty with all the potential of creative living still at the level of yolk and albumen. . . ."[7]

1. Ford, C. V.: A type of disability neurosis: The Humpty Dumpty syndrome: *Int. J. Psychiatry Med.*, 8:285–294, 1977-78.
2. Carroll: chap. 4, p. 262.
3. Morton, W. J.: Too bad for you, Humpty Dumpty: *J. MAG*, 69:901–902, 1980.
4. Organ, C. H., Jr.: General surgery and the Humpty Dumpty syndrome: *Aust. N.Z. J. Surg.*, 55:91–94, 1985.
5. Durham, p. 3.
6. Wilson, L.: *Talley's Folly*: New York, Hill & Wang, 1979, pp. 34–35.
7. Lonie, I.: From Humpty Dumpty to Rapunzel: Theoretical formulations concerning borderline personality disorders: *Aust. N.Z. J. Psychiatry*, 19: 372–381, 1985.
8. Orlin: Cartoon: *Am. Med. News*, July 13, 1984, p. 27.

Hygiene

Hygiene is defined as knowledge and practice relating to the maintenance of health.[1] Hygeia was the Greek goddess of health and the daughter of Aesculapius, although sometimes considered to be his wife.[2] She is represented in art as a virgin dressed in white and feeding a serpent from a cup. The Roman goddess of health or well-being was Salus.[3] The connection to the goddess of health with the god of medicine serves to reemphasize the truism that a division between the maintenance of health and the management of disease is artificial because they represent two extremes of a continuum.

Hygeia was the name of "A Journal of Individual and Community Health," published by

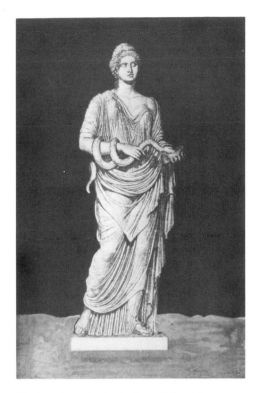

Hygiene Hygeia, the Goddess of Health.[5]

the American Medical Association beginning in 1923. In 1950, it was continued as *Today's Health*, and then absorbed in 1976 by *Family Health*, which now continues as *Health*.[4] Another but much earlier journal derived from the same Greek goddess of health is *Hygiea*, first published in Stockholm in 1839.

1. OED: IV:493.
2. Bulfinch, p. 482.
3. Boyce, A. A.: Salus and Valetudo: *J. Hist. Med. All. Sci.*, 14:79:81, 1959.
4. *Mayo Clinic Library List of Serials*: Rochester, Minnesota, 1971.
5. Nutting, M. A.: *A History of Nursing*: Vol. 1, New York, Putnam, 1907, frontispiece.

Hymen

The fold of mucous membrane which stretches across the vaginal introitus is named after Hymen of Greek mythology.[1] He was a beautiful youth, said to be the son of Apollo and a Muse. As the god of marriage and the personification of the wedding feast, he is usually represented as carrying a bridal torch.[2] Thus, one of the most uniquely feminine anatomical structures is named after a male god. In England of the eighteenth and nineteenth centuries there was a considerable amount of erotic literature on penetrating the hymen— "the delights of defloration [deflowering] of virgins."[3]

Hymenitis is the inflammation of this membrane.[4] The designation for the surgical incision of a thick, imperforated hymen is hymenotomy; for the instrument to incise the hymen, hymenotome; and for a plastic operation to close the vagina, hymenorrhaphy. The word hymen in classical Greece was applied more generally in anatomy to any kind of membrane, as, for example, serious membranes of the pericardial and peritoneal spaces.[5] The term became restricted to the vaginal membrane in the sixteenth century. Hymeno- is a generic combining form for membranous forms.[1] Thus, a hymenomycete is a type of fungus.

1. OED: IV:495.
2. Bulfinch, pp. 482–483.
3. Bloch, pp. 139–144.
4. Thomas, p. 792.
5. Skinner, p. 219.

Hypnosis

Hypnosis is an artificially induced trance state in which the subject places his ego structure in the control of the hypnotist.[1] The procedure is used medically in various situations, e.g., in behavior modification (smoking), anesthesia, psychotherapy, and labor. In Greek mythology, Hypnos (Sleep, Somnus), and Thanatos (Death) were the sons of Nox (Night) and lived in a cave in constant darkness.[2] Their cave had two gates; one of ivory through which false dreams and flattering visions issued, and the other of horn through which true dreams passed to mortals. Hypnos's function was to bring fair dreams to mortals.

Origination of the term hypnotism is usually credited to James Braid, a Scottish physician, in 1843. However, it was first proposed by the French scientist, de Cuvillers in 1821.[3] As defined in 1901 by William Osler,[4] it is "a sub-

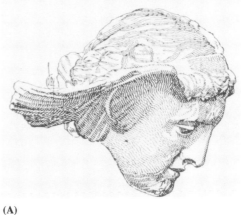

(A)

Hypnosis **A.** Hypnosis of Greek mythology.[2, p. 54] **B.** Svengali hypnotizing Trilby.[13, p. 437] (by du Maurier)

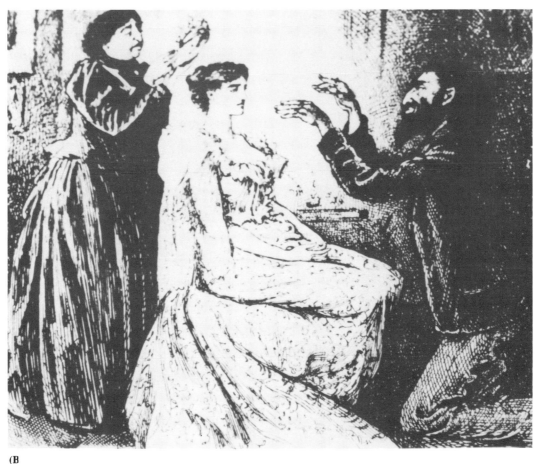

(B

105

jective physical condition . . . resembling somnambulism, in which, as Shakespeare says, in the description of Lady Macbeth, the person receives at once the benefits of sleep and does the effects of acts of watching or waking."[5] Hypnosis is a fairly common theme in literature with the hypnotist sometimes being credited with supernormal powers, often used for evil purposes.[6] The subject is also used to deal with the philosophical problem of mind versus body. Prime examples are Stoker's *Dracula* of 1897,[7] and Poe's *The Facts in the Case of M. Valdemar*.[8] The former is part of the folklore that believes vampires put their victims to sleep by means of a hypnotic ability.[9] In the latter,[8] M. Valdemar is kept on the brink of death from tuberculosis for seven months by being hypnotized.

The works of Conan Doyle include several stories based on this theme. In *The Parasite*[10] an evil, rejected woman uses her hypnotic powers to maintain continual control over a reluctant male. More humorous is his "The Great Keinplatz Experiment"[11] in which the professor inadvertently exchanges bodies with a student by means of hypnosis. Another literary eponym related to hypnosis is Svengali, a term used for a person of great and forceful powers.[12] He is described in du Maurier's *Trilby* as a sinister character, but a superb pianist.[13] Svengali transforms Trilby O'Ferrall, a tone-deaf artist's model, "who couldn't sing one single note in tune," into a magnificent and renowned singer by means of his mesmeric ability. She loses her priceless voice when Svengali's hypnotic control disappears on his death from heart failure.

The name of the god of sleep is also taken for the occurrence of nocturnal lumbosacral back pain in patients with diminished right heart compliance.[14] This is the Bane of Hypnos, also called "Vespers curse" night pain which arouses from sleep patients who have increased pressure in the right atrium. It is likely due to the pressure of venous distention on a presensitized nerve root lying within a rigid bony passage.

1. Hofling, C. K.: *Textbook of Psychiatry for Medical Practice:* Philadelphia, J. B. Lippincott, 1975, pp. 516–519, 1975.

2. Gayley p. 54.
3. Gravitz, M. A. & Gerton, M. I.: Origins of the term hypnotism prior to Braid: *Am. J. Clin. Hypnosis*: 27:107–110, 1984.
4. Schneck, J. M.: Sir William Osler and medical hypnosis: *Can. Bull. Med. Hist.*, 2:221–235, 1985.
5. Osler, W.: Medicine in the 19th century (1901): in *Aequanimitas with Other Addresses*: 3rd ed., Philadelphia, Blakiston, 1932, pp. 260–262.
6. Ludwig, A. M.: Hypnosis in fiction: *Int. J. Clin. Exp. Hypnosis*, 11:71–80, 1963.
7. Stoker, B.: *Dracula*: Modern Library, n.d.
8. Poe, E. .A.: "The Facts in the Case of M. Valdemar": in *The Annotated Tales of Edgar Allen Poe*, S. Peithman, Ed., New York, Doubleday, 1981, pp. 629–637.
9. Hill, D.: *The History of Ghosts, Vampires and Werewolves*: Ottenheimer, 1973.
10. Doyle, A. C.: *The Parasite*: London, Archibald Constable, 1894.
11. Doyle, A. C.: "The Great Keinplatz Experiment": *Belgravia Mag.*, 57:52–65, 1885.
12. Boycott, p. 119.
13. du Maurier, G.: *Trilby. A Novel*: New York, Harper & Bros., 1894.
14. LaBan, M. M.: "Vespers curse" night pain— The bane of Hypnos: *Arch. Phys. Med. Rehabil.*, 65:501–504, 1984.

I

Icarus Complex

An inner conflict caused by a disproportion between what is desired and what can be achieved is called the Icarus Complex.[1] It increases the risk and likelihood of failure. The psychological conflict is related to father-son rivalry, and may play a role in the double personality and paranoid megalomania.

Daedalus was the greatest architect and sculptor in Greek mythology. He had to leave his native town of Athens because he killed a young pupil. He and his son, Icarus, found a home in Crete where he built his famous labyrinth at Gnossus (Cnosus) for King Minos.[2] The king, however, imprisoned Daedalus and Icarus when they wanted to return to their native city. To escape, Daedalus made wings out of feathers which he fastened onto himself and his son with wax. Icarus ignored his father's warning not to go near the sun. He soared upward until the heat of the sun softened the wax which fastened his wings, and he plummeted into the sea.

The type-A aggressive, striving person has been compared to Icarus, each reaching for his nemesis, the former the obstructed coronary artery, and the latter the scorching sun.[3] The Icarus misadventure can be applied to other situations, as, for example, the victim of projects that are too ambitious. In this sense, it would be related to the Frankenstein Monster eponym. Waals equated icarusism with the narcissistic phase of adulthood.[4] Diel considers the Icarus myth as expressing two meanings: "the exalted desire for elevation and the inadequacy of the means to achieve it."[5]

Bertrand Russell used Icarus as an example of the dangers inherent in the progress of science in his long essay of 1924 on *Icarus, or the Future of Science*.[6] Just as Icarus was destroyed by his rashness, Russell fears that "the same fate may overtake the populations whom modern men of science have taught . . . while we retain our present political and economic institutions." ". . . the greater man's power to gratify his desires, the more destructive he will become."[6] How much more realistic this appears over a half century later when man has discovered how to split the atom and manipulate his very genes!

The name of Icarus's father, Daedalus, was taken to replace the title of the long-standing *Proceedings of the American Academy of Arts and Science*. However, the volume number was preserved, the first issue of *Daedalus* in May, 1955 being 86.[7] Justification for the eponymic derivation of the name of this journal is that Daedalus "enjoyed the composite reputation of being a scientist, a craftsman, a poser as well as a solver of riddles. . . ."[8]

1. Vaessen, M. L. J.: The Icarus complex: *Psychiatr. Neurol. Neurochir.*, 65:285–304, 1961.
2. Gayley, C. M.: pp. 246–247.
3. Pietroni, P. C.: The meaning of illness-holism dissected: *J. R. Soc. Med.*, 80:357–360, 1987.
4. Waals, H. G. van der: Problemen van het Narcisme: *Net. T. Geneesk.*, 94:1395, 1950.
5. Diel, p. 29.
6. Russell, B.: *Icarus, or The Future of Science*: New York, E. P. Dutton & Co., 1924, pp. 5–6.
7. Whitehill, W. M.: A Foreword to *Daedalus*: *Daedalus*, 86:3–5, 1955.
8. McCord, D.: Daedalus: *Daedalus*, 86:6–8, 1955.

Iris

The iris is a circular membrane which separates the anterior from the posterior chamber of the eye. It has a central opening (pupil) which enlarges or diminishes in size to control the amount of light transmitted through the lens to the retina.[1] Iris was the Greek goddess of the rainbow, the daughter of Thaumas and Electra, the granddaughter of Oceanus and Gaea, and the sister of the Harpies.[2] She was a messenger for Juno and Zeus, conveying divine commands to mankind, and thus being the female counterpart of Mercury. She also charged the clouds with water for fertilizing rains.

Iris is often represented as a beautiful virgin with wings of varied color and riding a rainbow. At times she wore a nimbus on her head which reflected the colors of the rainbow. In Greek the word iris was used for any bright-colored circle which surrounded a body.[3] The term was first applied to the eye membrane in 1721.[4] Any one iris of the eye does not have the varied colors of the rainbow, but it is circular as was Iris's nimbus.

The Yellow IRIS is an acronym for the International Remote Imaging Systems.[5] It is a method for urinalysis which uses automated intelligence microscopy coupled with a dipstick reader and specific gravity modules.[6]

1. OED: V:476.
2. Bulfinch, p. 484.
3. Editors of the American Heritage Dictionaries.
4. Skinner, p. 232.
5. Statland, B. E.: Automated urinalysis: *Med. Lab. Observer*, 17:13–14, 1985.
6. Roe, C. E. et al.: Evaluation of the Yellow Iris. An automated method for urinalysis: *Am. J. Clin. Pathol.*, 86:661–665, 1986.

Isis

Isis is the name of the official journal of the History of Science Society, which also includes medical history. The first volume appeared in 1912; by 1985 it had reached volume 76. Its aim is "to collect and publish the best information available, to coordinate the work of scholars scattered in many distant places . . . to organize the history of science as an independent and full-fledged discipline . . .;" and with a humanitarian orientation.[1]

Isis was an Egyptian goddess who was both the wife of Osiris and his counterpart.[2] She was equated with the earth and was the parent of all things born; and thus the beginning of all the ages and the parent of all the gods. According to G. Sarton, the founder of *Isis*, he chose the name because it was short and represented the beginning of mankind.[1] *Isis Revisited* is the title of a book published in 1877 by Helena Blavatsky, the founder of Theosophy, a movement in which several physicians were quite prominent.[3] It attempts to provide a scientific basis for Blavatsky's doctrine of mystical insight into the divine nature of the universe.

1. Sarton, G.: *The New Humanism*: Appendix I. The Publication of "Isis": *Isis*, 6:35–39, 1924.
2. Bulfinch, p. 484.
3. Oppenheim, J.: *The Other World. Spiritualism and Psychical Research in England, 1850–1914*: Cambridge, England, Cambridge University Press, 1985, pp. 159–199.

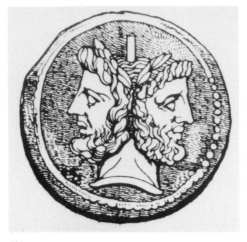

(A)

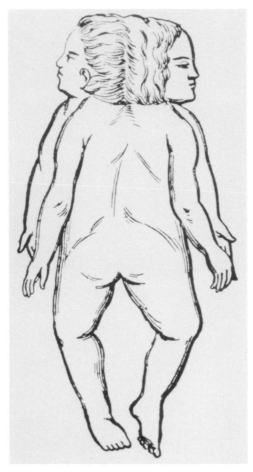

(B)

Janiceps Twins **A.** Ancient Roman coin with Janus head.[8] **B.** Janiceps Twins.[10]

J

Janiceps Twins

An unusual type of cephalothoracopagus is one in which the two heads are fused so that there is both an anterior and a posterior face.[1] By definition, lateral fusion of two heads does not constitute Janiceps twins because there are not front and rear faces; and neither do two-headed monsters (dicephalics).[2] The two faces may be similar in development, or one malformed[3] or rudimentary.[4] There is also fusion of the neck, thorax, and upper abdomen. Suggested causes are incomplete separation of two embryos from a single fertilized ovum,[5] or partial fusion of two embryonic axes in the embryonic disc.[6] The incidence of all types of conjoint twins is between 1/50,000 and 1/100,000 deliveries, and 1/600 in twin births.[7] Janiceps is one of the rarer types.

Janus was considered in Roman mythology to be the beginning of all things, including the change of years, seasons, and civilizations, and the vacillations of fortune. He is depicted as facing both ways;[8] or with two heads, one of a young (the beginning) and the other of an old man (the end).[9]

1. Herring, S. W. & Rolatt, W. F.: Anatomy and embryology of cephalothoracopagus twins: *Teratology*, 23:159–173, 1981.
2. Merwin, M. C. & Wright, J.: Lateral cephalothoracopagus: A case report: *Teratology*, 29:181–184, 1984.
3. Pack, G. T. & Berrey, I. C.: Janiceps asymmetros, with the report of a case: *Am. J. Obstet. Gynecol.*, 11:779–788, 1926.
4. Badawy, A. & Shehata, R.: Cephalothoracopagus: *Obstet. Gynecol.*, 18:106–112, 1961.

5. Grundfast, T. H. & Weisenfeld, S.: A case of cephalothoracopagus: *N.Y. State Med. J.*, 50: 576–579, 1950.
6. Sturrock, M. M. & McKenzie, J.: The abnormalities and genesis of cephalo-thoracopagus (janiceps) twins—Report of a case: *Anat. Anz. Bd.*, 133:350–362, 1973.
7. Wedberg, R. et al.: *Cephalothoracopagus (janiceps) twinning*: Obstet. Gynecol., 54:392–396, 1979.
8. Gayley, pp. 60–61.
9. Bulfinch, pp. 484–485.
10. Gould, G. M. & Pyle, A. M.: *Anomalies and Curiosities of Medicine*: Philadelphia, W. B. Saunders, 1896, p. 190.

Janus

There have been at least three medical journals named *Janus*, all related to the history of medicine.[1] The earliest was first published in Breslau in 1846. It was superseded in 1851 by another one also published in Breslau, but lasting only a few years. Volume one of the third *Janus* was published in Stockholm in 1896 with the subtitle "International Archives of the History of Medicine and Medical Geography."[2] It became an international journal with issues in German, French, and English.

The historical implication of this Roman god is that his two opposite-looking faces permitted him to look both backward as well as forward.[2] The implication for medicine is that it must have an "all-knowing vision of past, present, and future."[3] Such an interpretation of the two-faced god is similar to Montaigne's statement that "Youth sees ahead, old age looks back: was not this the significance of Janus' double face?"[4]

History of medicine journals first appeared in the eighteenth century, one example being the *Archives of the History of Medicine*, published in Nuremberg in 1790.

1. Stokvis, B. J.: Janus redivivus: *Janus*, 1:1–6, 1896.
2. Peypers, H. F. A., Ed.: Monsieur et tres Honoré Colligué: *Janus*, vol. 1, 1896.
3. Breo, D. L.: Tumult of '85 may presage triumphs: *Am. Med. News*, 29:4, 1986.
4. Sandblom, P.: *Creativity and Disease. How Illness Affects Literature, Art and Music*: Philadelphia, George F. Stickley, 1982, p. 67.

Janusian Thinking

The eponym Janusian Thinking has been used for creativity generated when an individual formulates two or more opposite or antithetic concepts which then coexist and operate simultaneously.[1] In this sense, Janus, whose two faces were in opposite directions, has been used to symbolize "man's ambience . . . the inner contrasts and opposites that beset man."[2] This eponym has also been defined as "two or more imaginative perspectives—conceptual, ideational, or perceptual—as existing side by side and/or equally operative or true."[3]

A prime example of Janusian Thinking is that given by Einstein. It is the contradiction of thought that provided the initial step toward his theory of relativity.[4] "Thus, for an observer in free fall from the roof of a house there exists, at least during his fall, no gravitational field . . . If the observer releases any objects, they will remain, relative to him, in a state of rest, or in a state of uniform motion. . . . The observer is therefore justified in considering his state as one of 'rest.' " Einstein's awareness of the contradiction of perception of falling and of being at rest at the same time generated the conflict that led to his seminal theory.

Janus-faced is a more colloquial term for a two-faced or deceitful person,[5] and janusmug for an intermediary in shady arrangements or transactions.[6] Thus, the physical configuration of this Roman god is used to designate the presence in a single individual of coexistent opposites in thinking or behavior, as exemplified by Stevenson's *Dr. Jekyll and Mr. Hyde*.[7]

1. Rothenberg, A.: The process of janusian thinking in creativity: *Arch. Gen. Psychiatry*, 24:195–205, 1971.
2. Meerlo, J. A. M.: Janus. The integration of man's inner antinomies: *Int. Rec. Med.*, 173:170–183, 1960.
3. McCarthy, J. J.: Janus: The gold of multiple perspectives: *Am. J. Psychiatry*, 136:992–993, 1979.
4. Rothenberg, A.: Einstein's creative thinking and the general theory of relativity: A documented report: *Am. J. Psychiatry*, 136:38–43, 1979.
5. Espy, p. 19.
6. Partridge, p. 612.
7. Stevenson, R. L.: *Dr. Jekyll and Mr. Hyde*: New York, Bantam, 1964.

Jekyll-and-Hyde Syndrome

Repeated deterioration of elderly patients after discharge from a hospital and improvement on readmission has been likened to the fictional description of alternating evil and good in one individual. The deterioration in capabilities away from the hospital is of greater magnitude than usual for disabled individuals.[1] Stevenson's Dr. Jekyll transformed himself into more base elements of his being, Mr. Hyde, by a chemical compound of his own making.[2] "[I] managed to compound a drug by which these [moral] powers should be dethroned from their supremacy, and a second form and countenance substituted, none the less natural to me because they were the expression, and bore the stamp of the lower elements of the soul."

The derivation of this eponym is somewhat stretched because Mr. Hyde was evil incarnate, which the patients at home are not. Both, however, undergo mental and physical deterioration.[3] Somewhat related to the Jekyll-and-Hyde Syndrome is the Diogenes syndrome derived from the fifth century B.C. Greek philosopher who kept himself in utter poverty.[4] It has been applied to elderly patients who are admitted to a hospital with acute illness and extreme self-neglect, including filthy personal appearance, dirty homes, hoarding of rubbish, and in 50% of cases higher than average intelligence but no psychiatric disorder.[5]

Dr. Jekyll's chemical compound has at least one property compatible with modern pharmacological knowledge.[6] Its gradual loss of power to transform him into Mr. Hyde is suggestive of drug tolerance. Jung has used the Jekyll and Hyde theme as a psychological symbol of the split in the inner, psychic state that causes neuroses.[7] On the folk level, the theme represents the striving of the forces of good and evil within a person for possession of the soul. The phrase a Jekyll and Hyde is used for a person who is alternately completely good or completely evil.[8] It is also used in the sense of crooked or counterfeit,[9] although only the doctor's alter ego was such.

1. Boyd, R. V. & Woodman, J. A.: The Jekyll-and-Hyde syndrome. An example of disturbed relations affecting the elderly: *Lancet*, 2:671–672, 1978.
2. Stevenson, R. L.: *Dr. Jekyll and Mr. Hyde*: New York, Bantam, 1964.
3. Roe, P. F.: Eponymous disorders: *Lancet*, 2:794, 1978.
4. *Encyclopaedia Britannica*: III:558.

5. Clark, A. N. G. et al.: Diogenes syndrome. A clinical study of gross neglect in old age: *Lancet*, 1:366–368, 1975.
6. An onlooker's notebook: One century of Jekyll and Hyde: *Pharmaceut. J.*, June 28, 1986, p. 819.
7. Jung, p. 7.
8. Espy, p. 140.
9. Partridge, p. 615.

Job's Syndrome

(granulomatous disease variant)

The designation of Job's Syndrome was first applied in 1966 to two girls who were afflicted with recurrent, staphylococcal skin abscesses since birth, with no known predisposing conditions.[1] In 1969, the syndrome was reported to be a variant of chronic granulomatous disease of males, both having recurrent staphylococcal infections with a normal defense system, except that neutrophils are unable to destroy some species of bacteria.[2] Job's Syndrome has only been reported in females, and chronic granulomatous disease usually only in males. The usual inheritance is sex linked.

Job was a God-fearing biblical "hero" who was inflicted with many disasters, including illnesses, by Satan or his representative in order to prove to God that there was no human who had absolute, enduring faith.[3] Of the many calamities which Job endured, the most painful were boils. ". . . My skin closeth up and breaketh out afresh."

The description of Job's skin disease is sufficiently vague to have generated many interpretations. A nineteenth century example was diagnosed as a severe case of varioloid (smallpox), especially as it lasted for seven days.[4] To support a diagnosis of yaws, Levin pointed out that boil is not an accurate translation of the Hebrew word shechin; more likely it is an ulcerative and suppurative lesion.[5] Job's disease has also been attributed to pemphigoid or parapemphigus.[6] Another interpretation is leprosy,[7] which has also been called St. Job's Disease.[8] Even Behçet's disease has been labeled as Job's Disease.[9] Other possibilities are the rare dermatitis herpetiformis,[10] and a syphilis-yaws complex, called Manes Ayoub (the malady of Job) in Egypt.[11]

Also incriminated as Job's skin condition have been vitamin deficiency diseases such as

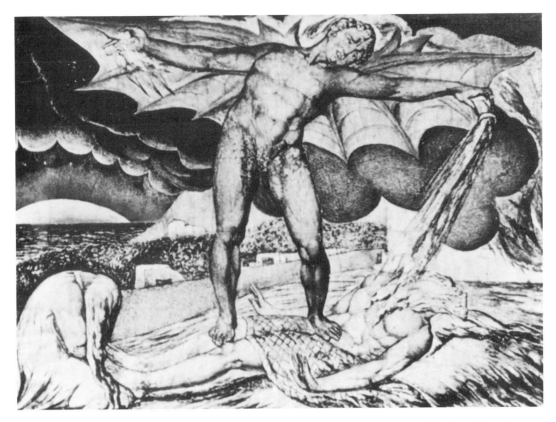

Job's Syndrome Job receiving boils from the devil. (by William Blake, 1826) (by permission of the Tate Gallery, London, England)

pellagra[12] and scurvy.[13] Proposed has been a psychosomatic dermatitis,[14] which may have contributed to Job's depression.[15] It was even suggested that Job suffered from syphilis.[16] Perhaps this is why the ward for venereal patients in St. Bartholomew's Hospital was called Job's Ward in the eighteenth and nineteenth centuries.[17] Kahn has written a book on the psychological interpretations of Job's illnesses.[18] He was certainly one of the first individuals in literature to be afflicted with a skin disease that caused considerable anguish.[19]

The Jobian theme has been transferred to our age in two plays, McLeash's *J. B.*[20] and Neil Simon's more humorous *God's Favorite*.[21] Anyone who patiently lives a life of affliction is called a Job.[22] For close concordance between the source and the eponym, a Job should also be "a wholehearted and upright man, one that feareth God, and shunned evil. . . ."[3] There is, however, the persisting connotation that illness is a punishment by God for sins.

Boils have been called Job's Comforters.[22] More generally this phrase refers to "anyone who tries to make you feel worse while purporting to make you feel better." The seeds of *Coix lachryma* are called Job's tears by natives of Papua because they are worn as a necklace by widows in mourning, presumably representing Job's separation from his family.[14] A jobation is a long, tedious scolding,[22] and a Job's wife one who does so.

Job is the name of a tapestry made from a painting by Chagall for the Rehabilitation Institute of Chicago.[23] It symbolized hope for him. Job, however, expressed little hope in the cure of his ailments by physicians. "But ye are plasterers of lies, Ye are all physicians of no value. Oh that ye would altogether hold your peace! And it would be your wisdom."[24]

1. Davis, S. D., et al.: Job's Syndrome. Recurrent, "Cold," staphylococcal abscesses: *Lancet*, 1: 1013–1015, 1966.
2. Bannatyne, R. M., et al.: Job's syndrome—A variant of chronic granulomatous disease: *J. Pediatr.*, 75:236–242, 1969.
3. OT: Job 7:5.
4. Letter to Editor: The case of Job medically considered: *Maryland Virginia Med. J.*, 14:255–256, 1860.
5. Levin, S.: Job's syndrome: *J. Pediatr.*, 76:326, 1970.
6. El-Gammal, S. Y.: Elecampane and Job's disease: *Hamdard*, 28:95–98, 1985.
7. Brown, M. W.: Was Job a leper?: *Med J. Rec.*, 138:32–33, 1933.
8. Murphy.
9. McGill, J.: Job and Behçet's disease with subsequent pellagra: *Southampton Med. J.*, 2:16–19, 1985.
10. Gwilt, J. R.: Biblical ills and remedies: *J. R. Soc. Med.*, 79:738–741, 1986.
11. Levin, pp. 19–80.
12. Brim, C. J.: Job's illness—Pellagra: *Arch. Dermatol. Syph.*, 45:371–376, 1942.
13. Swanson, J. H.: Evidence of scurvy among ancient Hebrews: *Bull. Hist. Med.*, 15:352–358, 1944.
14. Guy, W. B.: Psychosomatic dermatology circa 400 B.C.: *Arch. Dermatol.*, 17:354–356, 1955.
15. Kapusta, M. A. & Frank, S.: The Book of Job and the modern view of depression: *Ann. Int. Med.*, 86:667–672, 1977.
16. Rosebury, T.: *Microbes and Morals. The Strange Story of Venereal Disease*: New York, Viking Press, 1971, p. 102.
17. Partridge, p. 622.
18. Kahn, J.: *Job's Illness: Loss, Grief and Integration. A Psychological Interpretation*: Oxford, England, Pergamon Press, 1975.

19. Holubar, K.: Dermatology in biblical perspective. An illustration from the Book of Job: *Am. J. Dermatopathol.*, 7:437–439, 1985.
20. MacLeash, A.: *J.B.*: Boston, Houghton Mifflin, 1957.
21. Simon, N.: *God's Favorite*: New York, Samuel French, 1975.
22. Espy, p. 71.
23. Betts, H. B.: Job: Cover, *J.A.M.A.*, 255:3205, 1986.
24. OT: Job 13:4.

Jocasta Complex I, II

I   Jocasta of Greek mythology has been exemplified as the sexual desire of a mother for her son.[1] It is the converse of the Oedipus Complex in which the libido of the son (Oedipus) is directed toward his mother (Jocasta).[2] Oedipus was given by his father, Laius, the king of Thebes, to a herdsman to be killed because he was warned by an oracle that his throne would be in danger if his newborn son was allowed to grow up.[3] The herdsman took pity and left the infant tied by his ankles, hanging from a branch. There a peasant found and adopted him, giving him his name, which is translated as swollen-foot.

As a young man, Oedipus slew his unknown father for killing his horse. Shortly after, as a reward for besting the monstrous Sphinx of Thebes by solving its riddle, Oedipus was given the queen of Thebes, Jocasta, in marriage. He at least, was unaware that they were son and mother. In Gide's play *Oedipus*,[4] Jocasta bemoans, "Oh unhappy Oedipus! Why did you have to know? I did what I could to stop you from tearing aside the veil that protected our happiness. . . . If only I could turn back and undo what was done—forget our shameful bed. . . ."

Both the Jocasta and Oedipus Complexes relate to sexually directed love, one from the mother and the other to the mother.[5] It has been suggested that "Jocasta was entirely aware of events and had an active complicity in them."[6] Her crime was that her incest was a conscious act, unlike the ignorance of her son, Oedipus.[7] Such perverted mother love may vary from a mildly distorted maternal instinct to an overtly sexual attachment.[8] The related Phaedra Complex involves a stepmother and stepson.

II   The eponym Jocasta Complex was applied in a nonsexual sense by Besdine in a study of childhood origins of genius, using Michelangelo as a prototype.[9] Jocasta mothering occurs when the family "is dominated by the affect-hungry mother and by the absent, inept, distant, or aloof father. This constellation results in an unusual mothering process which is exclusive, intense and symbiotic."[10] The results in the son, as exemplified by Michelangelo, are masochistic and paranoid tendencies, unresolved Oedipus Complex, fear of love, homosexual feelings, marked egocentricity, exorbitant striving for recognition, and narcissism. Described as creative geniuses who had such a family background and who manifested its effects are Shakespeare, Freud, Christopher Marlowe, Goethe, Heinrich Heine, Balzac, Proust, Dostoievsky, and Sartre, among many others. Such an application of this eponym is somewhat inappropriate because Oedipus was given away by his father Laius at birth and did not relate to his mother until he became an adult.

The phrase bodies of countless Jocastas has been used to refer to women who have had radical mastectomies by surgeons who perform "procedures prescribed by their elders' paternal authority, to which they submit passively because they have not sufficiently resolved their conflicts with their biological fathers."[11] In this instance, Jocasta is used as a symbol of a passive wife, presumably because she allowed her newborn child to be given away by Laius.

1. Dickson, P.: *Words*: New York, Delacorte Press, 1982, p. 226.
2. Dudzinski.
3. Bulfinch, pp. 152–155.
4. Gidé, A.: *Oedipus*: J. Russell translator, New York, Vintage Books, 1950, p. 39.
5. Ober, p. 104.
6. Stewart, H.: Jocasta's crimes: *Int. J. Psychoanal.*, 42:424–430, 1961.
7. Raglan, L.: *Jocasta's Crime*: London, Metheun, 1933.
8. Kaltz, J.: *The Silent World of Doctor and Patient*: New York, Free Press, 1984, p. 174.
9. Besdine, M.: The Jocasta complex, mothering and genius. Part I: *Psychoanal. Rev.*, 55:259–276, 1968.
10. Besdine, M.: The Jocasta complex, mothering and genius. Part II: *Psychoanal. Rev.*, 55:574–600, 1968.
11. Campbell, p. 122.

Joseph Complex

Freud considered the motives for sibling

conflict to originate in infancy. "There is probably no nursery without violent conflicts between its intimates. The motives for these are rivalry for parental love, for common possessions, for living space."[1] Sibling rivalry may also represent a realistic conflict model over tangible goods because proprietary rights and divisions of labor are not made clear in the family.[2] It can also represent a preoedipal reaction of a sibling in response to another sibling who represents a threat to libidinal strivings for their mother.[3]

Jacob (Israel), a patriarch of the Old Testament, had twelve sons, of whom Joseph, the youngest, was the most favored. Symbolic of his special status was the gift of a coat of many colors from his father.[4] Joseph further antagonized his brothers by relating to them dreams in which his father's sheaf of wheat bowed down only to him, as did the sun, moon, and stars. On being cast out by his brothers, he eventually reached Egypt where he was imprisoned after being falsely accused of forcing himself on a captain's wife. His skills in interpreting dreams finally led to a position of great power in Egypt and eventual reconciliation with and respect by his brothers.

The eponym Joseph Complex was used by Freud to explain Napolean's drive as an unconscious striving to outdo his older brother, Lucien, although there may have been other more significant factors.[5] The Joseph story has also been used as an example of other familiar interactions. Thus Jacob's love for his son, and yet envy at his grandiose exhibitionism, is expressed in Joseph by being ingratiating at first and then assertive when rejected by his brothers. The pharaoh of Egypt then served as a father figure.[6]

Another variant of sibling rivalry is that engendered in some children by the presence of a handicapped sibling who receives considerable attention from the parents.[7] Joseph was handicapped by his father's greater love for him than for his brothers. Other biblical examples of sibling rivalry are Cain and Abel, and Esau and Jacob. The biblical Joseph story has been transformed into a theatrical musical, *Joseph and the Amazing Technicolor Dreamcoat*.[8]

Labeled as a Joseph Fantasy is Freud's identi-

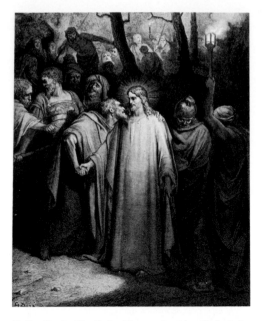

Judas Goat The Judas kiss received by Christ.[5] (by Gustav Doré, 1866) (by permission Dover Pubns., Inc.)

fication with this biblical figure, which was a prominent feature of his dreams.[9] Like Joseph, Freud moved from a rural environment (Freiburg) to an imperial city (Vienna). Both their lives were characterized by an extraordinary capacity for achieving success in the face of obstacles. Both were engaged in sibling rivalry, Freud with his brother, John.[10]

1. Freud, S.: Introductory lectures on psycho-analysis: *S.E.*, vols. 15 & 16, p. 205.
2. Felson, R. B.: Aggression and violence between siblings: *Social Psychol. Q.*, 46:271–285, 1983.
3. Neubauer, P. B.: Rivalry, envy, and jealousy: *Psychoanal. Study Child*, 37:121–142, 1982.
4. OT: Genesis 37–50.
5. Karlen, A.: *Napolean's Glands and Other Ventures in Biohistory*: Boston, Little, Brown & Co., 1984, p. 26.
6. Beebe, J.: The father's anima as a clinical and as a symbolic problem: *J. Analyt. Psychol.*, 29:277–287, 1984.
7. Israelite, N.: Sibling reaction to a hearing impaired child: *J. Rehab. Deaf*, 18:1–5, 1985.
8. Rice, T. & Webber, A. L.: *Joseph and The Amazing Technicolor Dreamcoat*: New York, Music Theatre International, 1970.
9. McGrath, W. J.: The dream of Joseph: in *Freud's Discovery of Psychoanalysis. The Politics of Hysteria*: Ithica, New York, Cornell University Press, 1986, pp. 26–39.
10. Shengold, L.: Freud and Joseph: in *Freud and His Self-Analysis*, Kanzer, M. & Glenn, J., Eds., New York, Jason Aronson, 1979, pp. 67–86.

Judas Goat

Satirized as a Judas Goat is the physician who betrays (Judas) foolishly (goat) his peers and the values of general practice, leading it "towards its own emotional and intellectual destruction in a closed system of education."[1] The context in which it is used relates to the incorporation of general practice into medical school curricula. The general practice of medicine then becomes changed to resemble the traditional academic departments. The consequent undesirable traits include rigid compartmentalization, increased orientation to technology (to the detriment of humanism), and weakening of the generalist orientation.

Judas Iscariot was the apostle who betrayed Christ for thirty pieces of silver.[2] The medical eponym relates only very generally to this biblical character, who is taken as the epitomy of any type of betrayal. The term as used here does not have a malicious connotation. In this vernacular, a Judas goat is an individual who leads others to destruction, as does a Judas kiss.[3] A judas is someone who betrays a friend, a traitor.[4] The judas tree of southern Europe is so called because it is reputed to be the species of tree from which Judas hanged himself.

1. Marinker, M.: The chameleon, the Judas goat, and the cuckoo: *J. R. Coll. Gen. Pract.*, 28:199–206, 1978.
2. NT: John.
3. Espy, p. 79.
4. Boycott, p. 62.
5. Doré, G.: *The Doré Bible Illustrations*: New York, Dover, 1974, p. 205

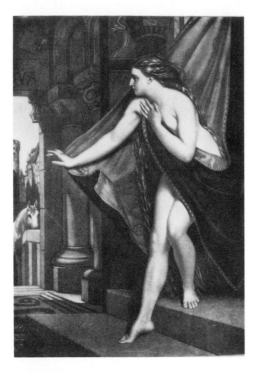

Lady Godiva Syndrome   Lady Godiva preparing for her ride.[7]

L

Lady Godiva Syndrome

(exhibitionism)

Lady Godiva has been used as an eponym for genital exhibitionism.[1] One motivation is an abnormal compulsion, usually in a male, to expose his genitals to the opposite sex.[2] Its development is related to a fear of castration and the need to reassure oneself that one is able to perform sexually.

Lady Godiva, the wife of Leofric, the earl of Mercia, made a horseback ride through the marketplace in Coventry, England, in order to get her husband to reduce his excessive taxes, which he then did.[3] She was completely nude except for her long hair which covered her body down to her legs. Although Lady Godiva may have been a historic individual in tenth century England, her ride is considered to be legendary. St. Agnes is another woman whose hair covered her nakedness, in this instance after she was stripped naked when persecuted as a Christian (see Agnus Castus).[4]

Lady Godiva is not a good example of exhibitionism because her primary motivation was not sexual, because she was as covered with hair as she would have been by clothes, and because the condition occurs predominantly in males. Jean Jacques Rousseau, in his *Confessions*,[5] described an episode of his own exhibitionism before several girls who came to a well. It was a time in his youth when "My heated blood incessantly filled my brain with girls and women." He was caught by a man with a sword, but released after pleading that he was a stranger "whose brain was affected." Another example of exhibitionism occurs in Hans Christian Andersen's *The Emperor's New Clothes*,[6] but this was involuntary because the Emperor believed he was the only one who couldn't see his supposed clothing.

1. Vaisrub, p. 22.
2. Freedman, pp. 1542–1543.
3. *Encyclopaedia Britannica*, IV:595–596.
4. Williams, p. 39.
5. Rousseau, J.-J.: *The Confessions of Jean Jacques Rousseau*: New York, Modern Library, n.d., pp. 90–92.
6. Andersen, H. C.: "The Emperor's New Clothes": in *Hans Christian Andersen, The Complete Fairy Tales and Stories*, E. C. Haugaard translator, Garden City, New York, Doubleday, 1974, pp. 77–81.
7. Brewer, 2:100.

Laius Complex

Fathers may be guilty of "psychic infanticide" in terms of the negative impact on their children of psychological and emotional inadequacies and aberrations.[1] According to Freud, there is a regressive potential in all men who have little children entrusted to them.[2]

Laius was the Greek mythological king of Thebes, who was the husband of Jocasta and the father of Oedipus.[3] He was warned by an oracle that his throne and life were in danger if his newborn son were allowed to grow up. He therefore gave Oedipus to a herdsman who tied the infant by the ankles and left him hanging from the branch of a tree. He was found by a peasant who took him to his master and mistress, who adopted him, giving him the name of Oedipus (swollen-foot). And, indeed, Oedipus as a young man did kill his father, but was unaware of their relationship.

Laius was certainly guilty of bad fathering, being concerned primarily with his own needs and perceptions to the detriment of his son. Oedipus is generally depicted as being quite virtuous in spite of his unwitting crime of incest. He had, however, an overwhelming pride and was narcissistic and aggressive with an inability to depend on others—all possibly related to the bad fathering he received.[1]

The Heracles (Hercules) Complex represents the extreme of bad fathering, being the hatred of a father for his children.[4] It is so named because Heracles, the mythological personi fication of strength, was visited by Lyssa, the Fury of madness, who had been sent by Hera because of her jealousy of Heracles's father, Zeus.[5] Heracles in his madness mistook his own children for those of his rival, Eurystheus, and slew them as well as their mother. This transgression of Heracles has been interpreted as the result of a psychotic episode with paranoid delusions and marked aggressive drives.[6] Because the hatred was not directed knowingly against his own children, the eponym Heracles Complex is somewhat inappropriate.

1. Ross, J. M.: Oedipus revisited. Laius and the "Laius complex": *Psychoanal. Study Child*, 37:169–200, 1982.
2. Freud, S.: "The Disposition to Obsessional Neurosis": *S.E.*, 12:317–326, 1913.
3. Bulfinch, pp. 152–155.
4. Campbell, p. 122.
5. Guirand, 1959, pp. 169–170.
6. Medlicott, R. W.: The sickness of Heracles: Some forensic aspects of the omnipotent narcissistic personality: *Aust. N.Z. J. Psychiatry*, 11:213–217, 1977.

Lasthénie de Ferjol Syndrome

Hypochromic anemia may result from chronic hemorrhages produced by self-inflicted injuries.[1] It has been described in twelve women of unstable personality, most working in medically related professions as nurses or laboratory assistants. They have a need to draw attention to themselves. All had masochistic tendencies. Hemorrhages were produced by injuring themselves at different sites—femoral arteries, ulnar veins, and hemorrhoidal veins. Such young women often have disturbed, withdrawn mothers. They are not suicidal but are borderline psychotic.[2] The act of self-mutilation has been symbolically linked to masturbation, menstruation, defloration, and vampiristic blood rituals. The fear of self-mutilation is considered as a phobia resulting from a hypersensitive mind.[3]

In D'Aurevilly's *The Story Without a Name*,[4] Lasthénie de Ferjol is the 16-year-old daughter of the widow Baroness de Ferjol. They lived in a hamlet at the foot of the Cévennes. Lasthénie was very innocent and girlish, and had never been separated from her mother. She was quite melancholy, with no companions, but became pregnant by someone whose name she would not reveal. The result was a stillborn baby. Thereafter she gradually became weaker and feeble. The medical diagnosis was a marasma of unknown cause; her mother's, the result of the girl's sin.

At the death of Lasthénie, the mother and her servant, Agathe, made a horrifying discovery—pins were stuck in the region of her heart. " 'Blood Agathe!' Her voice was horrible as she spoke . . . together they opened the waist. Horror seized them. Lasthénie had killed herself, slowly, little by little, each day a fraction more with pins. They drew out eighteen stuck in the region of the heart." Twenty-five years after her death, Lasthénie's mother discovered that it was a priest, Father Riculf, who had been befriended by the family who had gotten her daughter pregnant.

The concordance between the fictional character and the actual patients is excellent, except that the twelve patients did not have a suicidal intent as did Lasthénie.[1] She is an example of focal suicide on one part of the body which is subjected to self-mutilation and purposive accidents.[5] Related but not suicidal is the Lesch-Nyhan Syndrome in which there is compulsive biting of the lips, fingers, and hands.[6] It is a sex-linked syndrome of males that has as its basis faulty purine metabolism with resultant hyeruricemia, choreoathetosis, mental retardation, and cerebral palsy.

Jules-Amédée Barbey d'Aurevilly (1808–1889) was a French poet, novelist, and critic, who was born in Normandy, studied law, and lived in Paris. He was an arrogant, tempestuous, posturing, and flamboyantly romantic writer, who is now considered as a minor figure of nineteenth century French literature.[7] D'Aurevilly has been included with others as an example of a novelist who wrote about anemia.[8]

1. Bernard, J. et al.: Les Anémie Hypochromes dues a des Hémorragies Voluntairement Provoquées. Syndrome de Lasthénie de Ferjol: *Presse Med.*, 75:2087–2090, 1967.
2. Kwawer, J. S.: Some interpersonal aspects of self-mutilation in a borderline patient: *J. Am. Acad. Psychoanal.*, 8:202–216, 1980.
3. Langfeldt, G.: The hypersensitive mind in normals, neurotics, psychopaths and psychotics: *Psychiatr. Neurol. Scand.*, Suppl. 73, 1951, p. 73.

4. D'Aurevilly, B.: *The Story Without a Name*: New York, Bretano's, 1919.
5. Freedman, p. 1781.
6. Jablonski, p. 185.
7. Harvey, P. & Heseltine, J. E.: Barbey d'Aurevilly, Jules-Amédée (1808–89): in *Oxford Companion to French Literature*, Oxford, England, Clarendon Press, 1959, pp. 47–48.
8. Bernard, J.: Lasthénie de Ferjol, Marie de Saint-Vallier, Emilie de Tourville au le Romancier et l'Anémie: *Nouv. Rev. Fr. Hematol.*, 24:43–44, 1982.

Lazarus Complex

(Lazurus syndrome, near-death syndrome)

Experiences before resuscitation after cessation of vital signs due to cardiac arrest has been named after the biblical Lazarus.[1,10] Some patients have amnesia of the event, and some remember going into nothingness, fading out of lights, "feeling life flooding into you," and hearing someone say, "My God, his heart has stopped."[2] One patient felt his atheistic beliefs confirmed as "There is nothing there." Another had his faith vindicated as "There seemed to be music and angels singing on the other side." Moody's book on *Life After Life*[3] addresses the same situation, but finds that it is common to be outside of one's body, moving through a long tunnel, glimpsing the spirits of dead relatives and friends, and seeing a warm light at the end of the tunnel. Such perceptions have also been experienced by children.[4] Return to the land of living may be followed by symptoms of anxiety, depression, and a feeling of alienation.[5]

The study of near-death experiences has been considered important in determining the existence of survival after death.[6] A more pragmatic explanation is that the type of experience is influenced by "cultural and psychological factors, sensory deprivation and reflex adaptive responses to stress."[7] More specifically, the effects of hypercapnea and hypoxia on the temporal lobe have been suggested.[4] Ischemia of the occipital lobe can result in constriction of visual fields (tunnel vision).[8] There is no indication that the biblical Lazarus experienced such phenomena.

Lazarus of Bethany, the brother of Martha and Mary, died after an unspecified illness.[9] He was raised from the dead after four days by Jesus. "[Jesus] called out with a loud voice,

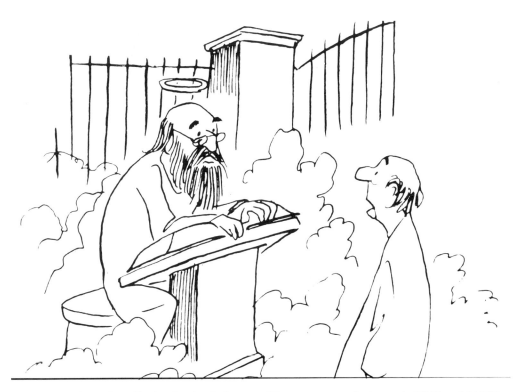

Lazarus Complex   "Sorry I'm late but they had me on a life support system for two weeks."[19] (Copyright 1985, *American Medical News.* By permission)

'Lazarus, come out!' Out came the one who had died feet and hands tied with grave clothes, and his face wrapped in a towel. Jesus told them, 'Unbind him and let him go.' " Jesus himself was raised from the dead. His immediate cause of death while being crucified has been attributed to hypovolemic shock and exhaustion asphyxia.[11]

There are two other instances of restoration of life by Jesus in the Bible. The only son of a widow in a town near Nain was brought back to life by telling him to rise.[12] Jesus performed a similar miracle for the daughter of Jairus, a ruler of a synagogue.[13] It has been suggested that some of these raisings of the dead may actually represent revival of patients suffering from catalepsy.[14] However, the effect of such therapy without drugs is not much less than miraculous.[15] Paul performed an even more remarkable miracle by reviving Eutychus, who had been killed by a fall from a third-story window after having fallen asleep on the ledge.[16] The cause of death is not given for Tabitha, a disciple in Joppa who was returned to the living by Peter through prayer and invoking "Tabitha, arise!"[17] Several dead biblical children were revived by a combination of physical efforts and prayer (see Elisha Method).

A nonbiblical variant of resuscitation after death is the zombie, related to the Haitian religion, vodoun, or voodoo.[18] A zombie is an individual raised by evil sorcerers from the grave in a trance and forced to work as a slave. The zombie condition may have had its origin from the effects of tetrodotoxin, a potent neurotoxin found in the tissues and organs of the blowfish. Poisoning can simulate death due to complete paralysis, although the individual may remain conscious.

1. Hackett, T. P.: The Lazarus complex revisited: *Ann. Int. Med.*, 76:135–137, 1972.
2. Dobson, M., et al.: Attitudes and long-term adjustment of patients surviving cardiac arrest: *Br. Med. J.*, 3:207–212, 1971.
3. Moody, R. A. Jr.: *Life After Life. The Investigation of a Phenomenon-Survival of Bodily Death*: Covington, Georgia, Mockingberg Books, 1975.
4. Morse, M. et al.: Childhood near-death experiences: *Am. J. Dis. Child.*, 140:110–114, 1986.
5. Vaisrub, p. 22.
6. Stevenson, I. & Greyson, B.: Near-death experiences. Relevance to the question of survival after death: *J.A.M.A.*, 242:265–267, 1974.
7. Greyson, B. & Stevenson, I.: The phenomenon of near-death experiences: *Am. J. Psychiatry*, 137: 1193–1196, 1980.
8. Watson, D. W. & Watson, M. E.: Exploring the phenomenon of near-death experiences: *Am. J. Dis. Child.*, 141:828, 1987
9. NT: John 11:11–44.
10. Dudzinski.
11. Edwards, W. D. et al.: On the physical death of Jesus Christ: *J.A.M.A.*, 255:1455–1463, 1986.
12. NT: Luke 7:11–15.
13. NT: Luke 8:40–55.
14. Caldwell, T.: *Dear and Glorius Physician*: Garden City, New York, Doubleday, 1959, p. 437.
15. Gwilt, J. R.: Biblical ills and remedies: *J. R. Soc. Med.*, 79:738–741, 1986.
16. NT: Acts 20:9–12.
17. NT: Acts 9:36–41.
18. American Scientist Interviews. Walde Davis: *Am. Sci.*, 75:412–417, 1987.
19. Cartoon: *Am. Med. News*, Nov. 22/29, 1985, p. 14.

Lazarus Illness

(Hansen's disease, Lazarus disease, leprosy)

The eponym Lazarus Illness has been applied to leprosy,[1] an infectious disease which has been recorded since biblical days.[2] There are two individuals in the New Testament who are called Lazarus, the name being the contracted form of the Hebrew Eleazar (God has helped). One is the brother of Mary, who was raised from the dead still wrapped in bandages (see Lazarus Complex), and the other the beggar full of sores in the parable of the rich man (see Abraham Ward).[3] There is some disagreement as to whether the two men were the same or different. Both are depicted as having skin diseases, although a leper in biblical times was more likely to have become a beggar.

Leprosy was also implied in earlier biblical times. ". . . if the hair in the plague be turned white, and . . . be deeper than the skin of his flesh, it is the plague of leprosy;"[4] " 'There seemeth to me to be as it were a plague in the house.' And the priest shall command that they empty the house, before the priest go in to see the plague, that all that is in the house be not made unclean."[5] "The Lord spoke unto Moses and unto Aaron, saying, 'When ye are come into the land of Canaan . . . and I put the plague of leprosy in a house . . . And the priest shall command that they empty the house . . . For the purifying of the house he shall take . . . hyssop.' "[6] Hyssop was the plant on which the penicillin-producing fungus was found in 1911.[7]

Whether Lazarus had leprosy or not is uncertain because many skin diseases were so-called in the biblical period.[8] In the Old Testament, the Lord told Moses to put his hand into his bosom, "and he put his hand into his bosom; and when he took it out, behold, his hand was leprous, as white as snow."[9] It has been pointed out that the description is not sufficient for a diagnosis of leprosy, and that the Hebrew word zaráath was arbitrarily translated as leprosy about A.D. 400.[8] A lazaret or lazaretto is a house or hospital for the diseased poor, especially lepers, and a lazar house is a leper hospital.[10] It is also a general term for a quarantine hospital for epidemics such as yellow fever.[11]

Other suggested diagnoses for the biblical

leprosy have been psoriasis,[12] vitiligo (leukoderma),[13] or even a skin disease that does not have a modern-day counterpart.[14] Hudson states that lazaret fever was one of the names for epidemic typhus, named after isolation hospitals of the Middle Ages.[15] St. Job's Illness was another designation for leprosy.[16] In antiquity, Jews were vilified by being called lepers, although the aspersion may have been to their keeping "as much apart from us as though they were lepers."[17] More recently, in 1792, Benjamin Rush considered the blackness of Negroes to be due to a mild form of congenital leprosy, which he called negritude.[18] The skull of Robert the Bruce, king of Scotland, who died in 1141, has been diagnosed as facies leprosa, consistent with his long terminal illness.[19]

From biblical days to the present leprosy has been a frequent theme in literature.[20] The afflicted characters have often been treated in an ambivalent manner, on the one hand being cursed because of sin and, on the other hand, blessed by special favor. Shakespeare used the words lazar and leprosy many times.[21] In *King Henry VI*, Part II, Queen Margaret implores, "What! dost thou turn away and hide thy face? I am no loathsome leper; look on me."[22] The phrase lazar kite was used by the bard for any beggar.[23] Leprosy is one of the several interpretations of the skin lesions of the Summoner in Chaucer's *The Canterbury Tales*.[24]

Coleridge's Ancient Mariner, on sighting the ghostly ship, described its sole occupant, a woman symbolic of death, as having "skin as white as leprosy."[25] Leprosy is also found in medieval art. An example is the graphic depiction in Hans Holbein's painting "St. Elizabeth Among the Lepers."[26] St. Elizabeth was a queen of Hungary who was canonized in 1231, four years after her death, because of her devotion to the sick, especially those with leprosy.[27] She is considered as the patron saint of lepers. Other protectors and healers of lepers were Saints Agatha, Giles, and Martin.[19] Leper hospitals were often dedicated to St. George.[28] The term elephantiasis was originally used by the Greeks for leprosy because the skin changes resembled an elephant's skin.[29]

In another painting, "The Fortune Teller"

by Georges La Tour (1593–1652),[30] the old gypsy is considered to be afflicted with leprosy because she is depicted with some of its effects — leonine facies, clawhand, and hypothenar atrophy.[31]

1. Cordero, F. A.: Leprosy in Guatemala 1982: *Acta Leprol.*, 94:19–37, 1984.
2. Walker, pp. 156–157.
3. NT: Luke 16.
4. OT: Leviticus 13:3.
5. OT: Numbers 5:2.
6. OT: Leviticus 14:33–49.
7. Levin, p. 69.
8. Gramberg, K. P. C. A.: Leprosy and the Bible: *Trop. Geogr. Med.*, 11:127–139, 1959.
9. OT: Exodus 4:6.
10. OED: VI:135.
11. Powell, J. H. : *Bring Out Your Dead. The Great Plague of Yellow Fever in Philadelphia in 1793*: Philadelphia, University of Pennsylvania Press, 1949.
12. Glickman, F. S.: Lepra, psora, psoriasis: *J. Am. Acad. Dermatol.*, 14:863–866, 1986.
13. McNiven, P.: The problem of Henry IV's health, 1403–1413: *Eng. Hist. Rev.*, 100:747–772.
14. Freilich, A. R.: Tzaraat—"Biblical leprosy": *J. Am. Acad. Dermatol.*, 6:131–134, 1982.
15. Hudson, R. P.: *Disease and Its Control. The Shaping of Modern Thought*: Westport, Connecticut, Greenwood Press, 1983, pp. 28–29.
16. Murphy.
17. Freud, S.: "Moses and Monotheism": *S.E.*, Vol. 23, p. 105.
18. Skultans, V.: *English Madness. Ideas on Insanity 1580–1590*: London, Routledge & Kegan Paul, 1979, p. 4.
19. Howell, M. & Ford, P.: "The Head That Wore the Crown": in *The Beetle of Aphrodite and Other Medical Mysteries*, New York, Random House, 1985, pp. 280–305.
20. Prioleau, E.: Leprosy. Reality and metaphor in literature: *Am. J. Dermatopathol.*, 5:377–380, 1983.
21. Kail, A. C.: The Bard and the body. 5. Disease: Its causes, diagnosis and cure: *Med. J. Aust.*, 2:568–577, 1983.
22. Shakespeare, *King Henry IV*: Part II, Act III,ii.
23. Kail p. 304.
24. Mandel, S. L.: Chaucer's vivid medical word pictures. (Reflections of yore afflictions): *Internat. J. Dermatol.*, 223:329–331, 1983.
25. Coleridge, S. T.: *The Rime of the Ancient Mariner* (1798): in *The Annotated Ancient Mariner*, M. Gardener, Ed., New York, C. N. Potter, 1965, p. 28.
26. Virchow, R.: A painting of lepers by Hans Holbein the Elder: S. M. Rabson & J. H. Drickx translators, *Am. J. Dermatopathol.*, 6:377–378, 1984.
27. Ohry, A. & Ohry-Kossoy, K.: St. Giles, St. Francis et al.: Medical patron saints: *Adler Museum Bull.*, 12:18–22, 1986.

28. Frey, E. F.: Saints in medical history: *Clio Med.*, 14:35–70, 1979.
29. Skinner, p. 157.
30. Harvey, M. J.: Cover: *J.A.M.A.*, 257:1559, 1987.
31. Wiebe, D. A.: Hansen's disease in *The Fortune Teller*: *J.A.M.A.*, 258:1176, 1987.

Lear Complex

The libido of a father toward his daughter has been named after Shakespeare's King Lear.[1] Lear divided his kingdom of England between his three daughters, but then disinherited Cordelia, his youngest, because she would not openly declare her love for him.[2] The other two daughters, Goneril and Regan, drove him away. Cordelia married the king of France who invaded Britain to help Lear. Father and daughter both died after a touching reunion.

There appears to be little justification for this eponym, at least no more than the familiar lack of understanding between a father and his young daughter, and then their later reconciliation. Freud discusses *King Lear*, not from the point of view of incestuous libido, but as having a deeper allegorical significance—one of an aged and dying man who "is not willing to renounce the love of women; he insists on hearing how much he is loved," but must renounce love and accept dying—as represented by his carrying the dead Cordelia on stage.[3] It has been suggested that Freud's attraction to the King Lear theme was the fact that he also had three daughters.[4] Like Cordelia, Freud's youngest daughter, Anna, provided him with considerable comfort and support during the latter part of his life.

King Lear has been analyzed as "a deserted child, left alone to howl his rage into the storm," because his abdication of power made him the dependent child of his daughters.[5]

1. Dudzinski.
2. Shakespeare, *King Lear*.
3. Freud, S.: "The Three Caskets": *S.E.*, Vol. 12, pp. 291–301.
4. Feeman, L. & Strean, H. S.: *Freud and Women*: New York, Frederick Ungar, 1981, p. 73.
5. Perry, R.: Madness in Euripides, Shakespeare, and Kafka. An examination of *The Bacchae, Hamlet, King Lear*, and *The Castle*: *Psychoanal. Rev.*, 65:253–279, 1978.

Leontes Syndrome

Pathological jealousy may be the cause of a

husband accusing his wife of unfaithfulness when he learns of her pregnancy.[1] This is a rare condition, more common being the feeling of neglect during the middle and third trimesters of pregnancy.

Leontes is Shakespeare's king of Sicily in *The Winter's Tale*.[2] He wrongly suspected Polixenes, king of Bohemia, of being the lover of his wife, Hermione, and the cause of her pregnancy. "She's an adulteress; . . . . Away with her to prison! . . . My child? Away with't. . . . The bastard brains with these my proper hands / Shall I dash out. Go, Take it to the fire. . . ." He tried to kill Polixenes and arrested Hermione after removing her son from her even though the Delphic oracle proclaimed her innocence. She delivered a daughter, Perdita, whom he ordered to be abandoned in a deserted spot. Leontes finally came to his senses.

Shakespeare's Othello also exhibited pathological jealousy toward his wife, but Desdemona was not pregnant and was murdered by her husband (see Othello Syndrome).

1. Measey, L. G.: Psychiatric problems in obstetrics: *Practitioner*, 220:120–122, 1978.
2. Shakespeare, *A Winter's Tale*: II:i.

Leprechaunism

(Donahue's syndrome)

This syndrome was first described by Donahue in 1948 under the term dysendocrinism for a female infant with peculiar elfinlike facies, hirsutism, and multiple endocrine abnormalities.[1] Another child with the same condition born to the same parents, was reported in 1954, and designated as leprechaunism, a rare familial disorder.[2] Other features include failure to thrive, resulting in a marasmic appearance, alteration of carbohydrate metabolism with hypoglycemia, and sexual precocity.[3] The major endocrinological findings have been hypoplasia of the adrenal and thyroid glands with large ovaries containing small follicular cysts.[4] The ovarian changes probably start in the seventh intrauterine month, with consequent hyperestrogenism, leading to enlarged nipples and external genitalia, hypertrichosis, increased excretion of 17-ketosteriods, hyperplasia of the islets of Langerhans, and large kidneys with tubular calcium deposits. There is

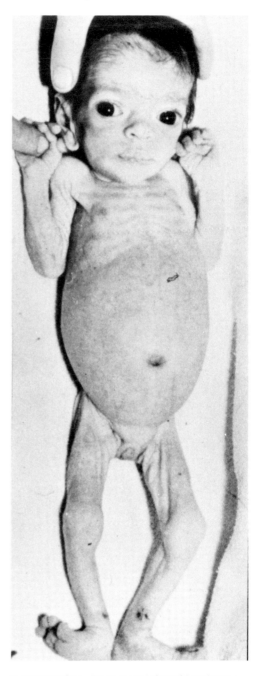

Leprechaunism Six week old infant with typical leprechaun appearance.[2] (by permission *J. Pediatrics*)

also suppression of growth hormone with consequent delay in bone growth.

The basic defect appears to be a primary insulin resistance owing to a defect in the target cell,[5] which is transmitted as a rare familial disorder.[2] The presence of ovarian cysts and increased estrogens suggests that Leprechaunism is the intrauterine and infantile equivalent of the Stein-Leventhal syndrome which occurs in adults.[4]

In Irish folklore, a leprechaun is a hairy, mischievous pigmy sprite who repairs shoes and carries a purse containing a shilling.[6] Although the facies are described as elfinlike, the syndrome is different than the Elfin Syndrome which is associated with hypercalcemia and supravalvular aortic stenosis. It has been pointed out that many marasmic infants from various causes result in a elfin appearance.[7] There appears to be some confusion between leprechauns and elves in this eponym, the former being found in Irish folklore and the latter in Teutonic mythology. Their facial appearance is quite variable in illustrations, but both are of dwarf size.

There has been an admonition that "terminologic vigilance must be exercised that the ponderous Leprechaunoid not be introduced on the scene of the charming Leprechaun."[8] Another related comment is that leprechauns of mythology are males and all patients with the syndrome have been females except one,[9] whose features, however, were not quite those of the syndrome.[3]

1. Donohue, W. L.: Clinicopathologic conference at the Hospital for Sick Children—Dysendocrinism: *J. Pediatr.*, 32:739–748, 1948.
2. Donohue, W. L.: Leprechaunism. A euphuism for a rare familial disorder: *J. Pediatr.*, 45:505–519, 1954.
3. Rogers, D. R.: Leprechaunism (Donohue's syndrome). A possible case, with emphasis on changes in the adenohypophysis: *Am. J. Clin. Pathol.*, 45:614–619, 1966.
4. Kálló, A., et al.: Leprechaunism (Donohue's syndrome): *J. Pediatr.*, 66:372–379, 1965.
5. Rechler, M. M.: Leprechaunism and related syndromes with primary insulin resistance: Heterogeneity of molecular defects: *Prog. Clin. Biol. Res.*, 97:245–281, 1982.
6. OED: VI:205.
7. Salmom, M. A., & Webb, J. N.: Dystrophic changes associated with leprechaunism in a

male infant: *Arch. Dis. Child.*, 38:530–535, 1963.

8. Senior, B.: Comment: Year Book Pediatr., 1963–1964, Year Book, 1963, pp. 340–341.
9. Patterson, J. H., & Watkins, W. L.: Leprechaunism in a male infant: *J. Pediatr.*, 60:730–739, 1962.
10. Balian, L.: *Leprechauns Never Lie*: Nashville, Tennessee, Abdington, 1980, title page.

Lilliputian Eyes

Quite small eyes, as in some animals, may occur in humans.[1] The height of the race of Lilliputians in Swift's *Gulliver's Travels*[2] was a little under six inches, but with all parts in the same proportion as that of ordinary humans. They are described as being able to see only nearby objects, but with great exactness.

Piggins has discussed the problem of Swift's description of the Lilliputians having myopia (nearsightedness).[1] Very small eyes are likely to have hyperopia (farsightedness) rather than myopia. One rationalization is that Lilliput is described as being near Australia, and thus in the same longitude as China, which has a very high incidence of myopia.[1] Such implied racial factors for this work of fiction is somewhat stretched. Related may be the fact that Swift himself probably was myopic. Another country in *Gulliver's Travels* contained a gigantic race of people who lived in Brobdignagian, the name of which is used for anything gigantic in size, in contrast to Lilliputian.[3]

1. Piggins, D.: Lilliputian eyes and vision: *Perception*, 7:609–610, 1978.
2. Swift, J.: *The Annotated Gulliver's Travels*: I. Asimov, Ed., New York, Clarkson N. Potter, 1980.
3. Espy, p. 130.

Lilliputian Syndrome

The Lilliputian Syndrome has been applied to an uncommon condition in which there are hallucinations of seeing minute people.[1] These hallucinations are usually motile and multiple, and only uncommonly auditory. The syndrome can occur in febrile delirium, chorea, infections, fasting, and dementia; and in intoxication by ether, alcohol, cocaine, and hashish.

Swift's Gulliver reached the land of Lilliput by sea, but was bound down by the minute natives.[2] The syndrome is accompanied by pleasurable feelings unlike those of Gulliver on awakening and finding himself captured by the little people. The Lilliputian Syndrome

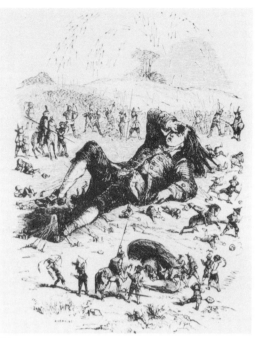

(A)

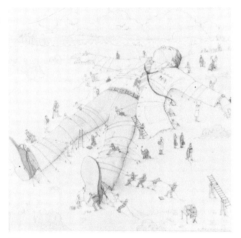

(B)

Lilliputian Syndrome **A.** Gulliver tethered by the Lilliputians. (by Alfred Crawquill, 1865) **B.** Medicine tethered by rules and regulations.[6] (Copyright 1985, American Medical News. By permission)

differs from the Alice in Wonderland Experience in which the perception is of one's own change in size rather than the size of others. It also differs from micropsia in which objects are perceived to be smaller than they actually are.[3] Micropsia can be due to psychopathological causes as well as eye lesions, unlike the Lilliputian Syndrome.[4] Its basis is a general sense of separation from people and the environment. Micropsia has also been described in fictional works.[5]

The Lilliputian theme of restraint by numerous little people has been applied to the physician bound down by the increasing number of governmental and third-party carrier regulations and restraints on health care delivery.[6]

Somewhat related to the Lilliputian Syndrome is the Invisible Man Syndrome in which we do not see what is present or we see what is not present.[7] This eponym relates not to hallucinations, but to the machinations of special effects in movies which achieve delusory end results. It is the methodology of the special effects themselves that are invisible, as was H. G. Wells's *The Invisible Man* of 1897.[8] The novel is more a statement of the misuse of science for selfish ends than is the eponym.

1. Leroy, R.: The syndrome of lilliputian hallucinations: *J. Nerv. Mental Dis.*, 56:325–333, 1922.
2. Swift, J.: *The Annotated Gulliver's Travels*: I. Asimov, Ed., New York, Clarkson N. Potter, 1980.
3. Bender, M. B. & Savitsky, N.: Micropsia and teleopsia limited to the temporal fields of vision: *Arch. Ophthalmol.*, 29:904–908, 1943.
4. Schneck, J. M.: Psychogenic micropsia: *Psychiatr. Q.*, 45:542–544, 1971.
5. Schneck, J. M.: Psychogenic micropsia in fact and fiction: *J.A.M.A.*, 251:2350, 1984.
6. Cover Drawing: Medicine84 The Year in Review: *Am. Med. News*, Jan. 4, 1985.
7. McConnell, F.: "Realist of the Fantastic: H. G. Wells About / In the Movies": in *H. G. Wells: Reality and Beyond*, Champaign, Illinois, Champaign Public Library, 1986, pp. 23–32.
8. Wells, H. G.: *The Invisible Man: A Grotesque Romance*: London, Arthur Pearson, 1897.

Lolita Complex

(pedophilia)

An overpowering desire for sexual relationships with young girls is not rare.[1] Pedophilia may be homosexual or heterosexual, and occurs in males. It is considered by some to be related to alcohol and a berating wife, leading to a desire to find other companionship and sexual satisfaction.

The complex is named after the novel, *Lolita*, by Nabakov.[2] Humbert Humbert was so obsessed by his attraction to the 12-year-old Lolita that he married her widowed mother. On discovering his reason for marriage, the mother ran hysterically out of the house and was killed by a car. Humbert and Lolita then lived and traveled together, engaging in frequent sexual activities until she was 15 years old.

Brigitte Bardot has been linked to Lolita because she presents in movies an image of both the innocence of childhood and considerable sexual allure.[3] Nabakov's Lolita was not "innocent" before Humbert, having had prior intercourse with a boy near her own age. The eponym might be more appropriately called the Humbert Complex, as it refers primarily to his pedophilia rather than to Lolita's sexual attractions as such. Edgar Allen Poe has been considered by some as being afflicted with the Lolita Complex[4] because he married Virginia Clemm when she was not quite 14 years old.[5] Lewis Carroll (Charles Dodgson) was not likely an example of the Lolita Complex. There is no evidence that his interest in photographing nude, young girls was manifested in explicit sexual overtures or relationships.[6]

The converse of the Lolita Complex is pederasty, the sexual attraction of men for young boys, being rather overt in ancient Greece. It is not unheard of in more modern times. Lord Byron was reputed to engage in such activities.[7]

1. Lief, H. I.: Normal and abnormal human sexuality: in *Comprehensive Textbook of Psychiatry*—II, Vol. 2, 2nd ed., A. M. Freedman et al., Eds., Baltimore, Williams & Wilkins, 1975, p. 1542.
2. Nabokov, V.: *Lolita*: New York, Putnam, 1955.
3. Beauvoir, S. de: *Brigette Bardot and the Lolita Syndrome*: New York, Arno Press, 1972.
4. Karlen, A.: "What Ailed Poor Poe": in *Napoleon's Glands and Other Ventures in Biohistory*, Boston, Little, Brown & Co., 1984, p. 88.
5. Symons, J.: "The Tell-Tale Heart" in *The Life and Works of Edgar Allan Poe:* New York, Harper & Row, 1978.
6. Bullough, V. L.: Profile: Lewis Carroll: *Med. Aspects Human Sexual.*, 17:139–140, 1983.

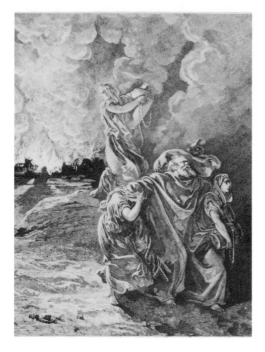

Lot Syndrome   Lot's wife looking back to Sodom.[5] (by Gustav Doré, 1866) (by permission, Dover Pubns., Inc.)

7. Bloch, pp. 187–191.

Lot Syndrome

(hypercalcinosis)

The term Lot Syndrome has been applied to patients with a considerable amount of calcium deposited in tissues as a result of increased concentration of calcium in the blood.[1] The most frequent cause of such metastatic calcification is release of a large amount of calcium by excessive bone resorption.[2] This occurs in hyperparathyroidism and in vitamin D intoxication.

Lot was the nephew of the biblical Abraham. He was warned to leave the sinful city of Sodom before it was destroyed by God, and not to look behind. "But his wife looked back from behind him, and she became a pillar of salt."[3] Although calcium is a metal, it is combined as a lime salt in the body. The biblical reference to a pillar of salt may, however, have been to sodium chloride. Southwest of the Dead Sea in Israel there are fantastically shaped masses of rock covered with salt.[4]

Unlike metastatic calcification, Lot's wife was completely transformed into salt. More compatible is the lithopedion, which refers to complete calcification of a fetus retained in the mother's body after it dies. Lot's Wife has been suggested as a more appropriate eponym, as it was she who looked back.[1] The phrase "Lot's Wife" has already been usurped, however, for yet another eponym (see Lot's Wife Syndrome).

1. Vaisrub, p. 22.
2. Berkow, p. 938–939.
3. OT: Genesis 19:26.
4. Krause, L.: Salt: *Maryland State Med. J.*, 1:277–281, 1952.
5. Doré, G.: *Doré's Bible Illustrations*: New York, Dover, 1974, p. 13.

Lot's Wife Syndrome

Chronic hypodipsic (decreased thirst) hypernatremia (excess blood sodium) with normal blood volume and kidney function is uncommon. Described as Lot's Wife Syndrome is the occurrence of such abnormalities in a patient with acute myeloid leukemia.[1] Her plasma sodium rose as high as 165 mmol / L (mEq / L), the normal range being 136 to 145. The condition may be caused by hypoplasia or destruction of the hypothalamic osmoreceptors that control thirst and vasopressin secretion.[2]

More commonly, increased sodium in the blood is associated with decreased body fluid volume resulting from water loss through the skins, lungs, or kidneys, unlike this syndrome. Other causes are excessive salt administration without water, and adrenal hyperfunction.[3] The Lot's Wife Syndrome is a suitable designation for an excess of sodium, unlike the Lot Syndrome which refers to an excess of calcium. Sodium commonly combines with chloride to form sodium chloride, which is the substance generally referred to as salt, and into which Lot's wife was transformed (see Lot Syndrome).

1. Barnett, M. M.: 'Lot's Wife' syndrome in acute myeloid leukaemia: *Bristol Med. Chir. J.*, 99:88–89, 1984.
2. Hammond, D. N. et al.: Hypodipsic hyernatremia with normal osmoregulation of vasopressin: *N. Engl. J. Med.*, 315:433–436, 1986.
3. Braunwald, pp. 203–204.

Lunacy

Lunacy is a term which was formerly used for intermittent insanity, supposedly brought about by changes in the moon, and now for any type of insanity.[1] In Greek mythology Helios was the charioteer of the Sun, Eos (Aurora) the goddess of the morning, and Selene the goddess of the moon.[2] A later name for Selene was Luna, from which the word lunacy is derived. She was worshiped as the moon. They were the children of Hyperion, the Titan.[3] Selene has been portrayed as having horns that supported the crescent of the moon.[4] She had been identified with Diana. Berserk, a word meaning an insanitylike rage, is derived from the name of a legendary Norse hero of the eighth century, so named after the bearskin that he wore.[5] He was noted for his reckless fury in battle.

Phases of the moon have been implicated in some studies of mental hospital admissions, criminal offenses, and psychiatric emergencies.[6] Results supporting a positive lunar / lunacy relationship may, however, be due to inappropriate analyses and failure to take other cycles into account.[7] Another factor may be a willingness to accept anything but chance as an explanation. Other possible biases in such a belief are selective attention, recall, and exposure.[8] The term lunar effect has been used for the supposed relationship between behavior and lunar phases.[9] There is even a *Lunar Newsletter* devoted to the subject.

Moon-related madness is a common theme in literature, as exemplified in the sixteenth century by the works of Marlowe[10] and Shakespeare. Hamlet warns that "Madness in great ones must not unwatch'd go."[11] Shakespeare has Othello refer to the lunar theory of madness when he learns of the murder of Roderigo by Cassio. "It is the very error of the moon; / She comes more nearer to earth than she was wont, / And makes men mad."[12]

In Jules Verne's *From the Earth to the Moon*,[13] of 1864 he refers to beliefs that the moon produces effects "that often hits the best minds" —great excitement, incredible behavior, nervous disorders, convulsions, vertigo, malignant fevers, somnambulism, the fainting spells of Bacon during an eclipse, and the madness of King Charles VI during the new moon or a full moon. Sherlock Holmes in *The Adventure of the Creeping Man* did not believe that Professor Presbury's intermittent insanity was related to the phases of the moon.[14]

Early Christianity did not neglect madness, Saint Dympna being the healer of insanity.[15] She was the daughter of a Celtic king who killed her when she refused his advances. Her relics were used for hundreds of years as cures for madness and insanity.

1. OED: VI:501.
2. Espy, p. 24.
3. Gayley, p. 39.
4. Schmidt, p. 92.
5. Espy, p. 167.
6. Coles, E. M.: Lunacy. The relation of lunar phases to mental ill-health: *Can. Psychiatr. Assoc. J.*, 23: 149–152, 1978.
7. Rotton, J. & Kelly, I. W.: Much ado about the full moon: A meta-analysis of lunar-lunacy research: *Psychol. Bull.*, 97:286–306, 1985.
8. Kelly, I. W. et al.: The moon was full and nothing happened. A review of studies on the moon and lunar beliefs: *Skeptical Enquirer*, 10:129–143, 1985/86.
9. Lieber, A. L.: *The Lunar Effect: Biological Tides and Human Emotions*: Garden City, New York, Doubleday, 1978.
10. Herring, H.: The self and madness in Marlowe's *Edward II* and Webster's *The Duchess of Malfi*: *J. Medieval Renaissance Studies*, 9:307–323, 1979.

11. Shakespeare, *Hamlet*: III,i.
12. Shakespeare, *Othello*: V,ii.
13. Verne, J.: *From the Earth to the Moon*: in *The Annotated Jules Verne*, W. J. Miller translator, New York, Thomas J. Crowell, 1978, pp. 125–126.
14. Doyle, A. C.: "The Adventure of the Creeping Man": *Strand*, 3:623–628, 1892.
15. Dewhurst, J.: Jest with saints. Second opinion: *Lancet*, 2:573–374, 1981.

Lycanthropy

Lycanthropy is a form of insanity in which the individual believes he is a wolf and exhibits depraved appetites and altered voice.[1] The condition was common in the middle ages, but is rare today.[2] Many of the victims suffered from paranoid schizophrenia. A variety of other psychiatric syndromes have been implicated as well as drug abuse and organic brain syndrome.[3]

Lycaon was a legendary Greek king of Arcadia.[4] He was impious and cruel.[5] When Zeus visited him in the form of a peasant, Lycaon served him food mixed with human flesh. Zeus, in a rage, killed all of Lycaon's sons, and changed him into a wolf. One of the several Babylonian kings named Nebuchadrezzar was afflicted with Lycanthropy.[2] In the middle ages such deluded individuals were feared and often hunted down and killed as a result of mass hysteria.

This type of insanity may have been stimulated by the formerly widespread belief that people could be changed into dangerous animals such as werwolves (werewolves).[6] The term wer, meaning man, is derived from twelfth century Anglo-Saxon.[7] The cruel King John of England was reputed to have arisen as a werwolf after being poisoned.[8] Paracelsus, the sixteenth century physician and iatro-chemist, stated that people who live bestial lives will return as wild beasts. The mythology of werwolves considers the transformation to be due to a pact between the individual and the Devil for strength and power, with the price being the individual's immortal soul (much as in the case of Faust) (see Faust Complex).[9] One method of change is by means of a salve which is rubbed over the body. It is reputed to have contained hemlock and opium.

Paré quoted Pliny in respect to "a man named Demarchus [who] was changed into a wolf,

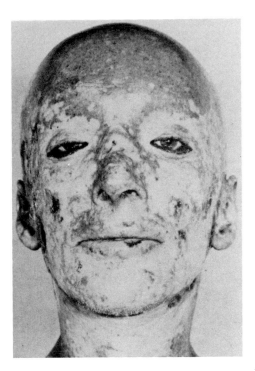

Lycanthropy   A patient afflicted with porphyria.[21] (by permission, Charles C Thomas)

having eaten the entrails of a sacrificed child."[10] Another supposed cause of Lycanthropy is the influence of the full moon.[11] Jules Verne, in his science fiction novel *From the Earth* of 1865,[12] refers to the "Wolves' sun." This is derived from the belief that certain men are transformed into wolves at full moon (the nighttime equivalent to the sun) (see Lunacy).

Legends of werwolves may have arisen from observation of several clinical conditions. These include individuals with a marked excess of hair (hypertrichosis) caused by genetic or endocrine conditions. In congenital porphyria the excess of porphyrins results in marked sensitivity to light which may lead to excess hair and, rarely, to the skin turning red.[13] These manifestations plus restriction of the affected individual's activities to night and periods of insanity could well have contributed to the werwolf legend. Isolated instances of lycanthropy continue to be reported (see Vampirism).[3, 14—16]

Unrelated to Lycanthropy is the "wolf-man" who was psychoanalyzed by Freud.[17] He was so-called not because of any supposed resemblance to a wolf, but because of the development of a severe wolf phobia at the age of four.[18] He was haunted by a recurring nightmare of seven wolves staring at him from their perch in a tree. The phobia evidently originated when he observed his parents copulating, with his mother on all fours.[17] The wolf-man became a landscape painter and wrote an autobiography.[19]

Related to the eponym Lycanthropy is lupus, the Latin word for wolf. Its first medical use was in the fourteenth century for an aggressive ulcerous disease of the skin which "is very hungry like unto a woolfe."[20] Examples are lupus vulgaris and lupus erythematosis.

1. OED: VI:521–522.
2. Freedman, p. 13.
3. Coll, P. G. et al.: Lycanthropy lives on: *Br. J. Psychiatry*, 147:201–202, 1985.
4. Espy, p. 37.
5. Schmidt, p. 164.
6. *Encyclopaedia Britannica*: VI:409.
7. Weekley, p. 1626.
8 Hill, D.: *The History of Ghosts, Vampires and Werewolves*: Memphis, Ottenheimer, 1973, p. 118.
9. McHargue, G.: *Meet the Werewolf*: Philadelphia,

J. B. Lippincott, 1976.

10. Paré, p. 101.

11. McDaniel, W. B.: The moon, werewolves and medicine: *Trans. Studies Coll. Phys.*, 18:113–122, 1950.

12. Verne, J.: *From the Earth to the Moon*: in *The Annotated Jules Verne* by W. J. Miller, translator, New York, Thomas Y. Crowell, 1978, p. 30, annot. 1.

13. Illis, L.: On porphyria and the aetiology of werwolves: *Proceed. R. Soc. Med.*, 57:23–26, 1964.

14. Surawicz, F. G. & Banta, R.: Lycanthropy revisited: *Can. Psychiatr. Assoc. J.*, 20:537–542, 1975.

15. Rosenstock, H. A. & Vincent, K. R.: A case of lycanthropy: *Am. J. Psychiatry*, 134:1147–1149, 1977.

16. Jackson, P. M.: Another case of lycanthropy: *Am. J. Psychiatry*, 135:134–135, 1978.

17. Freud, S.: "The Case of the Wolf-Man. From the History of an Infantile Neurosis": *S.E.*, Vol. XVII, pp. 7–22.

18. Gardiner, M., Ed.: *The Wolf-Man by the Wolf-Man*: New York, Basic books, 1971.

19. Loughman, C.: Voices of the wolf man: The wolf man as autobiographer: *Psychoanal. Rev.*, 7:211–225, 1984.

20. OED: VII:506.

21. Goldberg, A. & Rimington, C.: *Diseases of Porphyrin Metabolism*: Springfield, Illinois, Charles C Thomas, 1962, p. 122.

M

(A)

Mad Hatter Syndrome   **A.** The Mad Hatter at the teaparty. (by John Tenniel) (Dodgson)

Mad Hatter Syndrome

(erethism, Minamata disease)

Magalinia and Scrascia[1] have labeled mercury poisoning as the Mad Hatter Syndrome in their dictionary of medical eponyms. Its basis was the use of mercuric nitrate in the eighteenth and nineteenth centuries by English hat makers to soften the outer stiff hairs of felt.[2]

Chronic mercury poisoning is characterized by behavioral changes such as excessive embarrassment, timidity, withdrawal, fatigue, insomnia, hallucinosis, and despondency. Physical changes include gingivitis, tremor, renal damage, anorexia, hypertension, and peripheral neuritis.[3]

The behavior of the Mad Hatter, in Lewis Carroll's *Alice's Adventures in Wonderland*,[4] is suggestive of hallucinosis, but he was hardly easily embarrassed, timid or shy. "'If you knew Time as well as I do,' said the Hatter, 'you wouldn't talk about wasting *it*. It's *him* . . . I dare say you never even spoke to Time.'" His behavior was more that of "an eccentric extrovert with an obsession with time."[5] It is questionable whether Carroll knew the dangers of mercury poisoning, although he may have seen some "mad" hatters.[6] It is possible that the phrase was suggested to him by an article in *Punch* in 1862 entitled "Mad as a Hatter."[7] The word, erethism, which denotes a state of excitement or irritation, has been applied to the marked shaking of the Mad Hatter during the trial of the Knave of Hearts.[6] In this instance, it could be attributed to mercury poisoning. "Mad as a Hatter"[8] and "hatter's shakes" have been in common usage[9] for the same condition, although in the former instance, the derivation may have been from "mad as a nadder," a reptile.

Dentists also may be affected with the Mad Hatter Syndrome, especially if they frequently mix the dental amalgam of mercury between their fingers in a badly ventilated room.[10] Another example of mercury poisoning is Minamata disease, named after a city in Japan in which methyl mercury was released into a nearby bay from a factory manufacturing vinyl chloride. The result was poisoning from eating mercury-contaminated fish.[11]

Exposure to mercury in experiments has been suggested as the cause of Isaac Newton's brief period of insanity.[12] However, his symptoms of insomnia, anorexia, loss of memory, melancholia, and paranoia were not sufficiently typical for such poisoning.[13] Patient-staff meetings held in a psychiatric institute have been reported to be as bewildering as the Mad Hatter tea party.[14]

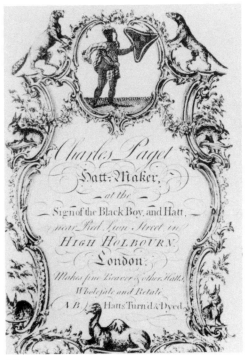

(B)

Mad Hatter Syndrome **B.** A London haberdasher's trade card of 1774.[2, pl. 56] (by permission, Dover Pubns., Inc.)

1. Magalini, S. I. & Scrascia, E.: *Dictionary of Medical Syndromes*: 2nd ed., Philadelphia, J. B. Lippincott, 1981, p. 513.
2. Heal, A.: *London Tradesmen's Cards of the XVIII Century. An Account of Their Origin and Use*: New York, Dover Pub., 1968, p. 79.
3. Freedman, p. 566.
4. Carroll, pp. 93–104, 148–150.
5. Waldron, J. A.: Did the Mad Hatter have mercury poisoning?: *Br. Med. J.*, 287:1961, 1983.
6. Price, T. M. L.: Did the Mad Hatter have mercury poisoning?: *Br. Med. J.*, 288:324, 1984.
7. Clark, A.: *Lewis Carroll. A Biography*: New York, Schocken Books, 1979, p. 134.
8. Partridge, pp. 711–712.
9. An onlooker's notebook: Hatters' shakes: *Pharmaceut. J.*, 232:433, 1984.
10. Dunlop, J. M.: The Mother Goose syndrome— A lighthearted look at paediatric literature: *Public Health*, 88:89–96, 1974.
11. Tedeschi, L. G.: The Minamata disease: *Am. J. Forens. Med. Pathol.*, 3:335–338, 1982.
12. Broad, W. J.: Sir Isaac Newton: Mad as a hatter: *Science*, 213:1341–1343, 1981.
13. Lieb, J. & Hershman, D.: Isaac Newton: Mercury poisoning or manic depression?: *Lancet*, 2: 1479–1480, 1983.
14. Klein, R. H.: The patient-staff community meeting: A tea party with the mad hatter: *Int. J. Group Psychother.*, 31:205–222, 1981.

Madonna-Harlot Syndrome

(madonna-prostitute split[1])

Some men expect women to display qualities that are divine or angelic.[2] If a woman behaves in a manner anything less than purity itself, she is considered to be an inferior beast, a whore. Such an either-or orientation does not acknowledge any behavior between these two extremes, and is thus aptly named the Madonna-Harlot Syndrome. Madonna is a term in Christian art which is associated with the Virgin Mary.[3] The name is used in a devotional sense rather than in a historical one. The word madonna is derived from the Italian for my lady and was originally used to address a queen.[4]

It has been postulated that Jack the Ripper murdered prostitutes and other "loose" women because he suffered from the Madonna-Harlot Syndrome.[2] The narrator in Gustave Flaubert's *Memories of a Madman* became enraged when he imagined his beloved Maria having bestial intercourse with her husband.[1] "I thought woman was an angel. Oh, how Molière was right to compare her to a soup!" Religious eponyms of the same derivation are the Madonna-Subconscious, defined as "the natural inclination of the human psyche toward a ready faith in God"; and the Satanic-Subconscious for the opposite.[5] Together these constitute the more psychological connotation of the Jekyll and Hyde Syndrome.

Madonna is the title of a poem by Valerie Berry which ennobles the dying moments of a woman. " . . . Awake, she fills the room with light,/ A bright flush on her face, her eyes a fevered glow,/ Her aching arms lie still against the white sheet,/ Palms up in supplication. She loves her pain/ With her saint's heart creaking in its cask,/ A relic worthy of beatitude . . . ."[6]

1. Baudry, F. D.: Adolescent love and self-analysis as contributors to Flaubert's creativity: *Psychoanal. Study Child.*, 35:377–416, 1980.
2. Johnson, W. S.: *Living in Sin: The Victorian Sexual Revolution*: Chicago, Nelson-Hall, 1979, p. 23.
3. *Encyclopaedia Britannica*: VI:472.
4. Weekley, p. 875.
5. Staehelin, B.: Das Marianische Unbewusste. The Madonna-Subconscious: *Schweiz. Rundschau Med.*, 71:881–886, 1982.
6. Berry, V.: Madonna: *J.A.M.A.*, 257:2642, 1987.

Matthew Effect

(halo effect)

The eponym Matthew Effect refers to "Eminent scientists [who] get disproportionately greater credit for their contributions to science while relatively unknown scientists tend to get disproportionately little credit for comparable contributions."[1] It has also been called the halo effect.[2] For example, if a paper is signed by both an unknown scientist and a Nobel laureate, the latter will be most likely to get credit for the discovery, no matter how little his actual contribution.

Matthew, the biblical tax collector, was one of the twelve disciples of Christ. He stated that "For to every one who has shall more be given, and he shall have abundance; but from him who has not, even what he has will be taken."[3] Thus, credit has been taken by eminent scientists (the haves), although not necessarily purposefully, from unheralded scientists (the have nots).

The Matthew Effect is related to the Ortega hypothesis which suggests that only a few scientists make a significant contribution to scientific progress.[4] Ortega y Gasset had written

that "the majority of scientists help the peripheral advance of science while shut up in the
narrow cell of their laboratory like the bee in
the cell of its hive . . . ."[5]

1. Merton, R.: The Matthew effect in science: in *The
   Sociology of Science*, N.W. Storer, Ed., Chicago,
   University of Chicago Press, 1973, pp. 439–459.
2. Cole, J. R. & Cole, S.: The Ortega hypothesis:
   Science, 178:368–375, 1972.
3. NT: 25:29.
4. Broad, W. & Wade, N.: *Betrayers of the Truth. Fraud
   and Deceit in the Halls of Science*: New York, Simon
   & Schuster, 1982, pp. 53–54.
5. Ortega y Gasset, J.: *The Revolt of the Masses*, New
   York, Norton, 1932, pp. 84–85.

Medea Complex

A mother may feel hatred and death wishes
toward her child, usually arising unconsciously
from a desire for revenge on her husband.[1] The
Medea Complex has been restricted to a
mother's death wish against her daughter, although Medea had only sons. Medea was, in
Greek mythology, a sorceress and the wife of
Jason, whom she helped to acquire the Golden
Fleece. When Jason put her away because he
wished to marry Creusa, she became so enraged that she killed her own children and fled
to Athens.[2]

The Medea Complex differs from some other
complexes related to family interactions, such
as those of Oedipus and Jocasta, in which
excessive love is the psychological problem. In
the Atreus Complex, it is the father who has
death wishes against his offspring. Colchicine,
a poisonous alkaloid used to treat gout, is named
after a crocus genus, *Colchicum*, which in turn is
named Colchis after the home of the sorceress
Medea.[3]

1. Campbell, p. 122.
2. Gayley, p. 235.
3. Espy, p. 313.

Medical Messiahs

The eponym Medical Messiahs has been
applied to health quacks.[1] Of particular concern are false claims through mail fraud and
false advertising, especially for cancer cures.
An early crusader against the intentional misleading of the public in health matters was
Morris Fishbein, a former editor of the *Journal*

of the American Medical Association. In his book on *Fads and Quackery in Healing*[2] of 1932, his targets were Perkins tractors, homeopathy, mind and faith healing, chiropractic, naturopathy, rejuvenation, and the therapeutic use of electricity. At the turn of the century, a compilation of articles on medical quackery was printed by the American Medical Association.[3] Highlighted were cures for consumption, "female weakness," asthma, cough, diabetes, obesity, and rheumatism.

Closely related to the eponym Medical Messiahs is another, the New Messiahs. It is used similarly for individuals who espouse their way to health for every conceivable type of illness, unrelated to any known or proven medical methods.[4] New Messiahs differ from Medical Messiahs in that some of the former are quite sincere about their belief in the efficacy of their cure-alls. Both differ from those afflicted with the Messiah Complex in that they do not have severe psychiatric conditions.

Examples of the nostrums promoted by these messiahs are natural nutrition, biofeedback, yoga, healing crystals, transcendental meditation, hypnotism, and self-affirmation courses as cure-alls. Successes can be attributed to faith in the messiah and his/her method, greatly enhanced by the healer's charisma and positivism. The influence of faith in healing is also quite effective when used by regular physicians who practice appropriate patient/doctor relationships.[4] In this sense the doctor becomes the therapeutic agent. Such placebo effects can contribute to the patient's well being, but is detrimental when used to promote and sell worthless nostrums.[5]

Of particular concern is the extensive promotion of unproven cancer cure-all drugs. Krebiozen (carcalon) was widely advertised and used in the 1960s, but its use gradually declined after analysis revealed the presence of creatine monohydrate, an amino acid of normal tissues that has not been shown to be of any value in cancer therapy.[6] In the following two decades, history repeated itself with a massive campaign for laetrile (amygdalin), which is a cyanogenic glycoside found in apricot seeds and claimed to be an anticancer vitamin.[7] It releases cyanide when exposed to beta-glycoside, but this enzyme is quite low in cancer tissue, and there is no evidence of an anticancer effect for laetrile. It is not harmless: Agranulocytosis[8] and death from cyanide poisoning[9] have been reported in certain individuals ingesting laetrile. On the one hand, vast fortunes have been made by its promoters, and on the other hand cancer patients and their families have had their financial resources depleted, all to no avail.[10] Also detrimental is the delay in receiving chemotherapy for malignant tumors on which an anticancer effect has been demonstrated.[11] It has been estimated that the cancer quackery of Medical Messiahs constitutes a two-billion-dollar-a-year business in the United States, and ten billion worldwide.[12]

Prior to the present century, quackery was even more rampant in both Europe and America. Major examples are mesmerism and cures for the then all pervasive syphilis.[13] The former was an astute mixture of hypnosis and pseudo-electricity which was widely practiced by Friederich Anton Mesmer as the answer to all health problems.[14] The extravagant medical quackery of eighteenth century England is well depicted in the engravings of William Hogarth.[15]

Messiah is the designation for the promised and expected deliverer of both Jews and Christians, the latter being Christ.[16] The name was derived from the Greek word messias by the translators of the Geneva Bible of 1560.[17] Thus, the eponym Medical Messiahs implies deliverance of humanity from all its ailments.

Another eponym that involves quackery is the Wizard-of-Oz Phenomenon.[18] It refers not to deceitful health care practices as such, but to the fact that a patient's power of belief alone can have good results, even with ineffective nostrums. The literary derivation is from the modernized fairy tale of the adventures of Dorothy in *The Wonderful Wizard of Oz*, published in 1900 by L. F. Baum, an American writer.[19] The great and terrible but fake Wizard succeeded through intimidation, flamboyancy, and challenges to give the straw Scarecrow the equivalent of a brain, the tin Woodman the equivalent of a heart, and the cowardly Lion the equivalent of courage. This children's tale has a moral (as most do) which is expressed by a chapter titled "The Magic Art of the Great Humbug"; anything can be accomplished with enough desire and belief, including some medical cures. As the Wizard of Oz said to himself, "How can I help being a humbug . . . . It was easy to make the Scarecrow and the Lion and the Woodman happy, because they imagined I could do anything."

1. Young, J. H.: *The Medical Messiahs. A Social History of Health Quackery in Twentieth-Century America*: Princeton, New Jersey, Princeton University Press, 1967.
2. Fishbein, M.: *Fads and Quackery in Healing. An Analysis of the Healing Cults, with Essays on Various Other Peculiar Notions in the Health Field*: New York, Blue Ribbon Books, 1932.
3. *Nostrums and Quackery. Articles on the Nostrum Evil and Quackery Reprinted from the Journal of the American Medical Association*: Chicago, American Medical Association Press, n.d.
4. Plainfield, S.: The healer within: *Mobius*, 5:58–69, 1985.
5. Shapiro, A. K.: A contribution to a history of the placebo effect: *Behavioral Sci.*, 5:109–135, 1960.
6. Miller, N. J. & Howard-Ruben, J.: Unproven methods of cancer management part I: Background and historical perspectives: *Oncol. Nursing Forum*, 10:46–52, 1983.
7. Greenberg, D. M.: The case against laetrile. The fraudulent cancer remedy: *Cancer*, 45:799–807, 1980.
8. Liegner, K. B. et al.: Laetrile-induced agranulocytosis: *J.A.M.A.*, 246:2841–2842, 1981.
9. Sadoff, L. et al.: Rapid death associated with laetrile ingestion: *J.A.M.A.*, 239:1532, 1978.
10. Lerner, I. J.: Laetrile: A lesson in cancer quackery: *CA*, 31:91–95, 1981.
11. Holland, J. C.: Why patients seek unproven cancer remedies: A psychological perspective: *CA*, 32:10–14, 1982.
12. Goldman, B.: A cure for cancer quackery needed, conference told: *Can. Med. Assoc. J.*, 136:1295–1296, 1987.
13. Rosebury, T.: *Microbes and Morals*: New York, Viking Press, 1971.
14. Mackay, C.: *Extraordinary Popular Delusions and the Madness of Crowds*: reprint 1852 ed., New York, Noonday Press, 1932, pp. 319–330.
15. Rodin, A. E. & Key, J. D.: Medicine in 18th Century London as Depicted in the Engravings of William Hogarth: *Medical Bull. U.S. Army*, PB-8-88-5:3–15, 1988.
16. Stein, p. 899.
17. OED: VI:375.
18. Weil, A.: *Health and Healing. Understanding Conventional and Alternative Medicine*: Boston, Houghton Mifflin, 1985, pp. 191–192.
19. Baum, L. F.: *The Wizard of Oz*: illustrated by M. Hague, New York, Holt, Rinehart & Winston, 1982.

Medical Nemesis

Medical Nemesis is the title of a book by Ivan Illich.[1] Its subtitle, "The Expropriation of Health," refers to the "disabling impact of professional control over medicine." Included under the broad title are the detrimental effects of professional monopoly (called the iatrogenic pandemic), which is responsible for the medicalization of life. Potential benefits are outweighed by clinical damage; political conditions that enhance an unhealthy society are obscured; and the mystification of medicine expropriates the power of the individual to heal himself and to shape his own environment. Recurring themes in the book are that medical enterprise turns pain into a technical matter, and thereby deprives suffering of its inherent personal meaning; undermines the continuation of old cultural programs for self-care and suffering; decreases coping mechanisms and encourages pampering; inhibits personal commitment by health professionals; replaces dying with medicalized death; is not responsible for decrease in sickness; and limits accountability for cost efficiency.

In Greek mythology, Nemesis was the daughter of Nox (Nyx, Night). She represented the righteous anger and vengeance of the gods toward the proud, the insolent, and the breakers of laws.[2] Current dictionary definitions of nemesis as a noun include an agent or act of retribution or punishment; that which a person cannot conquer or achieve; and an opponent whom a person cannot best.[3] Its common usage has the connotation of activities or situations that have an evil or devastating effect on any person, object, or activity. It is in this sense that Illich discusses the need to counteract a major threat to health, the medical establishment.

An abridged presentation given by Illich was printed in *Lancet* shortly before publication of his book.[4] In it he compares the medical establishment to "tantalizing hubris," a phrase which he coined after Tantalus, king of Phrgia, who stole from the gods their divine potion, Ambrosia, which gave them everlasting life.[5] Thus, "The members of this [medical] guild pass themselves off as disciples of healing Asklepios, while in fact they peddle Ambrosia."

Illich is following, in part, in the footsteps of George Bernard Shaw, who was even more scathing in his criticism of the medical profession, using a play, *The Doctor's Dilemma*, as his vehicle.[6] Even earlier are the plays of Molière which satirized seventeenth century French medicine.[7] One of his characters states that medicine is only for those fit enough to survive the treatment as well as the disease.

As might be expected, Illich's book has received an extensive reaction from the medical community. Articles in the *British Medical Journal* criticize his belief that effective treatment is usually simple and that suffering is an inescapable feature of humans;[8] that he does not delineate what health is;[9] that there is obscurity because of his fondness for exotic words, abstract nouns, and emotive phrases;[9] and that a return to the simple life would result in death of several hundred million people.[10] A letter in *Lancet* invokes Illich's ignorance of the role that medical knowledge has played in the control of epidemics.[11] There is a more extensive critique in the *International Journal of Health Services*.[12] Major points are that Illich seems to confuse care with cure; that the existing health care system is dependent on consumption which is intrinsically necessary for survival of a system based on commodity production; and that the basic cause of sickness or unhealth is not necessarily the individual himself.

The premise of Illich's book has been questioned because one of its major mythological references is to the punishment of Prometheus by Zeus for his giving fire to man—in itself a very beneficial act for man (unlike Illich's categorization of medicine).[13] To counterbalance the above negative reactions, there are a number of articles and letters that support Illich's concerns, if not in total, at least in the sense of pointing out some basic truths and serving as a stimulus for medicine and society to examine themselves for inherent evils.[14–21] Pointed out is that "the very clumsiness of [Illich's] words 'medicalization' and 'literature-ization' suggests the abstraction, the de-emphasis of the sick man, the new center of gravity on the printed page or the x-ray film."[22] "When I see a patient in consultation on a medical or surgical ward I often wonder if the physician has any idea of the patient's life . . . [which] may be far more relevant than sheaves of test reports."[14]

René Dubos, in a comment on Illich's book, has supported the role of the physician in health care.[23] ". . . the physician's appropriate behavior is based upon vast experience. Before seeing the course that the ailment takes, he knows that most symptoms involve no real problems, but he also knows how to spot those symptoms that sometimes . . . can reveal very serious problems." Dubos's concept of the importance of the physician's role, in contrast to the computer, is "to see the patient, listen to him, become familiar with his case history, learn about his general way of life, get to know his family circle, and then add the factor of his exclusively human judgement, so important in diagnosing and treating an illness."

It has been suggested that the intensity of antimedical literature may be proportional to the degree of medicalization.[24] This has been evident not only in the present century, but also in the works of such authors as Aristotle, Plato, and Molière. The more recent reaction against medicine as a guild (as represented by Illich's book) may well have been fostered by the infatuation of modern medicine with technology at the expense of the patient as an individual, one who is a human being with psychological and environmental influences that contribute significantly to both well being and illness. The massive counterresponse by physicians may be an indication of insecurity engendered by the increasing government regulation of medical practice.

1. Illich, I.: *Medical Nemesis. The Expropriation of Health*: New York, Pantheon Books, 1976.
2. Gayley, p. 38.
3. Stein, p. 957.
4. Illich, I.: Medical nemesis: *Lancet*, 1:918–921, 1974.
5. Gayley, p. 99.
6. Shaw, G. B.: *The Doctor's Dilemma. A Tragedy*: London, Constable, 1915.
7. Hall, H. G.: Molière satirist of seventeenth-century French medicine: Fact and fantasy: *Proc. R. Soc. Med.*, 70:425–431, 1977.
8. Editorial: Dream, mirage, or nemesis?: *Br. Med. J.*, 2:1521–1522, 1976.
9. Rhodes, P.: Indictment of medical care: *Br. Med. J.*, 4:576–577, 1974.
10. Discombe, G.: A romantic enthusiast: *Br. Med. J.*, 4:574–576, 1974.

11. Discombe, G.: Medical nemesis: *Lancet*, 2:584–585, 1974.
12. Navarro, V.: The industrialization of fetishism or the fetishism of industrialization. A critique of Ivan Illich: *Int. J. Health Serv.*, 5:351–371, 1975.
13. Vaisrub, S.: New chains for Prometheus: *J.A.M.A.*, 229:1213–1214, 1974.
14. Emanuel, E.: Musings: The physician's nemesis: *Can. Med. Assoc. J.*, 117:91–92, 1977.
15. Editorial: Medical nemesis: *Br. Med. J.*, 4:548–549, 1974.
16. Paton, A.: "Medicalization" of health: *Br. Med. J.*, 4:573–574, 1974.
17. Bradshaw, S.: Medical nemesis: *Lancet*, 1:1053, 1974.
18. Smith, R.: Medical nemesis: *Lancet*, 1:1160, 1974.
19. Keeve, J. P.: Medical nemesis: *Lancet*, 1:1160, 1974.
20. Mitchell-Fox, T. M.: Medical nemesis: *Lancet*, 2:232, 1974.
21. Bradshaw, J. S.: Medical nemesis: *Br. Med. J.*, 1:94, 1975.
22. Carter, A. H.: Esthetics and anesthetics: Nemesis, hermeneutics and treatment in literature and medicine: *Lit. Med.*, 5:141–151, 1986.
23. Dubos, R. & Escande, J.-P.: *Quest. Reflections on Medicine, Science, and Humanity*: P. Ranum translator, New York, Harcourt Brace Jovanovich, 1979, pp. 72–73.
24. Gelfand, T.: Medical nemesis, Paris, 1894: Léon Daudet's *Les Morticoles*: *Bull. Hist. Med.*, 60:155–176, 1986.

Medical Pickwick

The *Medical Pickwick*, a journal published in Saranac Lake New York, was established in 1915.[1] The foreword in the first issue was written by one of America's outstanding physicians, Fielding H. Garrison. He gave as its goal the cultivation of a "genial, humorous spirit in our profession, to consider medicine in a Pickwickian sense . . . . dedicated to the cause of peace and comity, good humor and good fellowship among medical men." It was intended to counteract the "preposterous omniscience, pompous infallibility" assumed as part of the professional dignity in medicine. In contrast to its stated purposes, the journal terminated its independent existence with volume 13 by merging into the *Urologic and Cutaneous Review* in July, 1927.

The title of this journal was taken from Charles Dickens's well-known book of 1836/7, *The Posthumous Papers of the Pickwick Club*.[2] The founder of the club was Mr. Samuel Pickwick, Esquire, a very naive and benevolent gentleman, who traveled about with his fellow club members, acting as their guardian and advisor. The major contribution of the book to medical terminology has been the Pickwickian Syndrome.

This journal's title, *Medical Pickwick*, is quite appropriate because the adjective, "pickwickian," is used in the vernacular to indicate remarks that are esoteric and not be taken seriously.[3] The journal was promoted as an "organ of the literary and cultural side" of medicine.[1] A more recent example of such a journal is *Medical Heritage*, established in 1985, 70 years later.[4]

1. F. H. G. (Garrison): Foreword: *Med. Pickwick*, 1: 2–3, 1915.
2. Dickens, C.: *The Posthumous Papers of the Pickwick Club*: New York, G. W. Carleton, 1883.
3. Espy, p. 138.
4. Goldwyn, R. M.: Introduction: *Med. Heritage*, 1: 1–2, 1985.

Medusa Locks Sign

(beehive, breadcrumbs, tangled thick cord signs, whirlpool)

Marked multiplication in the intestine of the nematode *Ascaris lumbricoides* (roundworm) may result in masses which cause intestinal obstruction.[1] On abdominal x-rays, these masses have translucent areas of gas trapped between the worms, giving an appearance suggestive of coiled locks of hair,[2] or a mass of worms.[3] Ascaris worms have been demonstrated in all parts of the bowel and stomach.[4] As many as 455 cases have been included in one report.[5] The comparison to Medusa, the mythical Greek Gorgon, is only on a supposed morphological resemblance of her hair to snakes (see Caput Medusa).

1. Ellman, B. A., et al.: Intestinal ascariasis: New plain film features: *Am. J. Roentgenol.*, 135:37–42, 1980.
2. Eisenberg, p. 61.
3. Isaacs, I.: Roentgenographic demonstration of intestinal ascariasis in children without using barium: *Am. J. Roentgenol.*, 76:558–561, 1956.
4. Bean, W. J.: Recognition of ascariasis by routine chest or abdomen roentgenograms: *Am. J. Roentgenol.*, 94:379–384, 1965.
5. Okumura, M., et al.: Acute intestinal obstruction by *Ascaris*. Analysis of 455 cases: *Rev. Inst. Med. Trop. Sao Paulo*, 16:292–300, 1974.

Medusa's Head

Freud has equated the terror of decapitation of the Gorgon Medusa of Greek mythology with the terror of castration, and her head being covered with snakes instead of hair a representation of the female genitalia, especially that of a male's mother.[1] The sight of her head turned the spectator as stiff as stone, in other words a penile erection. The Medusa Head is thus a symbol of castration.

"The Head of Medusa" has been used as the title for a series of three articles on "Contemporary Literature's Obsession with the Pathological."[2] Decried is the amount of sexual violence, perversions, greediness, selfishness, decadence, cruelty, and distortions of reality that present a distorted view of life. Popular literature and culture of today, such as comic books, contain fantasies of evil women, such as Medusa look-alikes and equivalents. They play a central role as images of sexuality.[3] Such "medusas" may have their origin in the earliest stages of infancy, especially in homes in which the father is absent, and where the mother has an intense but ambivalent relationship with her child. By confronting directly the monstrous Medusa found throughout much of literature, we may well become hypnotized and turned into stony insensitivity (see Caput Medusa).

1. Freud, S.: "Medusa's Head": *S.E.*, Vol. XVIII, pp. 273–274.
2. Scarlett, E. P.: The head of Medusa: *Arch. Int. Med.*, Part 1, 111:823–828; Part 2, 112:129–134; Part 3, 112:278–283, 1963.
3. Adams, A. A.: "Octopoid" genitalia and the medusal madonna: *J. Psychohist.*, 10:409–462, 1983.

Mercury

Mercury is an element that was widely used in past centuries for the treatment of syphilis,[1] even as early as 1501.[2] It is still used medically for some instruments of physiological measurement, such as blood and spinal fluid pressures. Mercury was the Roman name for Hermes, the Greek messenger of the gods. He was the son of Zeus and Maia.[3] Mercury was as swift as the wind, and bore the caduceus wand of two entwined snakes. He also conducted the souls of the dead to Hades. His speed was such that he flickered in and out of sight, being as volatile as quicksilver, which came to be called mercury.[4] Hermes (Mercury) has been considered as the father of alchemy. Hermetical was the alchemist's term for various procedures, especially the sealing of containers (thus hermetically sealed).[5] Mercurochrome is a more recent word for any dye obtained by substitution of mercury in the basic molecule.

Mercury was also the god of commerce, making the two-snaked caduceus a somewhat derogatory symbol of medicine, more related to Illich's view of physicians as the *Medical Nemesis* (see Medical Nemesis).[6] Mercury is also an important cause of environmental poisoning (see Mad Hatter).[7]

1. Dennie, C. C.: *A History of Syphilis*: Springfield, Illinois, Charles C Thomas, 1962, pp. 16–17.
2. Rosebury, T.: *Microbes and Morals*: New York, Viking Press, 1932, p. 47.
3. Gayley, pp. 19, 34–35.
4. Espy, p. 24.
5. Skinner, pp. 208, 271–272.
6. Illich, I.: *Medical Nemesis. the Expropriation of Health*: New York, Pantheon Books, 1976.
7. Eto, K. & Takeuchi, T.: A pathological study of prolonged cases of Minamata disease—with particular reference to 83 autopsy cases: *Acta Pathol. Jpn.*, 28:565–584, 1978.

Messiah Complex

(messiah delusion, messiah quest)

The Messiah Complex is a delusional identification with Christ which may occur during a psychotic episode, apparently arising from psychological conflicts related to parents.[1] The young boy (Puer) remains eternally (aeternus) between the maternal and paternal influences, even in old age (Senex). There may be feelings of a halo around the head, of obsession with a mission to save the world from impending doom, and of communication with God.[2] Messianic delusions also occur in Jews, but related to the Hebrew Messiah.[3] The word Messiah originated in the prophetic writings of the Old Testament to indicate a promised deliverer of the Jewish nation (see Medical Messiahs).[4] The eponym has also been applied to a charismatic character, Paul Atreides in Frank Herbert's science fiction *Dune* series.[5]

1. Rentrop, E.: Der Messias-Komplex beim Puer aeternus: *Analyt. Psychol.*, 9:284–301, 1978.
2. Zelt, D.: First person account: The messiah quest: *Schizophrenia Bull.*, 7:527–531, 1981.
3. Clark, R. A.: Religious delusions among the Jews: *Am. J. Psychother.*, 34:62–71, 1980.
4. OED: VI:374.
5. Garcia, G. D.: People: *Time Mag.*, June 11, 1984, p. 71.

Mickey Mouse Sign I, II

I   A resemblance to the head of the cartoon character Mickey Mouse is seen in the ultrasound transverse x-ray view of the main bile duct area.[1] The portal vein forms the head, the main bile duct the right ear, and the hepatic artery the left ear.

II   The head of Mickey Mouse is also suggested in plain abdominal radiographs of solid masses resulting from bilateral hydronephrosis.[2] Mickey Mouse is one of Walt Disney's most famous and popular animated characters, first introduced in the cartoon *Steamboat* of 1928.[3]

The phrase Mickey Mouse marketing has been applied to the need for nurse managers to apply one of the basic administrative principles used by Disney: That everyone needs to perform in a professional manner, whether their job requires interacting with the public or working "backstage."[4] A drawing of Mickey Mouse's face and ears on the cleansed area of the forearm has been used to reduce the unpleasantness of tuberculin immunization for children.[5] The inoculation is then given into Mickey's nose, and the child told that if he gets a cold his nose will turn red (positive reaction). In order to catch children's attention for dental health education, a Mickey Mouse suitcase is opened to reveal the cartoon character as well as various foods and a toothbrush.[6]

1. Bartrum, R. J. Jr. & Crow, H. C.: Inflammatory diseases of the biliary system: *Semin. Ultrasound*, 1:102–112, 1980.
2. Eisenberg, pp. 145, 448.
3. Daniels, L.: *Comix. A History of Comic Books in America*: New York, Outerbridge & Dienstfrey, 1971.
4. Reeves, D. M. & Underly, N.: Nurse managers and Mickey Mouse marketing: *Nursing Admin. Q.*, 7:22–27, 1983.
5. Mickey Mouse to the rescue: *Pediatr. Nursing*, 4:26, 1978.
6. Hassell-Bachman, C. & Hassell, T.: The Mickey Mouse suitcase: A novel dental health education device for children: *J. Am. Dent. Hyg. Assoc.*, 46: 362–363, 1972.

Mickey Mouse Syndrome

Intraoral and extraoral mouthguards have been developed to prevent dental damage in contact sports such as football and hockey.[1] The extraoral type has been rejected by participants because of its visibility. As one coach has said, "I don't want my team to look like a bunch of Mickey Mice." In this eponym Walt Disney's famous cartoon character is used for a concern with being considered sissified. Thus, the eponym refers more to the fear of exhibiting unmanliness than to the nature of the teeth of Mickey Mouse.

In common usage, the name Mickey Mouse has connotations of fake, useless, or expending much effort with little result.[2] It is also used to indicate anything trivial or gibberish.[3] Karl Menninger has called the change from the official psychiatric nosology developed during World War II to a much more complex one in 1969, a "sheer verbal Mickey Mouse" (see Mickey Mouse Signs).[4]

1. Wood, A. W. S.: The Mickey Mouse syndrome. "Full speed ahead and damn the scattering teeth": *Oral Health*, 60:5–7, 1970.
2. Espy, p. 337.
3. Ciardi, p. 249.
4. Menninger, K.: Sheer verbal Mickey Mouse: *Int. J. Psychiatry, 4:415, 1969.*

Midas Factor

A dispute between biological research institutions has occurred over the priority of credit for developing potentially profitable methods.[1] The example designated as the Midas Factor is a lucrative new way of producing synthetic vaccines. The method was published by two institutions within five days of each other, one the Scripps Clinic and Research Foundation and the other the La Jolla branch campus of the University of California and Salk Institute.

Midas was a Phrygian king in Greek mythology.[2] When Silenus, a satyr, wandered away from the god Bacchus (Dionysus) in an intoxicated condition, he was found by some peasants who took him to their king, Midas. Midas treated Silenus royally and then returned him to Bacchus, who offered Midas the choice of any reward. Midas asked that anything he touch be turned into gold. This was granted, and everything he touched did so. He beseeched the god to withdraw the gift because even his food and drink turned into gold. Bacchus did so by having him wash away his greediness in the Pactolus river (now in Turkey), in which thereafter gold has been found.

The term Midas has become, therefore, to mean selfish greed for wealth, and often with disastrous consequences for those so inflicted. It has a similar connotation to those of miser and Scrooge, which are somewhat harsher terms. On a more symbolic level, Midas's danger of "Physical death from starvation symbolizes the death of the soul from lack of spiritual food."[3] The eponym Midas Factor may be too ignoble a term to apply to two humanitarian research institutions.

MIDAS has been used as an acronym for an investigator-assisted computer analysis program of coronary patient data, using a software called, most appropriately, GOLD (Gathering of Laboratory Data).[4] MIDAS is also an automated computer system that can handle medical and other data of up to 30,000 people for purposes of correlations related to preventative medicine.[5]

1. Wade, W.: La Jolla biologists troubled by the Midas factor: *Science*, 213:623–628, 1981.
2. Gayley, pp. 157–158.
3. Diel, p. 106.
4. King, S. J. et al.: Midas: A program for investigator-assisted computer analysis of coronary patient data: *Comput. Programs Biomed.*, 3:36–44, 1973.
5. Kolouch, L. et al.: Midas-Aplikace Programu Ardis-Minsk V Lecebne-Preventivni Peci: *Cas. Lek. Cesk.*, 108:1166–1168, 1969.

Minerva Jacket

(Minerva plaster)

A Minerva Jacket is a special cast used for high cervical instability or fracture dislocation, often involving the odontoid process.[1] It extends from the top of the skull to the armpits on both sides, leaving the face exposed, but with barely enough room to chew.[2] Included are the abdomen, thorax, neck, forehead, and parietal regions of the skull.[3] Such an extensive cast is necessary because even minor cervical sprains may leave permanent disability.[4]

In Greek and Roman mythology, Minerva, also called Athena, sprang from the head of Jupiter, mature and in complete armor. The armor included a helmet, usually depicted as covering the entire head and forehead and extending over the posterior neck, as well as a breastplate of goatskin on which is fixed the

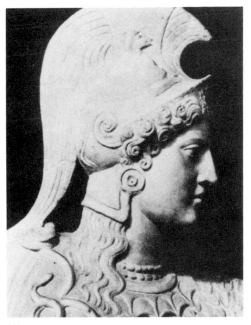

(A)

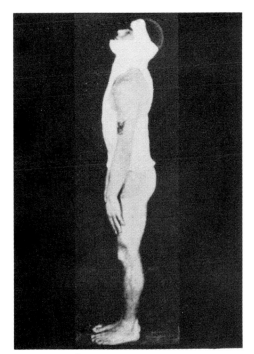

(B)

Minerva Jacket A. Minerva with head, neck and chest armor.[8] **B.** Minerva jacket cast.[3, p. 407] (by permission, W.B. Saunders Co.)

163

head of Medusa.[5] She was the virgin goddess of storms, war, health, wisdom, contemplation, and agriculture.

The Minerva Jacket bears resemblance to the goddess only in being quite extensive, with encasement of the head and neck. It has been both highly recommended[2] and strongly condemned[6] for whiplash injuries. A modification of the Minerva Jacket, the Minerva Pneumatica, has two layers to form a space which can be expanded by air.[7]

1. Sherk, H. H. et al.: Fractures of the odontoid process in young children: *J. Bone Joint Surg.*, 60-A:921–924, 1978.
2. Filius, J.: Whiplash injury or homage to Minerva: *Med. J. Aust.*, 2:1028, 1973.
3. O'Donoghue, D. H.: *Treatment of Injuries to Athletes*: 4th ed., Philadelphia, W. B. Saunders, 1984, p. 407.
4. Desijze, M. et al.: L'entrose cervicale: *Rev. Med. Brux.*, 2:951–954, 1981.
5. Gayley, p. 23.
6. Marshall, L. L.: Whiplash injury or homage to Minerva: *Med. J. Aust.*, 1:286, 1975.
7. Pavetto, G. C. & Zumaglini, G.: Un Nuovo Tipo di Apparecchio Ortopedica per il Rachide Cervicale: La "Minerva Pneumatica": *Minerva Ortoped.*, 17:687–689, 1966.
8. Bulfinch, p. 132.

Minerva Medica

Minerva Medica is an Italian medical journal published in Torino. The first volume appeared in 1909, and the journal is still being published.[1] Minerva was the daughter of Jupiter who sprang forth from his head, completely armed, and without a mother.[2] She was, among many other things, the goddess of wisdom and health. Justification of the use of her name is her other role as patroness of the guild of physicians.[3]

The *Index of National Library of Medicine Serial Titles* lists at least 46 medical journals with Minerva's name in the title.[1] Most are published in Italy and were inaugurated in the 1940s and 1950s. Most are related to various medical specialties or subspecialties. Another Italian medical journal is labeled with Minerva's Greek name, Athena. Minerva is also the pseudonym of the writer of the "Views" column in the *British Medical Journal*.[4] Minerva Press is the name of a book publisher (see Athena and Minerva Jacket).[5]

1. *Index of National Library of Medicine Serial Titles*.

2. Gayley, p. 7.
3. Neilson, W. A., Ed.,: *Webster's New International Dictionary of the English Language*: 2nd ed., Springfield, Massachusetts, G. & C. Merriam, 1955, pp. 1563–1564.
4. Minerva: Views: *Br. Med. J.*, 291:1207, 1985.
5. Blakey, D.: *The Minerva Press 1790–1820*: London, Bibliographical Society, 1939.

Miss Havisham Syndrome

A psychiatric syndrome has been described in which withdrawal from life occurs in order to maintain an illusion of a time in the past immediately prior to a traumatic emotional event. It occurs in young, aristocratic women of beauty and intelligence who suffer a catastrophic disappointment, such as bereavement or callous rejection by a lover.[1] The syndrome is characterized by the maintenance of the dress and immediate environment for a prolonged period of time.

The syndrome is named after a character in Charles Dickens's novel *Great Expectations* of 1862.[2] Miss Havisham, the spoiled child of a wealthy brewer, was jilted on her wedding day. Thereafter she lived as a recluse for many

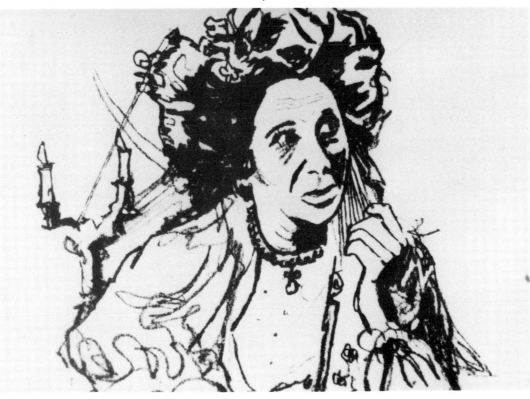

Miss Havisham Syndrome   Miss Havisham arrested in a time of the past.[1]

years, dressed in her wedding gown, and with her clock stopped at 8:40. Sunlight was not let in, cobwebs and dust accumulated, and she never left the house. According to the young hero, Pip:

I saw that the bride within the bridal dress had withered like the dress, and like the flowers, and had no brightness but the brightness of her sunken eyes. I saw that the dress had been put upon the rounded figure of a young woman, and that the woman upon which it now hung loose, had shrunk to skin and bone.

Such a reaction has been categorized as a psychological relapse, of which there are many in Dickens's fiction.[3] A well-known example of the Miss Havisham Syndrome is Queen Victoria. After the death in 1861 of her consort, Prince Albert, she withdrew into her suite of rooms in Windsor Castle. There she maintained everything as it had been at the time of her beloved husband's death.[4] The extent and length of her withdrawal may have been less than legend has it.[5] Various recluses have been proposed as the possible inspiration for Dickens's characterization of Miss Havisham, but not all match the criteria for the syndrome, as some were males.[6]

1. Critchley, M.: The Miss Havisham syndrome: *Hist. Med.*, 6:2–3, 5–6, 1969.
2. Dickens, C.: *Great Expectations*: New York, Greenwich House, 1982, p. 87.
3. Andrews, M.: Dickens and the medical profession: *N.Z. Med. J.*: 98:810–813, 1985.
4. Avery, G.: *Victorian People in Life and in Literature*: New York, Holt, Rinehart & Winston, 1970.
5. Hardy, A.: *Queen Victoria Was Amused*: New York, Tablinger Publishing Co., 1976.
6. Shatto, S.: Miss Havisham and Mr. Mopes the hermit: Dickens and the mentally ill (Part One): *Dickens Q.*, 11:43–49, 1985.

Mons Veneris

(mons pubis)

The eponym Mons Veneris can be translated literally as the mountain of Venus. It is located anterior to the pubic symphysis and superior to the labia.[1] Venus was the name of a Roman equivalent of Aphrodite, Greek goddess of love and beauty.[2] She was the daughter of Jupiter and Dione, although she is also said to have sprung from the sea.[3] Venus was given by Jupiter to Vulcan. Her son was Cupid, the god of love. Venus had an embroidered girdle (the cestus) which had the power of inspiring love.

The combination of being the goddess of love and having a love-inducing girdle is sufficient justification for the labeling of the mons, which is situated immediately above the female genitalia, as the girdle of Venus.

1. Jaeger, p. 89.
2. Schmidt, pp. 284–285.
3. Bulfinch, p. 9.

Moron

The word Moron was adopted in 1910 for a feeble-minded person by the American Association for the Study of the Feeble Minded.[1] Since then it has indicated a person with a mild mental retardation which is in the range of an IQ of 52 to 67.[2] The equivalent word in England is dullard. The moronic state falls within the category of arrested or incomplete development of the mind.[3] Its occurrence is determined by both genetic and environmental factors.

Moron was the name of a character in a Molière play of 1665, *La Princesse d'Elide* (The Princess of Elis).[4] He held the office of a bouffon for the princess of Elis. The French word "bouffon" is usually translated as a clown, and thus he was a court jester.[5] In the play, Moron is also called by the French word fou, which is translated as mad, crazy, or demented. In neither case is the connotation that of feeble-minded. In fact, Moron exhibited a considerable degree of cleverness and ingenuity in dealing with the princess, who was strongly opposed to romantic love. The prince of Ithaca, who was in love with the princess, stated that "You think you know him [Moron] well under his title of fool. But you must know that he is less one than he chooses to appear, and, in spite of the craft he practices today, he has more common sense than some who laugh at him."

Molière acted the part of Moron in the first production of "La Princess d'Elide." As a playwright he is best known for plays that satirize the medical profession, depicting medical practitioners as greedy, arrogant, and tyrannical.[6]

1. Hendrickson, p. 11.
2. Campbell, p. 304.
3. Leigh, D. et al.: *A Concise Encyclopaedia of Psychia-*

try: Baltimore, University Park Press, 1977, pp. 237–239.
4. Molière: *La Princesse d'Elide*: in *The Plays of Moliere in French with an English Translation and Notes by A. R. Waller*, Edinburgh, John Grant, 1926, pp. 306–371.
5. Stein, p. 1699.
6. Waterson, K.: Healers and patients in Molière's theatre: *Med. Heritage*, 2:462–469, 1986.

Morphine

Morphine is an alkaloid narcotic substance found in opium, which is prepared from the dried juice of the opium poppy.[1] It is used primarily as an analgesic. Effects also include drowsiness, changes in mood, respiratory depression, decreased gastrointestinal motility, vomiting, and changes in the endocrine and autonomic nervous systems.[2] Morpheus was the Greek god of dreams, and the son of the god of sleep, Somnus.[3] He could assume all forms of man in dreams.

A related eponym, the Morphine Abstinence Syndrome, is used for the narcotic withdrawal syndrome.[4] Sudden withdrawal of morphine from addicts can cause many distressful symptoms, the most serious of which are prostration, feeble pulse, and maniacal behavior.

Words derived from Morpheus for excessive use of morphine are morphinist and morphinomania.[1] There is some variability in the use of morphine-related words.[2] Opiate may refer to morphine or also to other drugs derived from opium, such as codeine. Opiod may have the same meaning as opiate, or it may refer to any drug with morphinelike actions.[4]

1. OED: VI:669–670.
2. Gilman, pp. 494–513.
3. Gayley, p. 177.
4. Durham, pp. 383–384.

Moses Complex

The Moses Complex denotes the desire of individuals to control and atone for their aggressive, homicidal drives, rather than to aggressive behavior as such.[1] Moses led the Tribe of Israel out of Egypt to Mount Sinai where he received the ten commandments, and then to the promised land, all in spite of his emotional reaction to the increasing resistance and frustration of his people.[2] The Moses Complex relates in good part to Freud's interpretation of the basis of religion.[3] " . . . I have never doubted that religious phenomena are only to be understood on the pattern of the individual neurotic symptoms familiar to us."

Freud's "Moses and Monotheism"[3] has been interpreted as reflecting Freud's strong Oedipal aggression because he describes Moses as struggling against his desire to take vengeance on his wayward people.[4] It may have been accentuated in Freud by the spread of anti-semitism in Germany.[5] Freud has been criticized for this work on Moses because of misquotations and inaccuracies related to his lack of knowledge of the Hebrew language and literature.[6] Freud's drive to write "Moses and Monotheism" has been called the Moses Motive, defined as Freud's identification with Moses whose people rebelled against him, as did Jung against Freud's preeminence in psychiatry.[4]

1. Szondi, L.: Thanatos and Cain: M. W. Webb trans., *Am. Imago*, 21:52–63, 1964.
2. OT: Numbers.
3. Freud, S.: Moses and Monotheism: *S.E.*, Vol. 23, pp. 1–37.
4. Wallace, E. R.: The psychodynamic determinants of *Moses and Monotheism*.: *Psychiatry*, 40:79–87, 1977.
5. Ater, M.: A new look at 'Moses and Monotheism': *Isr. J. Psychiatry Relat. Sci.*, 20:179–191, 1983.
6. Kagan, S. R.: Sigmond Freud on Moses and monotheism: *Med. Rec.*, 153:179–180, 1941.

Moses Syndrome

The eponym Moses Syndrome[1] is derived from the biblical description of Moses and his followers wandering in the desert for 40 years "until your carcasses be consumed in the wilderness."[2] It refers to the trials and errors that occur in trying to find a balance between cost, quality, and access to health care delivery. This literary eponym is not too appropriate, unless one considers the frustrations of physicians faced with the increasing and confusing governmental regulations as equivalent to the trials and tribulations of Moses in attempting to lead his people to the promised land.

Moses has been considered as a biblical physician even though he was not known as such.[3] An example is his cure of Israelites bitten by the fiery serpents sent by the Lord,[2] using a fiery serpent set on a pole. A modern interpretation is that the serpents were guinea worms.[3] Moses has also been called the father of preventative medicine because of his edicts on individual and group hygiene and dietary laws during the four decades of travel of the Jewish tribes.[4] Some of his edicts may have been based on nonhygienic factors, as their medical significance did not become apparent until the modern era.

Thirty-four years before the Moses Syndrome eponym was coined, a related book was published with the beguiling title of *Santa Claus, M.D.*[5] It is a polemic against socialized medicine. The focus of the book is the detrimental effects on health care delivery by governmental interference, and the denial that the population of the United States is in poor health. The United States government is labeled as Santa Claus, M.D. because it is offering all Americans "free" health care—but with monies that actually come from the very citizens who are receiving this supposedly free gift. It is evident that the concerns of some physicians about control by "big brother" have not changed in over three decades. This eponym is quite suitable because gifts from Santa Claus carry the connotation of rewards from parents (government) only if behavior of children (physicians) is appropriate.

1. Cost concerns overemphasized, physician says: *Am. Med. News*, May 11, 1984, p. 13.
2. OT: Numbers 14:33.
3. Levin, S.: Moses, physician for typhoid: *Practitioner*, 186:758–759, 1961.
4. Harrison, T. R.: If Moses could speak: *Chest*, 62:78–82, 1972.
5. Bauer, W. W.: *Santa Claus, M.D.*: Indianapolis, Indiana, Bobbs-Merrill, 1950.
6. Gwilt, J. R.: Biblical ills and remedies: *J. R. Soc. Med.*, 79:738–741, 1986.

Mother Goose Syndrome

The need to provide "A wide and stimulating range of experiences" for nursery education has been called the Mother Goose Syndrome.[1] It refers to the importance of nursery rhymes as a basis for health education at an early age. Thus, Humpty Dumpty teaches that our body cannot always be put back together again from a lot of little pieces; "Ring a Ring of Roses" illustrates the red rash of the plague; Jack Sprat may not have eaten fat because he had coeliac disease. The appropriateness of the Mother Goose Syndrome is questionable, as it is too much to expect the young child, let alone most parents, to read these implications into nursery rhymes. The author does point out that the rhymes provide a cultural orientation for children at an early age.

Mother Goose is the fictitious old woman to whom the traditional nursery rhymes were first ascribed in 1781.[2] She is often depicted as having a beak nose and sharp chin, and riding on the back of a goose. Mother Goose rhymes have been given as an example of the type of literature that pediatricians should recommend to mothers to read to their young children, in part to counteract the abundance of violence seen on television and the passive involvement of watching this medium.[3]

"Little Boy Blue," one of the Mother Goose nursery rhymes, has been used to study developmental, cross-cultural, and sex differences in the perception of situational causality in third and sixth grade children.[4] A significant increase in perception was found in the sixth grade in American children, but not in those from India. This suggests a developmental gradient in the former children.

1. Dunlop, J. M.: The Mother Goose syndrome—A lighthearted look at paediatric literature: *Public Health*, 88:89–96, 1974.
2. *Encyclopaedia Britannica*: VII:53.
3. Hall, C. B.: Rx: Mother Goose, hs: *Am. J. Dis. Child.*, 130:137–138, 1976.
4. Walker, C. et al.: A cross-cultural study of the perception of situational causality: *J. Cross-Cultural Psychol.*, 2:401–404, 1971.

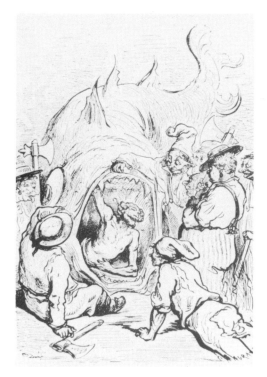

Munchausen Syndrome   Munchausen emerging from a whale.[9, p. 53] (by Gustave Doré)

Munchausen's Syndrome

(peregrinating problem patient,[1] Tomomania syndrome)

This well-known syndrome was first labeled as such by Asher in 1951,[2] and has given rise to other word forms, such as munchausenism and munchausenize.[3] The eponym refers to patients who present with an acute illness supported by a plausible and dramatic history, but which is largely made up of falsehoods, and which results in many hospital admissions. Varieties of the syndrome include acute abdominal, hemorrhagic, and neurological types. Somewhat whimsically named examples are laparotomophilia migrans, hemorrhagica historonica, and neurologica diabolica. A fourth type, cutaneous (dermatitis autogenetica), has also been suggested.[4] These patients are usually male. They are unlike malingerers, who have definite ends to gain, as did Sherlock Holmes on impersonating a dying man in order to trap a murderer.[5] Asher, however, listed several motives[1]—become the center of attention, satisfy a grudge against hospitals, escape from the police, appease a drug addiction, and get free board and room.

Personality defects found in Munchausen patients include hysteria, masochism, psychopathy, or schizophrenia. Another category is addiction to surgery, seen in maladjusted individuals who become laden with feelings of guilt and persecution after suffering mental or physical trauma in early childhood.[6] An example is a patient who after having one cardiac catherization feigned symptoms so that he would have many more.[7] Beggars in medieval times (and even today) feigned illness in order to arouse sympathy.[8]

The eponym is derived from *The Adventures of Baron Munchausen* by Raspe.[9] Baron Karl Friedrich Hieronymous Munchhausen was born in Germany in 1720 and became famous as a soldier, hunter, and raconteur.[10] Rudolph Erich Raspe retold some of Munchhausen's stories, added others, and published them anonymously in 1785 as satirical and ludricous accounts, with illustrations by Doré.[9] This small volume, and subsequent larger ones with additional tales by others, had little to do with the Baron's activities, but led to considerable notoriety before his death.[11]

Rudolph Eric Raspe (1737–1794) was a professor at Cassel, now in West Germany. He fled to England after being accused of stealing valuables from a collection of which he was the keeper.[10] It was there that he published *Baron Munchausen's Narrative of His Marvelous Travels and Campaigns in Russia*, spelling the Baron's name with one "h."[12] It has been claimed that the eponym should have two "h"s, as was true for the real baron.[13] However, the single "h" of the eponym is appropriate, as the eponym was named after the fictional baron of literature and not the historical one.[14]

The Munchausen Syndrome is one of three categories of chronic factitious disorders. It has physical symptoms, unlike the other two, which are psychological and atypical types.[15] Since Asher's designation of the syndrome in 1951,[3] the eponym has become quite popular, and many examples have been published. Included are coughing blood,[16] renal colic, hematuria,[17] crusted skin,[18] and even torsion dystonia.[19] There may be spontaneous remissions of the latter even when not factitious.[20]

Most striking is a 30-year-old woman who simulated acute spinal cord injury for nearly seven years while traveling over two continents.[21] She was found out when put under the influence of sodium pentathol. The true diagnosis was obscured by patient confidentiality requirements which prevented the transfer of critical medical data. Of similar interest is a Munchausen patient, the report of whom in the *British Medical Journal*[22] resulted in considerable correspondence from other physicians who had seen the same patient.[23] The difficulty in obtaining patient information by one institution from another appears to be a major factor in the perpetuation of some cases of the Munchausen Syndrome.

A variant of this eponym is the Munchausen Syndrome by Proxy,[24] which also has been called the Meadow Syndrome after the first describer.[25] These patients are children who are presented by their parents with fabricated disorders which require extensive medical investigation. In one study of 76 children, signs fabricated by parents included seizures, bleeding, rashes, fevers, abnormal urine and blood samples, renal stone, and feculent vomit.[26] Another example is that of bleeding from bruises and injuries to a child's mouth caused by the mother.[27] Other mothers have given their children various drugs which result in symptomatology.[28] The eponym Polle Syndrome has been suggested for the Munchausen by Proxy Syndrome on the basis that Baron Munchhausen's daughter, Polle, died in infancy.[29] This is quite inappropriate, as there is no historical basis for such an assumption,[30] nor did he have a child named Polle.[31]

Another variant of the Munchausen Syndrome occurs in females and not males. Females exhibiting this variant are more subtle and elaborate in their fabrication of illness, using undoubted abnormal laboratory findings, spurious pyrexia, and even symptoms induced by drugs.[32] The increasing availability and complexities of technological advances have contributed to the confusion in patients with this syndrome.[33] Yet another variant of the Munchausen Syndrome has been called the doctor impersonator.[34] It refers to a hospitalized patient who gave orders for his own care by telephone, including narcotic injections. Ahasuerus, Cinderella, and Albatross Syndromes are eponyms given to specific types of the Munchausen concept. In previous centuries the assumed maladies of such patients were designated as feigned complaints and morbus simulatus.[35]

The Munchausen Syndrome is considered to be one variety of imposture, other varieties being the great imposture syndrome, compulsive wanderers, literary imposture, transvestism, and imposture for gain.[36] In many cases, the behavior of impostors may originate from relationships with their mothers. The Munchausen Syndrome may have its origins in a mother who was both punishing and pleasing. It differs from hypochondriasis in which the patient is convinced he has a nonexistent disease, fears the disease, and is preoccupied with his body.[37]

In more common usage, munchausenism is a lie so outrageous as to be comical.[2] For example, in Conan Doyle's science fiction epic of 1912, *The Lost World*, Professor Challenger was called a "Professor Munchausen" because of his apparently outlandish stories of the existence of prehistoric animals on an isolated plateau in South America.[38]

A fitting statement of the Munchausen mystique is a verse by William Bean, the first lines being as follows.[39]

Baron Munchausen, a fabulous liar
The syndrome's eponym did inspire.
Richard Asher first used the name
For patients behaving much the same,
With strange warped minds and actions weird,
Vagrant gypsies, mentally queered.

1. Durham, pp. 376–377.
2. Asher, R.: Munchausen's syndrome: *Lancet*, 1: 339–341, 1951.
3. Espy, p. 132.

4. Chapman, J. S.: Peregrinating problem patients —Munchausen's syndrome: *J.A.M.A.*, 165:927–933, 1957.

5. Asher, R.: Malingering: *Trans. Med. Soc. Lond.*, 75:34–44, 1959.

6. Wright, M. R.: Surgical addiction. A complication of modern surgery: *Arch. Otolaryngol. Head Neck Surg.*, 112:870–872, 1986.

7. Shah, K. A. et al.: Munchausen's syndrome and cardiac catherization: *J.A.M.A.*, 248:3008–3009, 1982.

8. Paré, pp. 74–84.

9. (Raspe, R. E.): *The Adventures of Baron Munchausen*: New York, Grosset & Dunlap, n.d.

10. Ludwig, J. & Mann, R. J.: Munchhausen versus Munchausen: *Mayo Clin. Proc.*, 58:767–769, 1983.

11. *Encyclopaedia Britannica*: VII:99.

12. Rose, W.: Baron Munchausen: in *Men, Myths, and Movements* in *German Literature*, London, George Allen & Unwin, 1931, pp. 109–123.

13. Brugsch, H. G.: Munchhausen to Munchausen: *Ann. Int. Med.*, 86:833–834, 1977.

14. Golden, R. L.: Spelling of Munchausen: An "H" of a Mess: *J.A.M.A.*, 250:1975, 1983.

15. Hyler, S. E. & Sussman, N.: Chronic factitious disorder with physical symptoms (the Munchausen syndrome): *Psychiatr. Clin. North Am.*, 4:365–377, 1981.

16. Birch, C. A.: Munchausen's syndrome: *Lancet*, 1:412, 1951.

17. Armitage, G. H.: Munchausen's syndrome: *Lancet*, 1:743, 1951.

18. King, C. M. & Chalmers, R. J. G.: Another aspect of contrived disease: "Dermatitis simulata": *Cutis*, 34:463–464, 1984.

19. Batshaw, M. L. et al.: Munchausen's syndrome simulating torsion dystonia: *N. Engl. J. Med.*, 312:1437–1439, 1985.

20. Lang, A. E.: Munchausen's syndrome simulating torsion dystosia: *N. Engl. J. Med.*, 313:1088, 1985.

21. Lazar, R. B.: Munchausen syndrome presenting as acute spinal cord injury: *Arch. Phys. Med. Rehabil.*, 67:568–569, 1986.

22. Gawn, R. A. & Kauffmann, E. A.: Munchausen syndrome: *Br. Med. J.*, 1:1068, 1955.

23. Gawn, R. A. & Kauffmann, E. A.: Munchausen syndrome: *Br. Med. J.*, 1:1329–1330, 1955.

24. Meadow, R.: Munchausen syndrome by proxy. The hinterland of child abuse: *Lancet*, 1:343–345, 1977.

25. Warner, J. O. & Hathaway, M. J.: Allergic form of Meadow syndrome (Munchausen by proxy): *Arch. Dis. Child.*, 59:151–156, 1984.

26. Meadow, S. R.: Munchausen syndrome by proxy: in *Advanced Medicine*, A. Ferguson, Ed., Vol. 20, London, Pitman, 1984, pp. 243–252.

27. Amegavie, L. et al.: Munchausen's syndrome by proxy: A warning for health professionals: *Br. Med. J.*, 293:855–856, 1986.

28. McKinlay, I.: Munchausen's syndrome by proxy: *Br. Med. J.*, 293:1308, 1986.

29. Burman, D. & Stevens, D.: Munchausen family: *Lancet*, 2:456, 1977.
30. Strassburg, H. M. & Peuckert, W.: Not "Polle syndrome," please: *Lancet*, 1:166, 1984.
31. Meadow, R. & Lennert, T.: Munchausen by proxy or Polle syndrome?: *Pediatrics*, 74:554–556, 1984.
32. Bayliss, R. I. S.: The deceivers: *Br. Med. J.*, 288:583–584, 1984.
33. Shapira, J. D.: Munchausen's syndrome and the technologic imperative: *South. Med. J.*, 74:193–196, 1981.
34. Allegra, D. et al.: Munchausen as physician and patient: *Ann. Int. Med.*, 85:262–263, 1976.
35. Risse, G. B.: *Hospital Life in Enlightenment Scotland. Care and Teaching at the Royal Infirmary of Edinburgh*: Cambridge, England, Cambridge University Press, 1986, p. 168.
36. Wells, L. A.: Varieties of imposture: *Perspect. Biol. Med.*, 29:588–610, 1986.
37. Appleby, L.: Hypochondriasis: An acceptable diagnosis?: *Br. Med. J.*, 294:857, 1987.
38. Doyle, A. C.: *The Lost World*: London, Hodder & Stoughton, 1912.
39. Bean, W. B.: *Rarer Diseases and Lesions. Their Contributions to Clinical Medicine*: Springfield, Illinois, Charles C Thomas, 1967, p. 185.

Myth of Faust

Uriel has equated a theory of carcinogenesis to the Myth of Faust.[1] The theory states that cells can regress to a younger state which, if applied to the entire body, would constitute rejuvenation and immortality. However, the rejuvenated cells (Faust) are finally conquered by transformation into cancer cells (the devil) (see Faust Complex). The ability of mature cells to undergo retrodifferentiation (dedifferentiation) to a more immature form is contrary to long-held dogma that the differentiated state of mature cells is irreversible, but when exposed to carcinogenic agents can undergo transformation and altered growth characteristics.[2]

The basis for Uriel's converse proposal is that antigens found in tumors resemble those of fetal tissues, which are relatively undifferentiated; that the biological behavior of cancerous cells mimics those of developing cells; and that the simplified cytoplasmic organelles of cancer cells resemble those of immature cells.[1] "Cancer cells may thus be regarded as the myth of Faust on the cellular level, the cells' chimeric dream of rejuvenation and immortality, which, in the end, often turns into a fatal nightmare." The analogy is somewhat strained, as Faust sold his soul to the devil, not for immortality, but in exchange for knowledge, power, and Helen of Troy.[3]

1. Uriel, J.: Cancer, retrodifferentiation, and the myth of Faust: *Cancer Res.*, 36:4269–4275, 1976.
2. Robbins, S. L. et al.: *Pathologic Basis of Disease*: 3rd ed., Philadelphia, W. B. Saunders, 1984, p. 230.
3. Butler, E. M.: *The Fortunes of Faust*: Cambridge, England, Cambridge University Press, 1952.

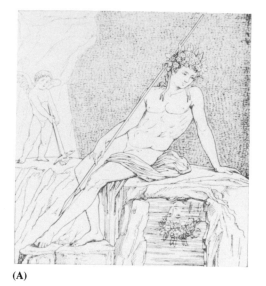

(A)

N

Narcissism

A superficial definition of narcissism is morbid self-admiration.[1] On a psychiatric level, it "denotes a personality disturbance characterized by an exaggerated investment in one's own

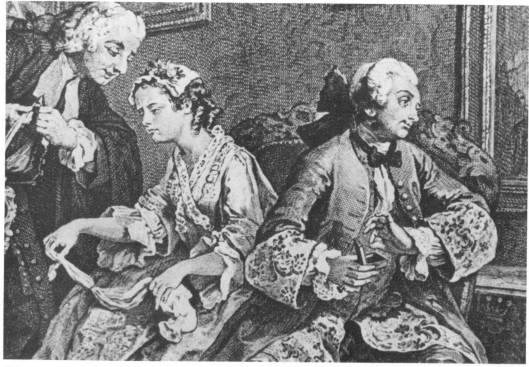

(B)

Narcissism **A.** Narcissus enraptured by his own image in the water.[6] **B.** A narcissistic groom enraptured by his own image in the mirror.[13] (by William Hogarth, 1745) (by permission, Dover Pubns., Inc.)

image at the expense of the self."[2] These individuals are more concerned with how they appear than with how they feel, and in essence deny their true self. For Freud, narcissism had a libidinal significance, with the sex object being internal instead of external.[3] It is an exaggeration of normal ego development which becomes predominant. Freud's orientation was developed in opposition to Adler's nonlibidinous concept of lack of social interest and "masculine protest" as major factors in neuroses.[4] The term narcissism has many different definitions and connotations, including selfish, self-centered, self-pity, self-esteem, self-continuity, and self-preservation (see Delilah Syndrome).[5]

Narcissus of Greek mythology was the son of the river god Cephissus, and the embodiment of self-conceit.[6] He fell in love with his own image reflected in the water of a river, to the extent of trying to talk to it and embrace it. He finally died of longing for his own image. His funeral pile disappeared. In its place a flower appeared, which bears his name. Narcissism as a psychological term was coined in the late 1890s, not by Freud but by Havelock Ellis to describe a specific sexual perversion.[7]

Lowen has extrapolated the concept of abnormal self-love to the cultural level. Narcissistic environments are those in which there is excessive concern for uniformity and material possessions to the detriment of quality and humaneness.[8] Under the phrase narcissism of the life cycle, Datan has suggested, from a review of fairy stories, that conflicts of interest between parents and children result in a narrow mindedness that leads to seeing one's present situation as more critical than any past or future problems.[9] Parents exhibit narcissism when they become overly involved in their child's achievements as a reflection of their own perfectionistic needs.[10] The phrase narcissistic attraction has been applied to a mutual attraction between two individuals who see themselves in each other, as suggested for Freud and his patient / student Marie Bonaparte.[11]

The narcissistic nature of essentially autobiographical films has also been elucidated.[12] Examples are films by such directors as Bob Fosse (*All That Jazz,*) Woody Allen (*Stardust*), and Fellini (*8 1/2*). These are interpreted as representation by the directors of narcissism expressed as mid-life crises and concern with death. Various forms of narcissism are depicted by various literary characters, as, for example, Albee's *Tiny Alice*, Sophocles's *Oedipus Rex*, and Giraudoux's *Judith*.[7]

1. Espy, p. 301.
2. Lowen, A.: *Narcissism. Denial of the True Self*: New York, Macmillan, 1983.
3. Freud, S.: "On Narcissism: An Introduction [1914]": *S.E.*, Vol. 14, pp. 73–102, 1975.
4. Ansbacher, H. L.: The significance of Alfred Adler for the concept of narcissism: *Am. J. Psychiatry*, 142:203–207, 1985.
5. Dyrud, J.: Narcissus and nemesis: *Psychiatry*, 46: 106–112, 1983.
6. Gayley, pp. 188–189.
7. Glenn, J.: Forms of narcissism in literary characters: *J. Clin. Psychiatry*, 5:239–258, 1983.
8. Bulger, R. J.: Narcissus, Pogo and Lew Thomas' Wager: *J.A.M.A.*, 245:1450–1454, 1981.
9. Datan, N.: The narcissism of the life cycle. The dialectics of fairy tales: *Human Devel.*, 20:191–199, 1977.
10. Harvey, J. C. & Katz, C.: *If I'm So Successful, Why Do I Feel Like a Fake? The Impostor Phenomenon*: New York, St. Martin's Press, 1984, pp. 157–159.
11. Freeman, L. & Strean, H. S.: *Freud and Women*: New York, Frederick Ungar, 1981, p. 93.
12. Gabbard, G. O. & Gabbard, K.: Vicissitudes of narcissism in the cinematic autobiography: *Psychoanal. Rev.*, 7:319–328, 1984.
13. Hogarth, W.: "Marriage-a-La-Mode": in *Engravings by Hogarth*, New York, Dover, 1973, plate 51.

Nemesis Feeling

An individual may have an all-prevading feeling that he or she is destined to repeat the same pattern of life as that of another, usually a father or mother, with tragic results, such as early death or psychosis.[1] The Nemesis Feeling arises from strong guilt feelings which are related to the death or psychosis of a parent during the patient's childhood. A related nemesis is the psychiatric breakdown that may occur when an individual reaches the age of death of his or her parent.[2] Nemesis was the avenging goddess of Greek mythology. She represents the righteous anger of the gods, especially toward the proud and insolent.[3] A current usage of the word nemesis is for any agent or act or retribution or punishment.[4] The Nemesis Feeling, in this sense, is the psychological punishment of the self by guilt feelings for supposed harm done to parents in particular. Unlike this all-prevading feeling is the "talion fear" of retribution related to a single act, such as an eye for an eye.[1]

The term nemesis has been evoked for other medically related conditions or situations in the sense of contributing to a downfall. Thus, exertional heat stroke is considered as the nemesis of a runner;[5] dysmenorrhea and premenstrual tension as that of women;[6] headache as that of industry;[7] inappropriate secretion of antidiuretic hormone as that of accurate treatment and management;[8] the existing concepts and treatment of drug abuse as that of psychiatry;[9,10] and legal need for evidence as that of psychotherapist confidentiality.[11]

Nemesis has also been invoked for the danger of dealing with narcissism on a superficial basis.[12] More recently, tuberculosis has been called an old nemesis because of its increase in incidence in patients with the acquired immune deficiency syndrome.[13]

1. Chapman, A. H.: The concept of nemesis in psychoneurosis: *J. Nervous Mental Dis.*, 129:29–34, 1959.
2. Birtchnell, J.: In search of correspondences between age at psychiatric breakdown and parental age at death—'Anniversary reactions': *Br. J. Med. Psychol.*, 54:111–120, 1981.
3. Bulfinch, p. 13.
4. Stein, p. 957.
5. Hart, L. E. et al.: Exertional heat stroke: the runner's nemesis: *Can. Med. Assoc. J.*, 122:1144–1150, 1980.
6. Dingfelder, J. R.: Prostaglandin inhibitors. New treatment for an old nemesis: *N. Engl. J. Med.*, 307:746–747, 1982.
7. Diamond, S. & Baltes, B. J.: Headache—An industrial nemesis: *Indust. Med. Surg.*, 36:585–587, 1967.
8. Snively, W. D. Jr. & Helmer, R.: Syndrome of inappropriate secretion of antidiuretic hormone (SIADH): Nemesis for the unwary: *J. Indiana State Med. Assoc.*, 74:514–518, 1981.
9. Wurmser, L.: Drug abuse: Nemesis of psychiatry: *Int. J. Psychiatry*, 10:94–107, 1972.
10. Dumont, M. P.: Comments on "drug abuse: Nemesis of psychiatry": *Int. J. Psychiatry*, 10:108–112, 1972.
11. Greenlaw, J.: Confidentiality—The psychotherapist's nemesis: *Nursing Law Ethics*, 1:7–8, 1980.
12. Dyrud, J.: Narcissus and nemesis: *Psychiatry*, 46:106–112, 1973.
13. Raymond, C. A.: Increase in AIDS—associated illness focuses new attention on an old nemesis: *J.A.M.A.*, 256:3323–3324, 1986.

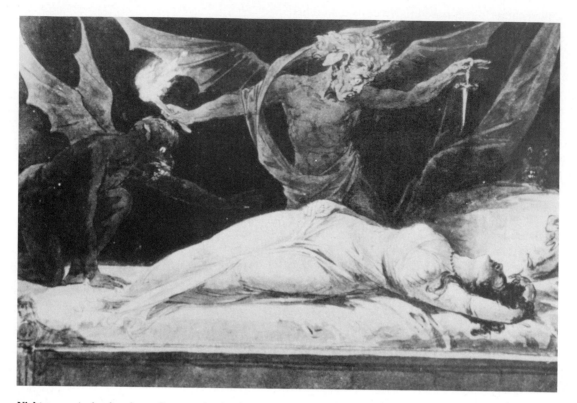

Nightmare An incubus descending on a sleeping female. (by Heinrich Fuseli, 1781)

Nightmare

(incubus, pavor nocturnus)

Nightmares are known to some as terrifying dreams accompanied by feelings of acute anxiety, terror, and helplessness.[1] The individual awakens with physical manifestations of an acute anxiety attack, including perspiration, heavy breathing, dilated pupils, and a facial expression of terror.[2] The nightmare is considered to be related to significant psychopathology, and may be associated with insomnia and somnambulism. There may be a familial association.

In the Middle Ages, "bad" dreams were attributed to demons, whose names were similar in various countries.[3] Examples include mare (Anglosaxon and Dutch), mahr (German), mara (Old Norse), and mora (Polish).[4] In Indian mythology, Mara is a Buddhist demon who was defeated by Bodhisattva, the future Buddha, even after Mara released a horde of horrible creatures who uttered inhuman cries and spread darkness.[5] Mara, along with his army of hideous demons and his seductive daughters, is identified as the enemy of the soul, endeavoring to damn it.[6] It is an integral part of Buddhism throughout Asia.[7] Night (Nox), in Greek mythology, was the sister of Erebus, born of Chaos, and in turn giving birth to Aether, Hemera (day), and also the Fates.[8]

Incubus is another term used for nightmare,[9] derived from the Latin, incubito (tum), to lie upon. An incubus is a legendary male demon, or evil spirit, who descends upon women during their sleep and has sexual intercourse with them.[10,11] A succubus is the female counterpart, who lies with men during their sleep. The term has also been used for a strumpet. As an incubus cannot produce semen, he obtains it from that deposited by a man in a succubus. These words are derived from late Latin words for nightmare.[4] In common usage, the incubus is a person or thing that oppresses or burdens like a nightmare.[12] Thus, medical malpractice suits have been considered as "an incubus upon the profession."[13]

Ambroise Paré wrote in 1573 that "such cohabitation (with incubi and succubi) is not done just while sleeping, but also while awake, which sorcerers and sorceresses have confessed and maintained several times, when they were being put to death."[14] In a later chapter, he defines the word incubus as a sickness manifested at night, and caused "most often from having drunk and eaten much too vaporous viands which have caused an indigestion, from which great vapors have arisen in the brain which fill one's ventricles . . . from which an imaginary suffocation arises, . . ."

Modern occultists consider nightmares to be occult attacks on the astral body by an evil spirit, but do not use the medieval terms.[15]

1. Stein, p. 966.
2. Kolb, p. 705.
3. Shipley, J. T.: *Dictionary of Word Origins*: New York, Philosophical Library, 1945, p. 225.
4. Weekley, p. 985.
5. Guirand, 1968, p. 352.
6. Bhattacharya, S.: *The Indian Theology. A Comparative Study of Indian Mythology from the Vedas to the Puranas*: Calcutta, Firma KLM Private Ltd., 1978, pp. 106–107.

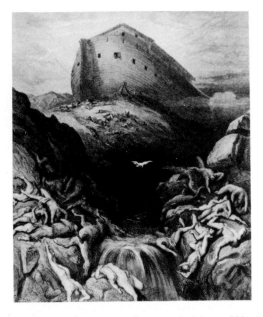

Noah Urge Noah's ark during the end of the world by flood.[1] (by Gustav Doré, 1866) (by permission, Dover Pubns., Inc.)

7. Hackin, J. et al.: *Asiatic Mythology. A Detailed Description and Explanation of the Mythology of All the Great Nations of Asia*: New York, Crescent Books, n.d., pp. 75, 206, 242.
8. Guirand, 1964, pp. 11, 13.
9. Stein, p. 722.
10. Espy, p. 225.
11. Fuseli, J. H.: The Dreams of Eleanor: in Powell, N. and Fuseli, J. H.: *The Nightmare*, New York, Viking Press, 1972, frontispiece.
12. Babcock, P., Ed.: *Webster's Third New International Dictionary*: Springfield, Massachusetts, Merriam-Webster, 1986, p. 1146.
13. King, L. S.: Medicine 100 years ago II. The doctor and the law: *J.A.M.A.*, 257:2204, 1987.
14. Paré, pp. 91–92, 105.
15. Walker, pp. 194–195.

Noah Urge

The Noah Urge has been defined by Rubinsky and Wiseman as "the desire to predict the End [of the world], to be right, and in so doing, to escape that End."[1] The believers do not recant when their prophecy fails, but exhibit an even greater intensity of conviction. Such continued fervor in the face of undeniable disconfrontation of a belief occurs when the belief is specific and the believer has social support.[2] A specific example of the Noah Urge is the attempted assassination of George III by Hatfield, who thought that the world was coming to an end, and that this act would hasten his own suicidal desires.[3]

Noah was about 500 years old when God warned him that He would send a flood to destroy all mankind.[4] "And the LORD saw that the wickedness of man was great in the earth. . . . And the LORD said, 'I will blot out man whom I have created from the face of the earth; ' . . . But Noah found grace in the eyes of the Lord." Thus was the ark built and a pair of every living creature saved, although mankind did not heed Noah's warning (and still does not in many ways). Perhaps nuclear bomb shelters are today's equivalent of Noah's ark.

There have been many predictions of the destruction of the world from biblical days to the present. Included have been flood, fire, cosmic bodies, earthquakes, and nuclear explosions—attributed by some to the wrath of God, to the Antichrist, or to science running wild (see Frankenstein eponyms). A universal flood is part of the tradition of many cultures and religions.[5]

A related eponym is Noah's New Flood, which has been invoked for the exponentially increasing world population.[6] Like the biblical flood, there is great danger that the lack of food, work, and law and order will lead, if not to the end of the world, at least to the end of the world as we know it.

Noah has been considered as the first example of a genetic condition, albinism.[7] An albino has very pale skin, white hair, and pink eyes.[8] According to the apocalyptic book of Enoch the Prophet, "His [Noah's] colour was whiter than snow: he is redder than the rose: the hair of his head is whiter than white wool: his eyes are like the rays of the sun. . . ."[9] There is no evidence, however, that he suffered from the photophobia which frequently accompanies the condition because of absence of protective pigment in the eye. If Noah was indeed an albino, then his father, Methuselah, or his mother was the first known carrier of this condition.[7]

1. Rubinsky, Y. & Wiseman, I.: *A History of the End of the World*: New York, William Morrow, 1982, p. 129.
2. Festinger, L. et al.: *When Prophecy Fails*: Minneapolis, University Minnesota Press, 1956.
3. Skultans, V.: *English Madness: Ideas on Insanity 1580–1890*: London, Routledge & Kegan Paul, 1979, p. 5.
4. OT: Genesis 6:5–8.
5. LaHaye, T. F. & Morris, J. D.: *The Ark on Ararat*: New York, Thomas Nelson, 1976.
6. Fox, T.: The multiplication of man or Noah's new flood: *Lancet*, 2:1238–1244, 1966.
7. Sorsby, A.: Noah—An albino: *Br. Med. J.*, 2:1587–1589, 1958.
8. Thomas, p. 52.
9. *The Book of Enoch the Prophet*: R. Laurence translator, 3rd ed., Oxford, J. H. Parker, 1838.
10. Doré, G: *Doré's Bible Illustrated*: New York, 1974, p. 8.

Nymphomania

The eponym Nymphomania is used for females with an uncontrollable, pathological desire for coitus.[1] The activity is not associated with sexual gratification or relief of tension. These patients have been described as narcissistic.

The nymphs of Greek mythology were daughters of Zeus and the sky, born from the springs caused by rains sent by the sky.[2] They served as female divinities of nature, providing fertilizing power. The nymphs were in love with not only the gods but also with mortals. Unions

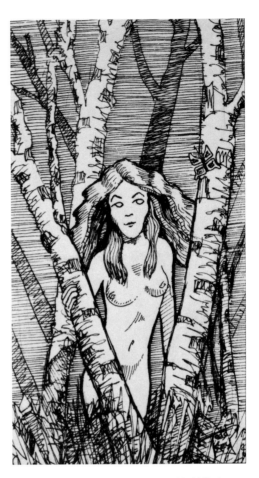

Nymphomania   A Wood Nymph (by Todd Key)

with the latter gave rise to demigods, the ancestors of the first human races.

The term nymphet (little nymph) designates a sexually attractive and alluring female in her early teens,[3] using Lolita, the young girl in the novel of the same name as the prototype (see Lolita Syndrome).[4] Her amorous activities were not sought out by her, although not resisted when offered. Different is the elation experienced by women during the first weeks of World War II which resulted in some going sexually berserk, the so-called war Nymphomania.[5] Androgens given therapeutically have been found to greatly increase the sex drive in both females and males (see Aphrodisiac).[6]

The two folds at the upper end of the labia minora of the female genitalia were called nymphes in the sixteenth century.[7] The term nymphs was once used for the clitoris. The Don Juan Syndrome and Satyriasis are the male equivalents of nymphomania.

1. Freedman, p. 1507.
2. Schmidt, pp. 193–194.
3. Espy, p. 225.
4. Nabokov, V.: *Lolita*: New York, Olympia Press, 1955.
5. Kern, S.: *Anatomy and Destiny. A Cultural History of the Human Body*: Indianapolis, Bobbs-Merrill, 1975, p. 200.
6. Greenblatt, R. B. et al.: Endocrinology of sexual behavior: *Med. Aspects of Hum. Sex. Behav.*, 6:119–131, 1972.
7. Paré, p. 188.

O

Oblomov Syndrome

(Oblomov sign, Oblomovism)

A special type of abulic and unstable psychopathy was first described under the term oblomovism in 1965.[1] It differs from other varieties in having a mania for remaining permanently in bed and being parasitic on society. These individuals usually have had a sadistical-masochistical symbiosis with their father or husband. In 1975, Wermut suggested the eponym Oblomov Syndrome, and related it to a passive depression.[2]

Oblomov[3] is the title of an 1859 Russian novel by Ivan Alexandrovich Goncharov, a prominent novelist in nineteenth century Russia.[4] Ilya Ilyich Oblomov, at the age of about 32, committed a small blunder at work and was sent home with a medical statement that he had lipomatosis of the heart, dilatation of the left ventricle, and hepatitis. He then spent the rest of his life at home, lying on a sofa until his death several years later following a left hemiplegia. "One morning there was lying in bed a gentleman named Ilya Ilyich Oblomov. . . . The prevailing lethargy was all consuming, all conquering—a true image of death . . . . from his eyes ennui peered forth like a disease." Perhaps Oblomov suffered from the chronic fatigue syndrome (see Raggedy Ann Syndrome).

The term oblomovism was used in nineteenth century Russia as a universal symbol of man's "propensity towards the line of least resistance, indolence, passivity and those daydreams which he cultivates in order to support his own sloth and comfort with a clear conscience."[4] Oblomov's behavior would now be characterized as an inadequate personality.[5]

1. Dietrich, H. von: Ein Besonderer Typ Willensschwacher Psycopathen (Oblomowisten): *Med. Wochenschr.*, 45:2225–2229, 1965.
2. Wermut, W.: "Oblomov syndrome"? (Oblomov sign): *J.A.M.A.*, 231:26, 1975.
3. Goncharov, I. A.: *Oblomov*: C. J. Hogarth translator, New York, Macmillan, 1915.
4. Lavrin, J.: *Goncharov*: New York, Russell & Russell, 1954.
5. Stone, A. A. & Stone, S. S.: *The Abnormal Personality Through Literature*: Englewood Cliffs, New Jersey, Prentice-Hall, 1966, p. 227.

Oedipus Complex

The Oedipus Complex was so-named and delineated by Freud.[1] "He [a son] begins to desire his mother herself . . . and to hate his father anew as a rival who stands in the way of this wish. He does not forgive his mother for having granted the favor of sexual intercourse not to himself but to his father, and he regards it as an act of unfaithfulness." The basis for this complex, according to Freud, is the discovery by the young boy that his parents engage in sexual intercourse. This "awakened memory-traces of the impressions and wishes of his early infancy."

In Greek mythology, Oedipus was rejected as an infant by his father, Laius, because of a warning from the Sphinx. He was then adopted and had no knowledge of his true parents.[2] As a young man he learned from an oracle that he was destined to kill his father, and therefore left his adopted father, Polybus. While driving on a narrow road he met Laius, his true but unknown father in another chariot. Oedipus slew Laius during an argument over the right of way. When he arrived in Thebes, Oedipus was challenged by the monstrous Sphinx to solve her riddle. "Tell me, what animal is that which has four feet at morning bright, two at noon, and three at night?" The Sphinx reacted in despair to Oedipus's correct answer, i.e., man, and killed herself. In gratitude for their deliverance, the Thebans made Oedipus their king. He then married Queen Jocasta, the widow of his father, Laius. Therefore Oedipus had married his own mother.

Oedipus remained unaware of his true relationship to Laius and Jocasta until many years later when his crimes of patricide and incest came to light through an oracle. When he discovered Jocasta's true identity the effects were devastating. In Gidé's play, Oedipus bewails, "This king whom I killed, tell me—No, don't speak. I see it all. I was his son . . . . And for me, who congratulated myself on not knowing my parents! Thanks to which I married my mother—alas! alas!"[3]

Freud referred to the Oedipus Complex frequently in his works, and gave it considerable importance in his psychoanalytic theories.[4] Thus, "the same complex constitutes the nucleus of all neuroses, as far as our present knowledge goes."[5] "The original animal sacrifice was already a substitute for a human sacrifice—for the ceremonial killing of the father; so that, when the father-surrogate once more resumed its human shape, the animal sacrifice too could be changed back into a human sacrifice."[6] He proposed an even broader significance to the Oedipus legend. "I should like to insist that its outcome shows that the beginnings of religion, morals, society and art converge in the Oedipus complex."[5]

Oedipus is the most widely known complex in our society today. Other literary eponyms which have implications derived from his saga are the syndromes of Don Juan and Othello; and the complexes of Cain, Clytemnestra, Electra, Griselda, Hamlet-Gertrude, Jocasta, Joseph, Moses, Orestes, Peter Pan and Wendy, Phaedra, and Ulysses.

There has been, however, some rejection of the universality of Freud's Oedipus Complex as an abnormal state. There is more emphasis on it as a normal transitory developmental phase which is usually replaced by the identification of the boy with his father's standards and goals.[7] The complex has also been placed in the context of all intrafamily relationships—". . . if society is to go on, daughters must be disloyal to their parents and sons must destroy (replace) their fathers."[8] Greek mythology contains several examples of the father/daughter variant of such familial difficulties, including Antigone (the daughter of Oedipus and Jocasta), and Electra (the daughter of Clytemnestra.[9] Of interest is that Freud identified his youngest daughter Anna with Antigone, referring to "my faithful Anna-Antigone."[10]

Literature has been pervaded by the Oedipus Complex, with various interpretations,[11] including the supposition that Oedipus was not the son of Laius and Jocasta,[12] with the exposition of related ramifications and implications. In Sophocles' play, *Oedipus Rex*,[13] Oedipus puts out his own eyes and wishes he was also deaf, presumably in the desire to return to the time before birth when he was guiltless.[14] Some of the works of Franz Kafka are considered to reflect his hostility toward his father.[15] The Oedipus Complex has been applied to Paul Morel, one of the sons in D. H. Lawrence's *Sons and Lovers*[16] in attributing his sexual difficulties to his maternal relationship.[17] There is, however, some objection to attributing such psychoanalytic motivation to Lawrence.[18]

The conflict between Coriolanus and his mother, Volumina, in Shakespeare's *The Tragedy of Coriolanus*, and its tragic outcome have been considered as an Oedipal mother-son relationship.[19] Both Shakespeare's Coriolanus and Sophocles' Ajax are considered to be individuals who have never fought out their Oedipal battles with their passive, defeated fathers. They project a hypermasculine defense reaction in response to intense identification with their domineering mothers.[20] Its role in the development of the superego has been called "the heir of the Oedipus Complex."[21]

Freud propounded a variant of his famous complex, the Inverted Oedipus Complex.[10] This refers to a boy with strong incestuous feelings toward his mother, but who is afraid to compete with his father. The result is a strong negative reaction to women and the idolization of men. Freud himself appeared to be oriented to the superiority of men. In some instances, a very strong mother fixation may result in homosexuality. In the adult, guilt feelings arising from being successful may originate from unresolved Oedipal wishes for incestuous desires toward the opposite-sex parent, success in one activity being equated subconsciously with the desire for success in the other.[22]

Diel posits a more drastic outcome for the neurotic with an Oedipus Complex.[23] "Tyrannized by excessive severity or love on the part of his parents, the child in turn becomes tyrannical towards them when they become the mutilators of his soul through their capricious and unjust demands. The man who has been maimed in this way in his childhood will ultimately be tyrannical towards the whole world: . . . ."

The Oedipus Complex is quite prominent in our current society. A comprehensive book has been published on the *Oedipus Myth and Complex*.[24] In 1984, there was a newspaper report of "A construction worker who claims he unwittingly married his mother [and] is negotiating a movie deal with a television production firm, his mother says."[25] A more trivial example of the application of the Oedipus complex is found in a commentary on Conan Doyle's novel *The Sign of the Four*. The collapse of Watson's wife-to-be, Mary Morstan, whenever the death of her father was mentioned, has been attributed to the Oedipus Complex,[26] — using the eponym inappropriately for the related Electra Complex, which is the desire of a girl for her father.

The concept of the Oedipus Complex has also been applied to the Finnish national epic poem, the Kalevala,[27] a poetic name for Finland meaning Land of the Heroes.[28] It was first compiled from folklore material in 1835.[29] The four heroes of this epic sought the Sampo, a mythical talisman that could bring happiness. The search for this charm has been equated psychoanalytically with the Oedipus Complex in two contexts.[27] First, the search for the Sampo represents the struggles of the adolescent "to free his own sexual body from the hegemony of his mother." Second, the Oedipal Complex is also symbolized in the struggle of a nation (son) to free itself from its rulers (mother).

1. Freud, S.: *S.E.*, Vol. IX, pp. 170–172.
2. Bulfinch, pp. 152–155.
3. Gidé, A.: *Two Legends: Oedipus and Thereus*: J. Russel translator, New York, Vintage Books, 1950.
4. Niederland, W. G.: The first application of psychoanalysis to a literary work: *Psychoanal. Qt.*, 29:228–235, 1960.
5. Freud, S.: *S.E.* Vol. 13, pp. 156–157.
6. Freud, S.: *S.E.* V.13, p. 151.
7. Kolb, pp. 72–73.
8. Leach, E.: *Claude Lévi-Strause*: New York, Viking Press, 1970, p. 83.
9. Wilner, D.: The Oedipus complex, Antigone

and Electra: The woman as hero and victim: *Am. Anthrop.*, 84:58–78, 1982.

10. Freeman, L. & Strean, H. S.: *Freud and Women*: New York, Frederick Ungar, 1981, pp. 52, 73, 82, 191.

11. Kanzer, M.: Oedipus: History, legends, plays, complexes: *Psychoanal. Psychother.*, 7:326–332, 1978–79.

12. Garma, A.: Oedipus was not the son of Laius and Jocasta: *Psychoanal. Psychother.*, 7:316–325, 1978–79.

13. Sophocles: "Oedipus The King": in *Plays of the Greek Dramatists*: G. Young translator, Chicago, Puritan Publishing, n.d.

14. Clair, M. St.: A note on the guilt of Oedipus: *Psychoanal. Rev.*, 48:111–114, 1961.

15. Probinsky, J.: The Oedipus complex or hey, mom, where is daddy?: *Int. J. Soc. Psychiatry*, 25:63–70, 1979.

16. Lawrence, D. H.: *Sons and Lovers*: New York, Modern Library, 1922.

17. Kern, S.: *Anatomy and Destiny*: Indianapolis, Bobbs-Merrill, 1975, pp. 185–187.

18. Macy, J.: Introduction: in *Sons and Lovers*, D. H. Lawrence, New York, Modern Library, 1922, p. VIII.

19. Putney, R.: Coriolanus and his mother: *Psychoanal. Q.*, 31:364–381, 1962.

20. Seidenberg, R.: For this woman's sake. Notes on the 'mother' superego with reflections on Shakespeare's *Coriolanus* and Sophocles' *Ajax*: *Int. J. Psychoanal.*, 44:74–82, 1963.

21. Campbell, pp. 609–610.

22. Harvey, J. C. & Katz, C.: *If I'm So Successful, Why Do I Feel Like a Fake. The Impostor Phenomenon*: New York, St. Martin's Press, 1984, pp. 163–166.

23. Diel, pp. 140–141.

24. Mullahy, P.: *Oedipus Myth and Complex. A Review of Psychoanalytic Theory*: New York, Hermitage Press, 1948.

25. *Dayton Journal Herald*, Sept. 14, 1984, p. 1.

26. Hunt, T. B. & Starr, H. W.: What Happened to Mary Marston: quoted in W. S. Barring-Gould, *The Annotated Sherlock Holmes*, Vol. 1, New York, Clarkson N. Potter, 1967, p. 626, note 32.

27. Hagglund, T. B.: The forging of the Sampo and its capture: The Oedipous complex of adolescence in Finnish folklore: *Scand. Psychoanal. Rev.*, 8:159–180, 1985.

28. *Encyclopaedia Britannica*: V:668.

29. Guirand 1968, pp. 299–300.

Old Sergeant Syndrome

(burnout, neurotic battle behavior)

A burnt-out state may occur in previously well-motivated and efficient soldiers after long periods of combat duty.[1] There is a personality change characterized by loss of self-esteem, dyspepsia, anxiety, tremulousness, depression, uncontrollable weeping, and rage reactions. Re-

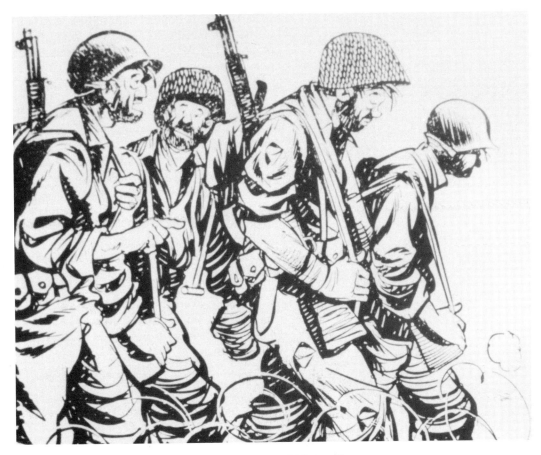

Old Sergeant Syndrome   Burnt out G.I.'s in France during WW II.[4, p. 143]

lated is the Da Costa syndrome, applied to World War I soldiers who developed fatigue, precordial pain, dyspnea, and palpitations, usually precipitated by emotional or physical strain.[2] This was first described as an irritable heart by Da Costa in 1871.[3]

The exhausted soldier is a common figure in folklore, being well depicted in cartoons by Bill Mauldin.[4] Such sergeants are featured in movie films such as *A Walk in the Sun* (1946). Considerable attention has recently been given to burnout of health care delivery professionals with major and critical responsibilities.[5] These individuals are initially highly competent and aggressive in respect to their work, but consequently suffer in their relationships with spouse and family. The three major components of burnout are emotional exhaustion, depersonalization of patients, and low productivity with feelings of low achievement.[6] These reactions to work stress lead to seeking even more work satisfaction to meet their high self-expectations and need for approval. The end result is an emotional breakdown and occasionally drug and alcohol dependence.

Burnout is a significant problem in neonatal intensive care units in which there are many major stresses: death of infants, ethical dilemmas, emotional reactions of parents, and the need to learn ever-increasingly complex technology.[7] The result is loss of motivation for creative involvement, depression, decreased energy, and questioning the value of one's efforts. This may be expressed as emotional or physical detachment, or as compensatory over-involvement as described above. Affected are physicians as well as nurses working in neonatal units. The results of a questionnaire sent to the former group revealed that 50% experienced moderate to severe stress and 20% suffered a stress-related illness in the prior five years.[8] One of the causes of stress was dealing with infant death.

1. Sobel, R.: The "old sergeant" syndrome: *Psychiatry*, 10:315–320, 1947.
2. Jablonski, S.: *Illustrated Dictionary of Eponymic Syndromes and Diseases and Their Synonyms*: Philadelphia, W. B. Saunders, 1969, p. 74.
3. Da Costa, J. M.: On irritable heart; A clinical study of a form of functional cardiac disorder and its consequences: *Am. J. Med. Sci.*, 61:17–32, 1871.
4. Mauldin, B.: *Up Front*: New York, Henry Holt, 1945.
5. Hall, R. C. et al.: The professional burnout syndrome: *Psychiatr. Opin.*: 16:12–17, 1979.
6. Mayou, R.: Burnout: *Br. Med. J.*, 295:284–285, 1987.
7. Marshall, R. E. & Kasman, C.: Burnout in the neonatal intensive case unit: *Pediatrics*, 65:1161–1165, 1980.
8. Clarke, T. A. et al.: Job satisfaction and stress among neonatologists: *Pediatrics*, 74:52–57, 1984.

Onanism

(Onan's act, Onania)

Onanism is defined variously as masturbation[1] or coitus interruptus.[2] The source is Genesis in which Judah indicated to his son, Onan, that he should have intercourse with Tamar, the wife of Onan's brother Er, who had been slain by the Lord for his wickedness.[3] "And Judah said unto Onan: 'Go in unto thy brother's wife, and perform the duty of a husband's brother unto her, and raise up seed to thy brother.' And Onan knew that the seed would not be his; and it came to pass when he went in unto his brother's wife, he spilled it unto the ground, lest he should give seed to his brother." Levirate marriage (by a man with his brother's widow)[4] was a requirement in the time of the Old Testament if the dead brother had been childless.[5] Because Onan did not comply, he was slain by the Lord, as had been his brother, Er.

It is not certain why Onan was slain by the Lord for what the rabbis call "threshing within and winnowing without," as this was not punishable by death.[6] In the sixteenth century, Paré opined that the seed (sperm) "if transported very little, or not at all, is immediately corrupted [and not suitable for reproduction] because the warmth and the spirit of the whole body is absent from it."[7] Freud considered the practice of coitus interruptus to result in anxiety neuroses in women.[8]

Onanism is more generally used to mean masturbation than coitus interruptus.[9] The biblical description is, however, undoubtedly that of the latter, Onan having first gone "in unto his brother's wife."[3] Even more inconsistent with the biblical account is the designation of masturbation by the female as female onanism.[10]

Puritic penile eruption due to masturbation in adult males has been labeled as frictional dermatitis of Onan.[11] During the nineteenth century, many so-called Onanist diseases were attributed to masturbation[12]—such as growth cessation, phimosis, epilepsy, and impotency.[13] More recently, masturbation was stated to be performed by men of feeble will and not dangerous, although "The loss of substance from frequent seminal ejaculations is also more or less weakening although the secretion from the prostrate plays a much greater part than the semen."[14]

An anticontraceptive book published in 1948 is called *The Cult of Onan*, and labels Onanism as the crime of self pollution.[15] The use of the term onanism for masturbation may have begun much earlier, in the eighteenth century.[16] Boswell, in a 1758 letter, asked Temple to buy him "the little pamphlet against Onania, a crime too little regarded. The title is curious. I should like to see it."[17] Both Rousseau and Ruskin admitted to masturbation.[18]

Mark Twain gave a very witty talk on Onanism to the Stomach Club in Paris in 1879.[19] He attributed related aphorisms to various historical figures. Homer: "Give me masturbation or give me death."; Queen Elizabeth: "It is the bulwark of virginity."; Cetewavo, the Zula: "A jerk in the hand is worth two in the bush."; Franklin: "Masturbation is the mother of invention." In another humorous vein, Dorothy Parker named her untidy canary Onan.[20] Old English phrases for masturbation are to mount a corporal and to fetch mettle (sperm).[21]

1. OED: VII:117.
2. Stein, p. 1005.
3. OT: Genesis 38:6–11.
4. Buttrick, G. A., Ed.: *The Interpreter's Dictionary of the Bible. An Illustrated Encyclopedia*: Vol. K–Q, New York, Abingdon Press, 1962, p. 602.
5. OT: Deuteronomy 25:5–10.
6. Brody, M.: Phylogenesis of sexual morality. Psychiatric exegesis on Onan and Samson: *N.Y. State J. Med.*, 1968:2510–2514, 1968.
7. Paré, pp. 92–93.
8. Freeman, L. & Strean, H. S.: *Freud and Women*: New York, Frederick Ungar, 1981, p. 205.
9. Waldman, G. D.: Onan's act: *J.A.M.A.*, 251:1026, 1984.
10. Kern, S.: *Anatomy and Destiny. A Cultural History of the Human Body*: Indianapolis, Bobbs-Merrill, 1975, p. 100.
11. Jorizzo, J. L. et al.: Frictional dermatitis of Onan: *J.A.M.A.*, 250:362, 1983.
12. Gilbert, A. N.: Doctor, patient, and onanist diseases in the nineteenth century: *J. Hist. Med. Allied Sci.*, 30:217–234, 1975.
13. Fishman, S.: The history of childhood sexuality: *J. Contemp. Hist.*, 17:269–283, 1982.
14. Forel, A. H. & Marshall, C. F.: *The Sexual Question. A Scientific, Psychological and Sociological Study*: Brooklyn, Physicians & Surgeons Book Co., 1926.
15. Manson, P.: *The Cult of Onan*: Glasgow, William MacLellan, 1948.
16. Ober, W. B.: Reuben's mandrakes: Infertility in the Bible: *Int. J. Gynecol. Pathol.*, 3:299–317, 1984.
17. Ober, chap. 1.
18. Johnson, W. S.: *Living in Sin. The Victorian Sexual Revolution*: Chicago, Nelson-Hall, 1979, p. 76.
19. Twain, M.: *Some Thoughts on the Science of Onanism or Mark Twain in Erection*: Privately Printed for the Trade, 1964.
20. Gordon, R.: *Great Medical Disasters*: New York, Dorset Press, 1983, p. 182.
21. Bloch, pp. 45–46.

Ondine's Curse

(central hypoventilation, Ondine's kiss, primary [idiopathic] alveolar hypoventilation)

The term Ondine's Curse was first applied in 1962 to three patients who experienced long periods of apnea even when awake, but who breathed on command.[1] This problem occurred during and after surgery involving the high cervical cord or brain stem.[2] Since 1962, Ondine's Curse has been used in the more general sense of primary (idiopathic) hypoventilation, assumed to be due to loss of chemoreceptor response of the central respiratory center.[3] It occurs most frequently in males between 20 and 60 years of age.

Several possible predisposing factors have been noted in some patients—a hypersensitivity to sedatives or hypnotic drugs given during surgery, an acute respiratory infection, a past history of encephalitis, neurosyphilis, and schizophrenia. Ondine's Curse has also been reported to occur after carotid endarterectomy.[4] One instance has been described in a three-and-one-half-year-old with signs of hypothalamic disease.[5] At least five newborns with idiopathic Ondine's Curse have been reported.[6–10] One was also afflicted with Hirshprung's disease and multiple neuroblastomas (neurocristopathy).[10]

The name Ondine was taken for this syndrome from the version of the German myth described in Giraudoux's 1939 play, *Ondine*.[11] Ondine was a water nymph who was jilted by her husband for a mortal woman. For punishment, she took away his autonomic functions, including that of breathing, so that he had to consciously remember in order to breathe.

Hans: Since you left me, Ondine, all the things my body once did by itself, it does now only by special order . . . A single moment of inattention, and I forget to breathe. He died, they will say, because it was a nuisance to breathe.

Hans did finally fall asleep and died.

There has been some negative reaction to Ondine's Curse as a diagnostic term. One objection is that there are other versions of the Ondine myth in which she does not afflict her husband by a curse,[12] although this should not negate its use based on one version. A some-

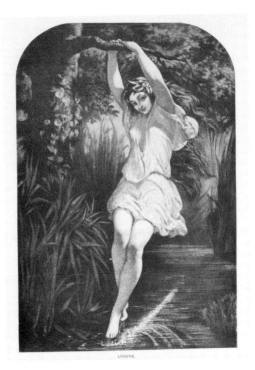

Ondine's Curse   The Bewitching Ondine.[18]

what more cogent objection is that Hans exhibited other effects of loss of autonomic function, such as disorders of his five senses and muscles, unlike patients with this syndrome.[13] Sleep apnea can occur in other conditions, such as the Shy-Drager syndrome, which is associated with generalized autonomic insufficiency and extrapyramidal derangement caused by a degenerative process of autonomic neurons.[14] However, the original description of Ondine's Curse was based on failure of automatic breathing even while awake.[1]

A suggestion has been made to change the eponym to Ondine's Kiss because in one version of the myth she killed her unfaithful husband by squeezing him to death during their farewell kiss.[15] Others have recommended that the eponym be discarded,[16] and even that "Scientists who introduce new terminology should, by law, be required to post a $1,000 bond, to be forfeited if the terminology is both misleading and used."[17]

1. Severinghaus, J. W. & Mitchell, R. A.: Ondine's curse—Failure of respiratory center automaticity while awake: *Clin. Res.*, 10:122, 1962.
2. Fielding, J. W. et al.: "Ondine's curse." A complication of upper cervical-spine surgery: *J. Bone Joint Surg.*, 57A:1000–1001, 1975.
3. West, J. B.: Disorders of ventilation: *Harrison's Principles of Internal Medicine*, R. G. Petersdorf et al., Eds., New York, McGraw-Hill, 1983, pp. 1589–1590.
4. Beamish, D. & Wildsmith, J. A. W.: Ondine's curse after carotid endarterectomy: *Br. Med. J.*, 2:1607–1608, 1978.
5. Fishman, L. S., Samson, J. H. & Sperling, D. R.: Primary alveolar hypoventilation syndrome (Ondine's curse): *Am. J. Dis. Child.*, 110:155–161, 1965.
6. Mellins, R. B. et al.: Failure of automatic control of ventilation (Ondine's curse). Report of an infant born with this syndrome and review of the literature: *Medicine*, 49:487–504, 1970.
7. Wells, H. H. et al.: Control of ventilation in Ondine's curse: *J. Pediatr.*, 96:865–867, 1980.
8. Coleman, M. et al.: Congenital central hypoventilation syndrome. A report of successful experience with bilateral diaphragmatic pacing: *Arch. Dis. Child.*, 55:901–903, 1980.
9. Taitz, L. S. & Redman, C. W. G.: Ondine's curse with recovery: Alveolar hypoventilation: *Proc. R. Soc. Med.*, 64:1222, 1971.
10. Bower, R. J. & Adkins, J. C.: Ondine's curse and neurocristopathy: *Clin. Pediatr.*, 19:665–668, 1980.
11. Giraudoux, J.: "Ondine": in *Jean Giraudoux. Four*

Plays, adapted, and with an Introduction by Maurice Valency: Vol. 1, New York, Hill & Wang, 1958.

12. Sugar, O.: In search of Ondine's curse: *J.A.M.A.*, 240:236–237, 1978.
13. Keelan, P.: Of Pickwick and Ondine: *Irish Med. J.*, 74:339–340, 1981.
14. Lehrman, K. L. et al.: Sleep apnea syndrome in a patient with Shy-Drager syndrome: *Arch. Int. Med.*, 138:206–209, 1978.
15. Topliss, D.: Ondine's kiss: *Lancet*, 2:147, 1980.
16. Vaisrub, S.: The kiss of death: *J.A.M.A.*, 245: 1152, 1981.
17. Comroe, J. H. Jr.: Frankenstein, Pickwick and Ondine: *Am. Rev. Respir. Dis.*, 111:689–692, 1975.
18. Brewer, 4:172.

Ophelia Complex

Death by drowning is a distinct type of suicide that is more common in females, especially in literary works.[1] The prime example of the complex is Ophelia, a character in Shakespeare's *Hamlet*.[2] She was the young and innocent daughter of Polonius, who obeyed her father's request to spurn Hamlet's advances. After Hamlet killed her father in error, she became mad, and "Fell into the weeping brook ... Till that her garments, heavy with their drink, / Pull'd the poor wench from her melodious lay / To muddy death."[3]

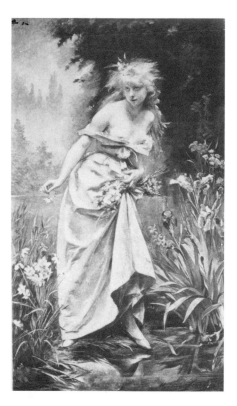

Ophelia Complex The Mad Ophelia.[10]

There is doubt as to whether Ophelia committed suicide or accidently fell into the brook from a "pendent bough."[3] The priest at her burial considered the cause of her death to be doubtful,[4] and this may have been the reason why she was buried in consecrated ground, but not accorded all the sacred rites.[5] In England, the coroner was often consulted by clergymen regarding the possibility of suicide.[6] Bachelard considers that "Water is the element of young and beautiful death, of flowery death, and in the dramas both of life and literature, it is the *element* of death with neither pride nor vengeance, of masochistic suicide."[1]

The Charon Complex is a related eponym which has been applied to the persistence in traditions and dreams of ancient myths of the relationship of death to a voyage in a boat over water.[1] Charon was the ferryman of Greek mythology who conveyed the shades of the dead across the rivers of the lower world.[7] The death by drowning of Shakespeare's Ophelia is one example of the persistence of this theme.[2]

More modern is the use of the sea as a symbol of death in the poetry of the poet-physician William Carlos Williams.[8]

1. Bachelard, G.: The Charon complex, the Ophelia complex: in *Water and Dreams*, E. R. Farrell translator, Zurich, Spring Publications, 1983, pp. 171–193.
2. Shakespeare, *Hamlet, Prince of Denmark*.
3. Shakespeare, *Hamlet*, IV,vii.
4. Shakespeare, *Hamlet* V,1.
5. Faber, M. D.: Ophelia's doubtful death: *Lit. Psychol.*, 16:103–108, 1966.
6. Adelson, L.: The coroner of Elsinore. Some medicolegal reflections on Hamlet: *N. Engl. J. Med.*, 262:229–234, 1960.
7. Bulfinch, pp. 328–330.
8. Breslin, J. E.: *William Carlos Williams. An American Artist*: Chicago, University of Chicago Press, 1985, p. 223.
9. Brewer, 4:126.

Ophelia Syndrome

Described has been the loss of recent memory in a patient with Hodgkin's disease, possibly related to metastases or a cancer associated demyelinating lesion of the limbic system of the brain.[1]

The daughter of the author had a severe loss of memory and hallucinations leading to a diagnosis of schizophrenia before Hodgkin's disease became evident.[1] Hodgkin's is a rare cause of this complication,[2] and even rarer is the successful therapy of her disease with return of memory. There is little concordance with Shakespeare's Ophelia, who died after becoming mad following the murder of her father, rather than due to a physical ailment (see Ophelia Complex).[3]

1. Carr, I.: The Ophelia syndrome: Memory loss in Hodgkin's disease: *Lancet*, 1:844–845, 1982.
2. Kaplan, H. S.: *Hodgkin's Disease*: Cambridge, Massachusetts, Harvard University Press, 1980.
3. Shakespeare, *Hamlet*: IV,iv, v.

Orestes Complex

(matricide)

The Orestes Complex is defined as the son's desire to kill his mother.[1] It may be the result of an Oedipus reaction, which can lead to feelings of frustration and rejection by one's mother.[2] This complex has been considered by some to be universal. It has also been suggested that excessive attachment to a mother can become directly transformed into violent hostility toward her.[3] These sons are usually quite young, with no past criminal records, very fond of their mothers, and with little interest in the female sex.

In Greek mythology, Orestes, the brother of Electra, killed his mother, Clytemnestra, and her paramour, Aegisthus, after Clytemnestra and Aegisthus had killed his father, Agamemnon.[4] He was then pursued by the Furies for his crime of matricide until his acquittal by the command of Minerva. The mythological story of Orestes is told in a drama by Aeschylus. Orestes says, "And still, while I have some self-control, / I say to my friends in public: I killed my mother, / not with a little justice. She was stained / with father's murder, she was cursed by god. / and the magic spells that fired up my daring?"[5]

The matricidal legend has existed since ancient times. More recently, it has been proposed that in Lewis Carroll's Jabberwocky poem,[6] the boy and the Jabberwocky which he killed represent son and mother (see Electra, Oedipus, and Clytemnestra Complexes).[7]

1. Campbell, p. 123.
2. Rubinstein, L. H.: The theme of Electra and Orestes: A contribution to the psychopathology of matricide: *Br. J. Med. Psychol.*, 42:99–108, 1969.
3. Wertham, F.: The matricidal impulse: Critique of Freud's interpretation of Hamlet: *J. Crim. Psychopathol.*, 2:455–464, 1941.
4. Gayley, pp. 315–317.
5. Aeschylus: "Orestes": in *The Oresteia*: R. Eagles translator, New York, Viking Press, 1975, p. 236.
6. Carroll, pp. 191–197.
7. Halpern, S.: The mother-killer: *Psychoanal. Rev.*, 52:71–74, 1965.

Orphan Annie Eyes

One of the morphological features of the fetal alcohol syndrome is shortened, more open palpebral fissures, giving the eyes a circular appearance.[1] Round, blank eyes are a feature of the cartoon character, "Little Orphan Annie," her dog Sandy, and her enormously wealthy stepfather, Daddy Warbucks.[2] This long-standing cartoon was created by Harold Gray, making its debut on August 5, 1924. After Gray's death in 1968, a succession of artists and writers continued the strip.

The relatively round eyes of the fetal alcohol

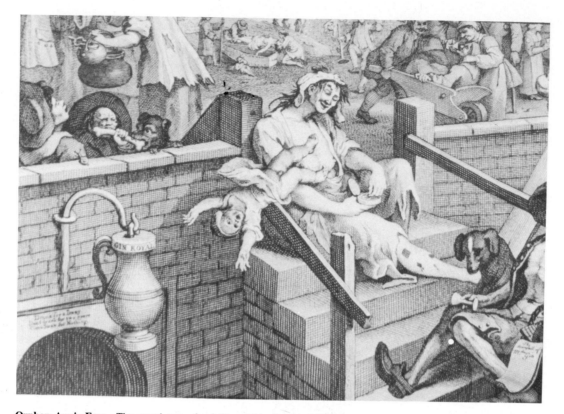

Orphan Annie Eyes The round eyes of a falling child of an alcoholic mother.[4, pl. 76] (by William Hogarth, 1751) (by permission, Dover Pubns., Inc.)

syndrome have only recently been described.[3] They are evident, however, in a satirical engraving, "Gin Lane," drawn by William Hogarth in 1751.[4] Depicted are various detrimental effects of gin, at that time the scourge of the lower classes in England. The most dominant figure in the engraving is that of an unkempt stupified woman whose unattended child is falling from her lap to his death. The child is depicted with round eyes, which are not a feature of other drawings by Hogarth.[1]

Other reported ophthalmic findings in the fetal alcohol syndrome are tortuosity of arteries and veins of the retina, optic nerve hypoplasia or atrophy, exotropia, blepharophimosis, and hypertelorism.[5] Less frequent are epicanthus (47%) and thickened brows (41%). Markedly widened palpebral fissures are also found in some children with positive serological tests for the AIDS virus subsequent to exposure to the virus as a fetus in utero.[6]

1. Rodin, A. E.: Infants and gin mania in 18th-century London: *J.A.M.A.*, 245:1237–1239, 1981.

2. Horn, M., Ed.: *The World Encyclopedia of Comics*: New York, Chelsea House, 1926 p. 459.
3. Jones, K. I. et al.: Pattern of malformation in offspring of chronic alcoholic mothers: *Lancet*, 1:1267–1271, 1973.
4. Shesgreen, S., Ed.: *Engravings by Hogarth. 101 Prints*: New York, Dover Pub., 1973, plate 76.
5. Rabinowicz, I. M.: New ophthalmic findings in fetal alcohol syndrome: (as reported by E. R. González in Medical News) *J.A.M.A.*, 245:108, 1981.
6. Marion, R. W.: Fetal AIDS syndrome score. Correlation between severity of dysmorphism and age at diagnosis of immunodeficiency: *Am. J. Dis. Child.*, 141:429–431, 1987.

Osiris

A journal titled *Osiris* is published in Belgium and devoted to the history of science, including medicine.[1] Volume 1 was published in 1936. The journal is available in English, French, or German. Osiris was the most beneficent of Egyptian gods.[2] He was identified with the life-giving powers of the sun and the waters of the Nile river. He was the son of Seb, and waged war against his brother Seth, who represented the principle of evil. Osiris was defeated by the latter, who cut him into small pieces. Osiris's wife, Isis, found and wrapped the pieces of his body to form the first mummy. He then became the judge of the underworld and the chief deity of the Egyptians. The re-formed Osiris was given the name of Onnophoris. He is usually depicted with two horns.

The use of the name Osiris for a scientific and medical journal can be justified on the basis that the Osiris myth was identified with life-giving qualities and is related to the course of human life and to life after death.

The Osiris story may also be the origin of the name of the bone below the last vertebra, the sacrum.[3] It is a Roman name derived from the Greek word for sacred or holy. In one version, when the pieces of Osiris's body were found a temple was set up to venerate each part. The sacral bone was especially important to ancient Egyptians, who considered it as sacred to Osiris, the god of resurrection, possibly because of its proximity to the generative organs.

1. *Index of NLM Serial Titles*.
2. Gayley, p. 554.
3. Sugar, O.: How the sacrum got its name: *J.A.M.A.*, 257:2061–2063, 1987.
4. Bulfinch, p. 367.

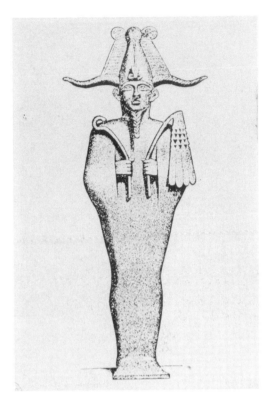

Osiris   Osiris, the Egyptian god.[4]

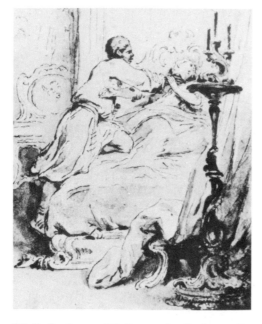

Othello Syndrome Othello strangling Desdemona.[11]

Othello Syndrome

(erotic jealousy syndrome,[2] morbid jealousy,[3] Othello psychosis[1])

The delusion of infidelity of a spouse is a dangerous type of paranoic psychosis.[1] It may appear in pure form, but more commonly during the course of paranoid schizophrenia, cyclophrenia, epilepsy, and the psychoses of senility and chronic alcoholism. Addiction to cocaine is an aggravating factor.[3] Such cases of sexual jealousy have a strong familial tendency, and there is frequently a marked difference in the sexuality of the married partners. It can occur in either sex. Consequences may include a disruptive effect on marriage, homicide, and suicide.[4] Narcohypnotic suggestion and sexual guidance have been recommended as therapy.[5]

In Shakespeare's play *Othello*, the Moor was craftily encouraged by Iago to become enraged over supposed infidelity of his wife, Desdemona, with Cassio.[6] The result was Othello's murder of Desdemona by smothering. His remorse resulted in his own suicide by his sword. ". . . then must you speak / Of one that loved not wisely but / too well; / Of one not easily jealous, but being wrought, / Perplex'd in the extreme; / of one whose hand / Like the base Indian, threw a pearl away / Richer than all his tribe; . . . ."

It has been suggested that Othello's murderous behavior originated as Oedipal conflicts.[7] Another extrapolation is that Othello's pleasure in war resulted from sublimation of self-destructive death wishes to the enemy; and when he was recalled from command in Cyprus, he turned to Desdemona as the enemy to protect himself from his own self-injuring impulses.[8] A severe case of paranoid jealousy is found in Eduardo Mallea's *The Heart's Reason*,[9] in which Montuvio finally convinces himself that the unfamiliar woman he saw with Bordiguera was actually his wife having a tryst.

The Othello Syndrome has also been evoked for the acceptance of a medical statement without checking it out properly.[10] Examples are blind acceptance of advertised "cures," acceptance without reservations by a junior staff member of a diagnosis made by a senior physician, and in 1726, the belief of the surgeon St. André that Mary Tufts had given birth to rabbits. Presumably the relationship to the tragedy of Othello is his implicit belief in Iago's slanderous statements about Desdemona.

1. Todd, J. & Dewhurst, K.: The Othello syndrome. A study in the psychopathology of sexual jealousy: *J. Nerv. Ment. Dis.*, 122:367–374, 1955.
2. Langfeldt, G.: Hypersensitive mind in normals, neurotics, psychopaths, psychotics; prevention and treatment: *Acta Psychiatr. Neurol. Scand.*, 26(suppl.73):3–147, 1951.
3. Shepherd, M.: Morbid jealousy. Some clinical and social aspects of a psychiatric syndrome: *J. Ment. Sci.*, 107:687–753, 1961.
4. Famuyiwa, O. O. & Ekpo, M.: The Othello syndrome: *J. Natl. Med. Assoc.*, 75:207–209, 1983.
5. Gajwani, A. K. et al.: The Othello syndrome: *Can. J Psychiatry*, 28:157–158, 1983.
6. Shakespeare, *Othello*: V,ii.
7. Reid, S.: Othello's jealousy: *Am. Imago*, 25:274–293, 1968.
8. Reid, S.: Othello's occupation: Beyond the pleasure principle: *Psychoanal. Rev.*, 63:555–570, 1976–77.
9. Malea, E.: *The Heart's Reason*: excerpted in Stone A. A. & Stone, S. S., *The Abnormal Personality Through Literature*, Englewood Cliffs Place, New Jersey, Prentice-Hall, 1966, p. 143.
10. The Othello syndrome: *N. Zeal. Med. J.*, 88:496, 1978.
11. Shakespeare, W.: *The Annotated Shakespeare*, A-L. Rowse, Ed., New York, Clarkson N. Potter, 1978, p. 332.

P

Pac-Man Phalanx

Intense pain and stiffness in the interphalangeal joint of the thumb have occurred while playing the Pac-Man video game.[1] This requires sustained hyperextension and flexion of the thumb. The symptoms subside after cessation of play. Pac-Man is one of the most popular of the video games, requiring frequent and rapid manipulation of images through a maze.[2]

Another joint disorder related to video games is Space-invaders Wrist.[3] This game requires many rapid flexions and extensions of the wrist with consequent ligamentous strain of the joint. The pathogenesis of photocopier thumb is similar.[4]

Another nonliterary eponym for yet another injury of the thumb is the gamekeeper's thumb, so-called because it has been described in British gamekeepers, but also may occur in skiers.[5] It is due to rupture of the ulnar collateral ligament of the metacarpophalangeal joint of the thumb, and is usually caused by falling on the abducted thumb.

1. Gibofsky, A.: Pac-Man phalanx: *Ann. Rheum.*, 26:120, 1983.
2. Uston, K.: *Mastering Pac-Man*: New York, New American Library, 1981.
3. McCowan, T. C.: Space-invaders wrist: *N. Engl. J. Med.*, 304:1368, 1981.
4. Rosner, F.: Pac-Man tendinitis: *Ann. Int. Med.*, 4:571, 1983.
5. Sternback, G. & Campbell, C.S.: Gamekeeper's thumb: *J. Emerg. Med.*, 1:345–347, 1984.

Pac-Man Tendinitis

Severe pain over the biceps muscle may occur after prolonged use of the Pac-Man game.

Play requires the gripping of a lever by the wrist and manipulation with considerable force.[1] The pain disappears several days after cessation of use. Related to Pac-Man tendinitis is slot-machine[2] and typist tendinitis.[1] Another medical danger of video games are the seizures that can be caused by flashing lights.[3] Examples are Dark Warrior epilepsy and Astro Fighter's epilepsy.

Joystick digit is another result of tendinitis from playing video games frequently and for long periods of time.[4] The condition consists of locked trigger fingers caused by the small computer joystick pressing directly against the flexor sheath of the finger. It is seen most frequently in boys ages 11 to 14 years.

1. Rosner, F.: Pac-Man tendinitis: *Ann. Int. Med.*, 4:571, 1983.
2. Neiman, T. C. & Ushiroda, S.: Slot-machine tendinitis: *N. Engl. J. Med.*, 304:1368, 1981.
3. Gordon, R.: *Great Medical Disasters*: London, Arrow Books, 1983, p. 107.
4. Osterman, L. A.: Joystick digit: *J.A.M.A.*, 257: 782, 1987.

Panacea

A panacea is a remedy or cure-all claimed to be curative of all diseases.[1] Panacea was one of three daughters of Aesculapius, the mythological father of medicine,[2] She healed all illnesses by use of herbs. The word panacea is used more generally for any solution of problems or difficulties.[1] In the field of medicine, Panacea has been invoked in conjunction with the phrase Pandora's Box, from which the ills of mankind were released when opened by Pandora (see Pandora's Box). The eponym is used to contrast benefits (Panacea's curative powers) versus ill effects of various treatments (the ills released from Pandora's Box). Thus, the third generation of cephalosporins are quite active against bacteria of the family Enterbacteriaceae (panacea), and yet not against enterococci, *Clostridia difficile*, and *Bastersides fragilis* bacteria (Pandora's Box), not to mention the expense of this antibiotic (Pandora's Box).[3]

Malpractice prescreening panels have been mandated in several states of the U.S.[4] These may reduce expensive and time-consuming professional liability actions by eliminating some claims early (panacea); but more cost and

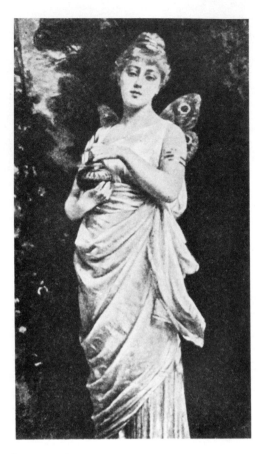

Pandora's Box Pandora holding her vase of mixed blessings.[6]

time may result because the parties involved can still resort to the courts, no matter what the findings of the prescreening boards (Pandora's Box). The use of arbitration boards can quickly resolve disputes between health care employees and management, thus avoiding strikes that would remove essential services for long periods of time (panacea). However, these same arbitration boards tend to give away management rights that could have long-term detrimental effects on health care delivery (Pandora's Box).[5]

1. Stein, p. 1041.
2. Schmidt, p. 206.
3. Moellering, R. C., Jr.: The third generation cephalosporins: Panacea or Pandora's box: *Pharmacotherapy*, 2:169–171, 1982.
4. Kilroy, J. M.: Malpractice pre-screening panel—Panacea or Pandora's box?: *Missouri Med.*, 74:11–15, 17, 1977.
5. Carew, W. L.: Interest arbitration in health care—A Panacea or Pandora's box?: *Dimensions*, 61:17–18, 1984.

Pandora's Box

The eponym Pandora's Box is often used to express the evils that afflict mankind, such as disease,[1] untoward effects of treatment,[2] research,[3] and health care delivery (see Panacea).[4,5]

In Greek mythology, Pandora was the first mortal woman, comparable to Eve. She was created by Jupiter (Zeus) as punishment for mankind because Prometheus had stolen fire for man from the chariot of the sun.[1] She was given gifts of beauty, charm, and music by the gods, who sent her to earth to become the wife of Epimetheus, Prometheus's brother. She had also been given a vase which she was forbidden to open. Overcome by curiosity, Pandora lifted the lid and there escaped a multitude of ills which were released upon mankind—plagues, gout, rheumatism, colic, envy, spite, and revenge. She quickly closed the lid, but only hope remained within. In another version, Pandora was made by Jupiter to bless man, and given a box of marriage presents consisting of blessings.[6] When she opened it all the blessings escaped and were lost except for hope. It is the former version of released ills that is used for the medical applications of this eponym.

Pandora's Box has become an overworked

eponym in medicine. It has been applied to the numerous cerebral problems in patients with lupus,[7] the many disorders of the autonomic system in patients with heart disease,[8] the detrimental effects of industrial air pollutants on the respiratory system,[9] and to a family of several generations with a multitude of diseases.[10] Psychiatry has not been exempt. Designated as Pandora's Box are the many psychic problems of adolescent girls with secondary amenorrhea,[11] the relationship of a woman's dreams to the fear that her sexuality is uncontrollable and poisonous,[12] and the many troubling fantasies of an autisticlike child during therapy.[13]

Therapeutic Pandora Boxes include the complexity and possible deleterious effects of treating sexual dysfunction in alcoholics,[14] the mixed blessings of antenatal surgery,[15] the side-effects of increased serum acetate concentration which occur with dialysis,[16] the mixed blessings of continuous ambulatory peritoneal dialysis,[17] possible complications of treatment with barbiturates following cardiac arrest,[18] and the pros and cons of combination antibiotic therapy.[19]

In dentistry, faulty planning of Social Security legislation without consulting dentists has been equated with Pandora's Box,[20] as have expanded duties of dental auxiliaries.[21] Compulsory continuing education has been described as a Pandora's Box of impeding regulations and paperwork.[22]

Other extrapolations from Pandora's Box are the difficulties engendered by the complexities of chemical carcinogenesis,[23] the regulation of hematopoiesis,[24] and the public perception of cancer as a Pandoran Curse.[25] Medicine in general has been equated with Pandora's role in releasing evils on human society because it has not sufficiently warned the public about health problems produced by technological alterations of the environment.[26] A lid is considered as needed for the Pandora's Box which released the dangerous evils of exponential growth in population and technology.[27]

Day care for young children has been designated as a Pandora's Box as it carries with it benefits, such as being a socializing force, as well as evils, such as possible poor health care and abdication of parental responsibility.[28] And finally, a binocular range finder used for measurement of apparent depth perception has been called Pandora's Box.[29] References to illness and diseases in poetry has been reviewed under the title of Pandora's Box,[30] the connotation being that of a varied mixture.

1. Gayley, p. 11.
2. Moellering, R. C. Jr.: The third generation of cephalosporins: Panacea or Pandora's box: *Pharmacotherapy*, 2:169–171, 1982.
3. Louderback, A. L.: Enzymes and isoenzymes: A new Pandora's box?: *Can. J. Med. Technol.*, 29:42–51, 1967.
4. Kilroy, J. M.: Malpractice screening panel—Panacea or Pandora's box?: *Missouri Med.*, 74:11–15, 17, 1977.
5. Carew, W. L.: Interest arbitration in health care—A Panacea or Pandora's box: *Dimensions*, 61:17–18, 1984.
6. Bulfinch, p. 22.
7. Bernstein, R. M.: Cerebral lupus: A peep into Pandora's box: *J. Rheumatol.*, 9:817–818, 1982.
8. González, E. R.: Pandora's Box of autonomic ills found in some heart patients: *J.A.M.A.*, 245:107–108, 1981.
9. Salvaggio, J. E.: Hypersensitivity pneumonitis: "Pandora's box": *N. Engl. J. Med.*, 283:314–316, 1970.
10. Dickinson, K. G.: A difficult case. Pandora's box: *Br. Med. J.*, 287:954–955, 1983.
11. Mozley, P.: Forced femininity. Opening Pandora's box: *Obstet. Gynecol.*, 34:414–417, 1969.
12. Harris, H. E.: Pandora: *Psychiatr. Commun.*, 10:19–21, 1969.
13. Durham, M. S.: Pandora's box. The fantasies of an autisticlike child: *J. Am. Acad. Child. Psychiatry*, 11:255–269, 1972.
14. Thiel, D. H. Van & Lester, R.: Therapy of sexual dysfunction in alcohol abusers: A Pandora's box: *Gastroenterology*, 72:1354–1356, 1977.
15. Soper, R. T.: President's address. The Pandora's box of antenatal surgery: *Am. Surgeon*, 49:285–289, 1983.
16. Novello, A. C.: Pandora's box revisited: A second look at the acetate story: *Int. J. Artif. Organs*, 3:255–257, 1980.
17. Swainson, C. P.: Continuous ambulatory peritoneal dialysis—Pandora's gift to nephrology?: *N. Z. Med. J.*, 96:424–425, 1983.
18. Rockoff, M. A. & Shapiro, H. M.: Barbiturates following cardiac arrest: Possible benefit or Pandora's box?: *Anesthesiology*, 49:385–387, 1978.
19. Schwartz, R. H.: Opening Pandora's box!: *J. Pediatr.*, 91:165–166, 1977.
20. Seldin, J. B.: Pandora's box: *N.Y. J. Dent.*, 38:60–62, 1968.
21. Whitney, R. G.: Opening Pandora's box: *J. Am. Dental Assoc.*, 94:424, 1977.

22. Kennedy, L. M.: The Pandora's box: Why compulsory continuing education?: *Ohio Dent. J.*, 44:317–319, 1970.

23. Bresnick, E.: The price of progress or Pandora's purse: *Biochem. Pharmacol.*, 32:1331–1336, 1983.

24. Eaves, C. J. & Eaves, A. C.: Factors and hemopoiesis: Pandora's box revisited: Aplastic anemia: in stem cell biol, advances treat., *Prog. Clin. Biol. Res.*, 148:83–92, 1984.

25. Weinhouse, S.: Prometheus and Pandora—Cancer research on our diamond anniversary: Presidential address: *Cancer Res.*, 42:3471–3474, 1982.

26. Glass, B.: Prometheus and Pandora—1971: *Bull. N.Y. Acad. Med.*, 47:1045–1058, 1971.

27. Fawcett, N. G.: A lid for Pandora's box: *J. School Health*, 41:292–295, 1971.

28. Almy, M.: Day care: Pandora's box?: *Am. Med. Woman's Assoc.*, 28:252–255, 1973.

29. Berbaum, K. et al.: Depth perception of surfaces in pictures: Looking for conventions of depiction in Pandora's box: *Perception*, 12:5–20, 1983.

30. Lowbury, E.: Pandora's box. Thoughts on health and illness in poetic literature: *Ann. R. Coll. Surg. Eng.*, 53:355–369, 1973.

Panglossian Paradigm

The Panglossian Paradigm is an eponym applied with a critical connotation to the evolutionary school of thought which has been predominant for the past half century. This school "regards natural selection as so powerful and the constraints upon it so few that [it considers] adaptation . . . [as] the primary cause of nearly all organic form, function and behavior."[1] Thus, organisms have traits or structures which are optimally designed by natural selection for their functions. However, the theory ignores nonadaptive forces, such as the fixation of genes in species by random genetic drift.[2]

In the study of animal behavior (ethology), the dominant intentional theory is similar in concept to the traditional adaptionist approach to evolution.[3] Intentional theory makes the assumption that all animal behavior is developed on the basis of intentional optimal solutions to problems. This may ascribe more intelligence to some species or individuals than actually exists.

The intentional theory of animal behavior and the adaptionist theory of evolution both imply that what happens is always for the most optimal and for the best, as did Dr. Pangloss.

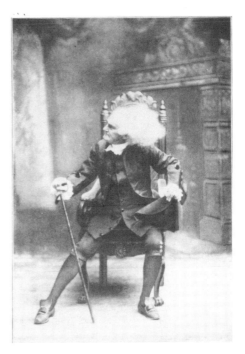

Panglossian Paradigm   Doctor Pangloss as played by Jefferson.[8]

Pangloss is one of the major characters in Voltaire's novel, *Candide, ou L' Optimisme*, of 1750.[4] He is the tutor of Candide, who accepted all his teachings on "metaphysico-theologo-cosmonigology." "He proved admirably that in this best of all possible worlds, His Lordship's castle was the most beautiful of castles, and Her Ladyship the best of all possible baronesses." Pangloss maintained that ". . . individual misfortunes create general welfare, so that the more individual misfortunes there are, the more all is well." He used such optimistic reasoning to rationalize that all untoward calamities happened for the best, including personal disastrous adventures and natural upheavals.

An example of Pangloss's great ability to rationalize, and Voltaire's to satirize, is the conclusion that " . . . if Columbus, on an American Island, hadn't caught that disease [syphilis] which poisons the source of generation, which often even prevents generation, and which is obviously opposed to the great goal of nature, we would now have neither chocolate nor cochineal." Such outrageous optimism was Voltaire's reaction to Leibniz's creed that "All is for the best in this best of all possible worlds."[5] Another eponym for an unduly optimistic outlook is Pollyannism.[6]

The adaptionist panglossian view of evolution, if taken to its extreme, would support the view that the nose developed its present shape so that man could wear glasses! Charles Darwin would have been sympathetic with the satiric eponym Panglossian Paradigm because he did not consider natural selection to be the exclusive means of modification of the species.[7]

1. Gould, S. J. & Lewontin, R. C.: The spandrels of San Marco and the Panglossian Paradigm: *Proc. R. Soc. Lond.*, 205:581–598, 1979.
2. Lewontin, R. C.: Elementary errors about evolution: *Behav. Brain Sci.*, 6:367–368, 1983.
3. Dennett, D. C.: Intentional systems in cognitive ethology: The "Panglossian paradigm" defended: *Behav. Brain Sci.*, 6:343–355, 1983.
4. Voltaire: *Candide ou L' Optimisme*: L. Bair translator, New York, Bantam Books, 1959.
5. Benét, W. R.: *The Reader's Encyclopedia*, p. 163.
6. OED: Supp. III:631, 1981.
7. Darwin, C.: *The Origin of the Species*: New York, Modern Library, n. d.
8. Brewer, 3:154.

Panic Terror

Panic terror is defined as "a state of extreme, acute, intense anxiety accompanied by disorganization of personality and function."[1] There is a marked discharge of the autonomic nervous system with increased respiration, heart rate, sweating, and dryness of the mouth accompanied by trembling and marked weakness. It is a greatly exaggerated reaction which may function as a warning of impending emotional decompensation, possibly derived from fearful experiences in the individual's remote past.[2] Panic terror is an extreme reaction of fear. Attacks may occur in homosexuals accompanied by assaults and hallucinations induced by feelings of dependency and weakness.[3] Panic episodes have also been reported with the organic brain syndrome and drug-induced behavior disturbance.

The word panic is an eponym derived from Pan, the ancient Greek god of woods, fields, shepherds, and flocks.[4] He was the son of Mercury and a wood-nymph (dryad), distinguished by a human torso and the hoofs, horns and ears of a goat and very hairy skin (see Esau Lady).[5] Pan was also considered a symbol of fertility, as he made goats and ewes prolific; he became the Priapus of Mysia in Asia Minor.[6] Pan lived in the woods and mountains of Acadia where he amused himself by giving lonely travelers sudden fright;[7] and thus the origin of the eponym Panic Terror.

1. Freedman, pp. 809–810.
2. Hofling, C. K.: *Textbook of Psychiatry for Medical Practice*: 3rd ed., Philadelphia, J. B. Lippincott, 1975, pp. 63–66.
3. Glick, R. A. et al., Eds.: *Psychiatric Emergencies*: New York, Grune & Stratton, 1976, pp. 56, 252.
4. Boycott, p. 87.
5. Gayley, p. 45.
6. Guirand 1968, p. 161.
7. Bulfinch, pp. 211–213.

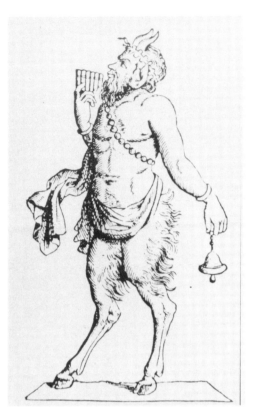

Panic Terror   Pan with goat's hoofs and horns.[7]

Peeping Tom Syndrome

(scopophilia, voyeurism)

Peeping Tom, the archetypic voyeur, represents a common social problem, occurring most frequently in males.[1] It consists of obtaining sexual gratification by watching other people when they are undressing, naked, or engaging in sexual activity.[2] It may be accompanied by masturbation. Like exhibitionism, voyeurism may originate from the emotional effects on a young child on seeing parents engaging in sexual intercourse. He then attempts to regain the excitement of seeing his mother undress, but may also develop aggressive and murderous fantasies against women.[3] It has been considered as the visual manifestation of a compulsive neurosis.[4] Some success has been reported with behavioral treatment in severe cases.[5]

Peeping Tom is part of a British legend in which Tom the tailor opened the window to watch Lady Godiva as she rode naked on her horse through the streets of Coventry.[6] In some accounts, he was struck blind and in others struck dead. Lady Godiva's ride apparently occurred in the eleventh century and was first recorded in the thirteenth, but the Peeping Tom legend was not added until the seventeenth century, (see Lady Godiva Syndrome).

Today, the punishment of the voyeurist is more legal than physical. When voyeurism occurs to a lesser degree, it may be a manifestation of normal sexual curiosity. A literary Peeping Tom is found in Bernard Malamud's *The Assistant*,[7] in which Frank's secretive observation of Helen's nakedness raised a multitude of feelings, including guilt, passion, greed, loss, shame, fear, and finally joy.

1. Stone, A. A. & Stone, S. S.: *The Abnormal Personality Through Literature*: Englewood Cliffs, New Jersey, Prentiss-Hall, 1966, p. 342.
2. Chapman, p. 233.
3. Kolb, p. 530.
4. Manhaes, M. P.: Importancia do Fator Visual Na Neurose Compulsiva—"Peeping Tom": *Rev. Bras. Psican.* 11:5–14, 1977.
5. Stoudenmire, J.: Behavioral treatment of voyeurism and possible symptom substitution: *Psychother. Theory Res. Pract.*, 10:328–330, 1973.
6. *Encyclopaedia Britannica*: VII:832.
7. Malamud, B.: *The Assistant*: New York, Farrar, Straus & Giroux, 1957.

Persephone Syndrome

A woman may be unable to adjust to marriage because of incomplete emancipation from a childhood dependency on her mother.[1] Anxiety, depression, and stress reactions to separation from mothers have been described in married Greek immigrant women living in the United States. Aggravating these feelings is a superficial interest in their marriage, which is based on custom, and failure to adapt to a new cultural environment. In Greek society, the mother-daughter relationship is very intimate, whereas the husband-wife relationship is more formal. They may leave their husbands and return to their homeland.[2]

In Greek mythology, Persephone (Proserpina in Roman mythology) was the goddess of earth and daughter of Ceres (Demeter) and Jupiter. Venus asked her son, Cupid, to send a dart into Hades (Pluto), the god of the underworld. This was to make him fall in love with Persephone, as revenge on her mother (Ceres) who threatened to defy Venus.[3] Hades fell in love with Persephone and abducted her to his underworld kingdom. Ceres searched for her daughter throughout the entire world. In rage at not finding her daughter, she inflicted drought, famine, flood, and plague upon the earth until Zeus intervened and made a compromise. Persephone would live half her time on earth with her mother, and the other half with Hades. The earth bloomed during the former period and withered during the latter (see Queen of Hell Syndrome).

This mythological explanation of the marked contrast between winter and summer does show strong attachment between mother and daughter, although it is the former who takes the initiative of making a change, unlike the related psychiatric syndrome in which it is the daughter who does so. A poem by William Carlos Williams, *Spring and All*, invokes Persephone as the spirit of spring, which represents the emergence of life (spring) out of death (winter) and of ecstacy out of despair.[4] In Jungian psychology, Persephone is one of the many goddesses who exemplify the great mother female archetype.[5]

1. Dunkas, N. & Nikelly, G.: The Persephone syndrome. A study of conflict in the adaptive process of married Greek female immigrants in the U.S.A.: *Social Psychiatry*, 7:211–216, 1972.
2. Vaisrub, pp. 18–19.
3. Gayley, pp. 159–163.
4. Breslin, J. E. B.: *William Carlos Williams. An American Artist*: Chicago, University of Chicago Press, 1985, pp. 62–63.
5. Martin, P. W.: *Experiment in Depth. A Study of the Work of Jung, Eliot and Toynbee*: London, Routledge & Kegan Paul, 1955, pp. 99–100.

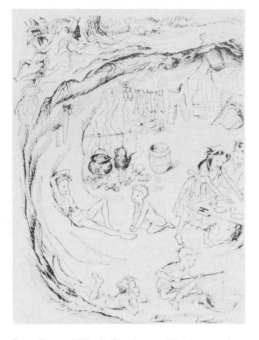

Peter Pan and Wendy Syndrome Wendy preparing a
meal for the indolent Peter Pan.[2, p. 105] (by permission,
George Thieme Verlag)

Peter Pan and Wendy Syndrome

One type of a marital situation is that of an
unfaithful and narcissistic husband and a long-
suffering and depressed wife.[1] The couple are
usually in their middle thirties. The husband
has a relationship conflict and anxiety, and
devotes considerable time to studies, sports,
and other women.

In Barrie's *Peter Pan and Wendy*, Peter Pan is
the leader of the lost boys who have been
abandoned by their parents, all of whom live in
Neverland along with Tinker Bell and Tiger
Lily. Peter helps Wendy to overcome her fear of
flying by sprinkling her with pixie dust, and
off they go to the magic Neverland.[2] The pirate
leader, Captain Hook is the major protagonist.
To consider Peter Pan as the narcissistic husband and Wendy as the depressed wife may be a
gross extrapolation.

Closely related to the Peter Pan and Wendy
Syndrome is the Wendy Dilemma. The latter applies to women who feel trapped into
mothering their husbands, even though they
realize that this encourages immature behavior
in men.[3] They have conflicts with the traditional feminine role versus personal freedom,
with self-sacrifice versus self-promotion, and
with short-term goals versus long-term goals.
There is also fear of rejection if the mothering
is abandoned. The suggested resolution of the
dilemma is developing into a loving, responsible, and mature individual through self-exam-
ination.

A study of essays written by teenagers revealed that girls were much more oriented
toward marriage and family life than a career.[4]
This is consistent with Freud's views on the
subject.[5]

One might consider characterizing femininity psychologically as giving preference to passive aims.
This is not, of course, the same thing as passivity; to
achieve a passive aim may call for a large amount of
activity. It is perhaps the case that in a woman, on
the basis of her share of sexual function, a preference for passive behavior and passive aims is carried
into her life . . . . But we must be aware in this of
understanding the influence of social customs, which
similarly force women into passive situations.

Barrie's Peter Pan has received considerable

psychoanalytic study. Wendy, in effect, punishes her parents by running away from her wonderful but controlling mother and her childlike, ineffectual father.[6] Captain Hook, represents the evil father whom Peter symbolically castrated by cutting off his hand.[7] The Oedipus Complex has been evoked for Peter Pan's hostile relationships with Hook, the father figure, and for the warm caring of Wendy, the mother figure for the lost boys.[8]

The relationship of the Peter Pan myth to Barrie's own life has not been neglected. Peter, the boy who lives forever, may be Barrie's own older brother whose death was a severe shock to his mother.[9] Children flying through the air in their nightgowns are "obviously" dead children. Flying in through a window is considered symbolic of returning from the dead. Barrie's own father was severe in nature, as is the literary Captain Hook.

The author had many infatuations with women, possibly represented by Tinker Bell, Tiger Lily, and Wendy.[1] The story of Peter Pan also has been considered as a representation of pedophilia, "peter" being a slang name for penis, and "Pan" being the Greek god of sexual libertinism.[10] Flying is a psychological symbol of sexual activity, and the pixie dust sprinkled on Wendy by Peter Pan has been interpreted as sperm.[1]

Green has commented on the significance of relating Barrie's life (or that of any author) to his works.[11] "Writers of the greatest works for children seem to have become the natural prey of the psychoanalysts, and Barrie even more than Lewis Carroll or Kenneth Grahame has proved an irresistible target for their attentions. . . . But while the psychological background may help to form a work of art, it is false logic to assume that the work of art is rendered unhealthy by any oddness in the spiritual equipment of the author . . . it is not the past [childhood] that is morbid, but the desire to escape too often into it."

1. Quadrio, C.: The Peter Pan and Wendy syndrome: A marital dynamic: *Aust. N.Z. J. Psychiatry*, 16:23–28, 1982.
2. Barrie, J. M.: *Peter Pan and Wendy*: London, Hodder & Stoughton, 1911.
3. Kiley, D.: *The Wendy Dilemma. When Women Stop*

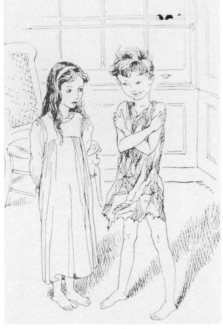

(A)

(B)

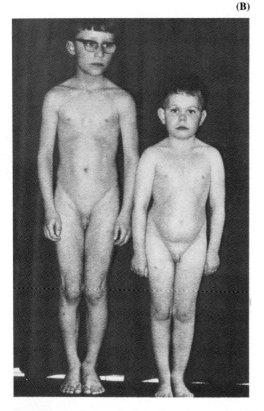

Peter Pan Syndrome **A.** Peter Pan, the eternal child, with Wendy.[2, p. 41] **B.** Hypopituitary dwarf with child of the same age.[9] (by permission, Georg Thieme Verlag)

Mothering Their Men: New York, Arbor House, 1984.

4. Humphrey, M. & Lenham, C.: Adolescent fantasy and self fulfillment: The problem of female passivity: *J. Adoles.*, 7:295–304, 1984.
5. Freud, S.: *S.E.* Lecture 33, Vol. 22.
6. Jacobs, E. L.: Neverland: *Issues Ego Psychol.*, 1:22–27, 1978.
7. Meisel, F. L.: The myth of Peter Pan: *Psychoanalyt. Study Child.*, 32:545–563, 1977.
8. Faigel, H. C.: The Barrie syndrome. Peter Pan as the dramatization of emotional retardation: *Clin. Pediatr.*, 4:343–347, 1965.
9. Karpe, M.: The origins of Peter Pan: *Psychoanal. Rev.*, 43:104–110, 1956.
10. Ober, p. 111.
11. Green, R. L.: *J. M. Barrie*: New York, Henry Z. Walck, 1961, pp. 48–49.

Peter Pan Syndrome I, II

I   The presence of dwarfism and microphallus in congenital hypopituitarism results in an appearance that is much younger than the actual chronological age, as represented by the eternally young Peter Pan.[1] The diagnosis is strongly suggested by the presence of a very small penis, from 0.5 to 2.5 cm in size, and of hypoglycemia. Phallic growth can occur with testosterone treatment, suggesting a hypothalamic hormone deficiency rather than a primary pituitary defect. Thus, the Peter Pan Syndrome I is based primarily on morphology—the underdevelopment of the secondary, extragonadal sexual structures which are equivalent to those of a younger child.[2]

II   Another Peter Pan Syndrome has a psychological basis rather than a morphological one. It has been used to label men who refuse to grow up,[3] as did Barrie's Peter Pan. "Wendy: 'Peter, how old are you? . . . .' Peter: 'I don't know, but quite young Wendy. I ran away the day I was born . . . [b]ecause I heard my father and mother talking of what I was to be when I became a man. I want always to be a little boy and to have fun.' "[2] Suggested as an example of this syndrome are men who postpone maturity and the fathering of children.[4]

Development of this syndrome is enhanced by parental permissiveness, an atmosphere of tension at home, loneliness, and sex role conflict, all of which enhance magical thinking, narcissism, and chauvinism.[5] They put on a pretense of being happy-go-lucky, but actually cry for attention, and snicker at ones who do care. The related Peter Pan Profile is a measure of the degree of such reluctance of adolescents to grow up.[6] It consists of forty-eight items with six subscales. Test validity was indicated by successful differentiation between high and low scoring groups. It can serve as an indication of the eventual success in resolving the conflict between the desire for the freedom of childhood and the responsibilities of adulthood.

Barrie's *Peter Pan or the Boy Who Never Grew Up*[2] owes its enormous and perpetual success to its depiction of the wonder of never having to grow up, of being able to believe forevermore in magic, and of taking part in dangerous and exciting adventures. Peter Pan, the leader of the lost boys, flew into Wendy's bedroom and then they flew to a never-never land of adventure and freedom from parents except allegorically for the pirates. Peter Pan has become a universal symbol of the eternal child, essentially without libido and living in a world of adventure and magic.[7]

There is yet another connection between J. M. Barrie's classic tale of immortal youth and medicine.[8] He assigned the copyright of its play to the Great Ormond Street Sick Children's Hospital in London, thus providing it with a considerable amount of funds in the form of royalties.

1. Lovinger, R. D. et al.: Congenital hypopituitarism associated with neonatal hypoglycemia and microphallus: Four cases secondary to hypothalamic hormone deficiencies: *J. Pediatr.*, 87:1171–1181, 1975.
2. Barrie, J. M.: *Peter Pan or the Boy Who Would Not Grow Up*: New York, Charles C. Scribner's Sons, 1928, p. 32.
3. Roe, P. F.: Eponymous disorders: *Lancet*, 2:794, 1978.
4. Goodman, E.: Maybe menopause gives a better focus on life: *Dayton Daily News J. Herald*, Nov. 6, 1986, p. 15.
5. Kiley, D.: *The Peter Pan Syndrome*: New York, Dodd, Mead, 1983.
6. Randolph, E. M. & Dye, C. A.: The Peter Pan profile. Development of a scale to measure reluctance to grow up: *Adolescence*, 16:841–850, 1981.
7. Hallman, R. J.: The archetypes in Peter Pan: *J. Analyt. Psychol.*, 14:65–73, 1969.
8. Dunlop, J. M.: The Mother Goose syndrome—A lighthearted look at paediatric literature: Public Health, 88:89–96, 1974.
9. Moll, H.: *Atlas of Pediatric Diseases*: Philadelphia, W. B. Saunders, 1976, p. 79.

Phaedra Complex

Romantic love of a mother for her son has

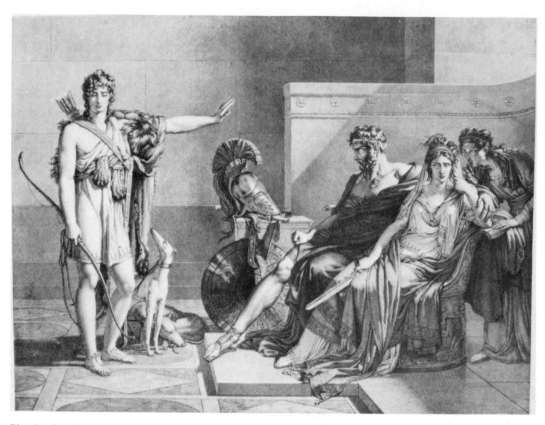

Phaedra Complex   Phaedra and Hippolytus.[3]

been designated as the Jocasta Complex. The Phaedra Complex, however, is used more specifically to refer to an attraction between a stepmother and a male step-child.[1] It is now encountered more frequently because of the increasing number of divorces and remarriages.

Phaedra was the daughter of Minos, king of Crete.[2] She married Theseus, the son of Aegeus, king of Athens, but fell in love with her husband's son, Hippolytus, who was nearer her own age. When he rejected her, Phaedra's love turned to hate and she made Theseus jealous of his son, Hippolytus. The father then invoked on his son the vengeance of Neptune, who had Hippolytus killed in a chariot accident caused by a sea monster. But Aesculapius restored Hippolytus to life and placed him under the protection of the nymph Egeria.

Both the Jocasta and Phaedra Complexes could be considered as the counterpart of the Oedipus Complex. The Jocasta and Oedipus Complexes have, however, their origin in the relationship of the infant to his parents; unlike the Phaedra Complex, in which the relationship originates in an older son on remarriage of his father to a different woman.

1. Campbell, p. 123.
2. Bulfinch, p. 196.
3. Brewer, 3:198.

Pickwickian Syndrome

(cardiopulmonary syndrome, obesity heart syndrome,[1] reversible cardiopulmonary obesity–hypoventilation syndrome with extreme obesity)

In 1906, William Osler called obese, sleepy people pickwickians[2] in reference to such a character in Dickens's novel *The Pickwick Club*.[3] "An extraordinary phenomenon associated with excessive fat in young persons is an uncontrollable tendency to sleep—like the fat boy in Pickwick."[4] This was more fully delineated in 1956 by Burwell as the Pickwickian Syndrome of extreme obesity associated with alveolar hypoventilation.[4] Clinical features are marked obesity, somnolence, twitching, cyanosis, periodic respiration, secondary polycythemia with apnea, and right ventricular hypertrophy and failure. In fifty patients with these criteria, Alexander found an increased incidence of hypertension, dyspnea, edema, and increased pulmonary wedge pressure suggestive of both right and left sided heart failure.[5] Elevated pressure of blood carbon dioxide (PCO_2) and decreased pressure of oxygen (PO_2) are caused by a reduction in lung volumes, vital capacity, and compliance of the chest cage secondary to the enormous amount of fat.[6]

Some patients with the Pickwickian Syndrome have a diminished sensitivity of the respiratory center to carbon dioxide; others have an increased upper respiratory obstruction during sleep.[7] Weight loss may result in a dramatic cure if instituted before permanent cardiac damage. An autopsy on a patient with this syndrome revealed myocardial hypertrophy and marked replacement of the sinus node by fat.[8] Although most common in adults between the ages of 30 and 50, some instances have been reported in children of various ages, the youngest being four years of age,[9,10] and others seven, eleven,[11] and thirteen years of age.[12]

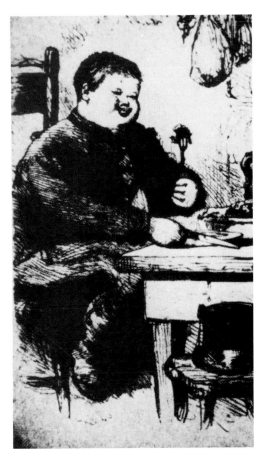

Pickwickian Syndrome Fat Boy Joe indulging.[9] (by permission, copyright 1960, Amer. Med. Assoc.)

Fat Boy Joe is Mr. Wardle's page, who has a huge appetite in Dickens's *The Posthumous Papers of the Pickwick Club*,[13] first published in 1837. In Chapter 4, he raises the ire of the old gentleman. " . . . the fat boy waddled to the same perch and fell asleep instantly. 'Joe! — the damn boy, he's gone to sleep again . . . Sleep . . . he's always asleep. Goes on errands asleep and snore as he waits on tables.' " In Chapter 28 " . . . the fat boy laid himself affectionately by the side of the cod-fish and placing an oyster-barrel under his head for a pillow, fell asleep instantaneously. . . . . 'Come, wake up young dropsy!' But as young dropsy evinced no symptoms of returning animation, Sam Weller sat himself down in front of the cart . . . ." The unctuous fat boy Joe did have, however, considerable temptation put in his way because picnics and banquets are prominent in the book.[14]

The Pickwickian Syndrome has become one of the most popular of medical eponyms derived from literary characters. The designation is not, however, without its detractors. One etymological objection has been that Mr. Pickwick himself did not exhibit these signs and symptoms,[15] although one must admit that his name is more euphonious than "Fat Boy Joe Syndrome." Justification may be that the syndrome is named after the book, rather than its main character, Mr. Pickwick himself (although this is contrary to most literary eponyms). Scientific objections have been based on the absence of symptoms in Joe of hypoventilation, such as apnea, irregular respiration, slow breathing, or cyanosis.[15] He is called young dropsy by Sam Weller, which might be indicative of heart failure with edema,[16] but the term dropsy was also used in the eighteenth century to mean an insatiable thirst or craving.[17]

An apparently tongue-in-cheek suggestion has been to rename the Pickwickian Syndrome the Fee-Fi-Fo-Fum Syndrome because the giant in *Jack and the Beanstalk* was grossly obese, and exhibited not only excessive daytime sleepiness and snoring, but also ill temper, which can be a feature of sleep apnea syndromes.[18] It has been noted, however, that the giant's sleep apnea was secondary to the hypertrophic changes in tongue and pharyngeal tissues that accompany acromegaly.[19] In fact, such a patient has been called an Acromegalic Pickwickian.[20] Sleep-induced apnea has also been described in non-obese patients,[21] and may be associated with cardiac arrhythmias.[22] A hypochondriacal example is Thurber's literary character Briggs Beall, "who believed that he was likely to cease breathing when he was asleep," and consequently set his alarm clock to ring at intervals during the night.[23]

Cases similar to the Pickwickian Syndrome have been described long before the twentieth century.[24] The first known was in 1614 by Felix Patter of Basel of an enormously fat man who fell asleep all the time even when talking or eating.[25] Also a hypoventilation syndrome is Ondine's Curse, but its basic cause is failure of central autonomic control of ventilation rather than the more peripheral pathophysiological elements of the Pickwickian Syndrome.[26] Sleep-induced breathing disorders have been classified as sleep apnea syndromes, primary alveolar hypoventilation, irregular breathing patterns, and nocturnal hypoxemia.[27] The Pickwickian Syndrome is compatible with the first two categories (see Rip Van Winkle Syndrome).

The fifteen physicians and seven surgeons mentioned in works of Dickens have been put in a positive light as compared to other professions.[28] The many diseases in works of Charles Dickens have not been overlooked,[29] nor has the possible association between his literary children and his own suffering as a child.[30] There is no evidence that Dickens himself or Mr. Pickwick were obese as boys, although Dickens may well have observed such an individual. Another possible literary example of the Pickwickian Syndrome occurs inthe same book.[31] The obese Mr. Justice Starlight fell asleep twice during a trial, only to be awakened by the silence. Not to be overlooked is Shakespeare's cowardly and very obese knight, Sir John Falstaff, who had inappropriate somnolence and intermittent mental confusion (see Falstaff Obesity).[32]

1. Estes, E. H., Jr. et al.: Reversible cardiopulmonary syndrome with extreme obesity: *Circulation*, 16:179–187, 1957.
2. Osler, W.: *The Principles and Practice of Medicine*: 6th ed., New York, Appleton, 1905, p. 431.
3. Tucker, W. S. Osler and sleep apnea: *Arch. Int. Med.*, 144:1085, 1984.

4. Burwell, C. S. et al.: Extreme obesity associated with alveolar hypoventilation—A Pickwickian syndrome: *Am. J. Med.*, 21:811–818, 1956.

5. Alexander, J. K.: Observations on some clinical features of extreme obesity, with particular reference to cardiorespiratory effects: *Am. J. Med.*, 32:512–524, 1962.

6. Olefsky, J. M.: Hypoventilation syndrome (Pickwickian syndrome): in *Harrison's Principles of Internal Medicine*, 10th ed., R. G. Petersdorf et al., Eds., New York, McGraw-Hill, 1983, p. 443.

7. Gastaut, H.: Polygraphic study of the episodic diurnal and nocturnal (hypnic and respiratory) manifestations of the Pickwick syndrome: *Brain Res.*, 2:167–186, 1966.

8. James, T. N.: De sumbitaneis mortibus III. Pickwickian syndrome: *Circulation*, 48:1311–1320, 1973.

9. Spier, N. & Karelitz, S.: The Pickwickian syndrome. Case in a child: *A.M.A.J. Dis. Child.*, 99:822–827, 1960.

10. Ward, W. A. & Kelsey, W. M.: The Pickwickian syndrome: A review of the literature and report of a case: *J. Pediatr.*, 61:745–750, 1962.

11. Metzl, K. et al.: The Pickwickian syndrome in a child. An extreme example of psychoneurotic obesity: *Clin. Pediatr.*, 8:49–53, 1969.

12. Cayler, G. G.: Pickwickian syndrome in children: *J. Dis. Child.*, 98:663–665, 1959.

13. Dickens, C.: *The Posthumous Papers of The Pickwick Club*: New York, G. W. Carleton, 1883, pp. 63, 370.

14. Montgomery, D. W.: The Fat Boy: *Med. Pickwick*, 6:67–68, 1915.

15. Comroe, J. H., Jr.: Frankenstein, Pickwick, and Ondine: *Am. Rev. Respir. Dis.*, 111: 689–692, 1975.

16. Robin, E. D.: Of sleep and seals and many things: Pickwickians—1978: *West. J. Med.*, 129: 419–421, 1978.

17. OED: III:682.

18. Phillipson, E. A.: Pickwickian, obesity-hypoventilation, or fee-fi-fo-fum syndrome?: *Am. Rev. Respir. Dis.*, 121:781–782, 1980.

19. Bass, J. B., Jr.: To The Editor: *Am. Rev. Respir. Dis.*, 122:657, 1980.

20. Romanczuk, B. J., Potsic, W. P., & Atkins, J. P., Jr.: Hypersomnia with periodic breathing (an acromegalic Pickwickian): *Otolaryngology*, 86: 897–903, 1978.

21. Tilkian, A. G. et al.: Sleep-induced apnea syndrome. Prevalence of cardiac arrhythmias and their reversal after tracheostomy: *Am. J. Med.*, 63:348–358, 1977.

22. Miller, W. P.: Cardiac arrhythmias and conduction disturbances in the sleep apnea syndrome. Prevalence and significance: *Am. J. Med.*, 73:317–321, 1982.

23. Thurber, J.: "The Night the Bed Fell": in *The Thurber Carnival*, New York, Harper & Row, 1945, pp. 176–181.

24. Markel, H.: In defense of the Pickwickian syndrome: *Henry Ford Hosp. Med. J.*, 33:24–26, 1985.

25. Schiller, F.: A note on the Pickwickian syndrome and Felix Platter (1536–1614): *J. Hist. Med. Allied Sci.*, 40:66–67, 1985.
26. Keelan, P.: Of Pickwick and Ondine: *Irish Med. J.*, 74:339–340, 1981.
27. Hall, J. B.: The cardiopulmonary failure of sleep-disordered breathing: *J.A.M.A.*, 255:930–933, 1986.
28. Literature and medicine: *MD*, August, 1962.
29. Brain, R.: Dickensian diagnoses: *Br. Med. J.*, 2:1553–1556, 1955.
30. Markel, H.: The childhood suffering of Charles Dickens and his literary children: *Pharos*, 48:5–8, 1985.
31. Kryger, M. H.: Fat, sleep, and Charles Dickens: Literary and medical contributions to the understanding of sleep apnea: *Clin. Chest Med.*, 6:555–562, 1985.
32. Sullivan, J. S.: The medical history of Shakespeare's Sir John Falstaff: *Med. Herit.*, 2:391–401, 1986.

Pied Piper Phenomenon

Societies contain forces which entice children away from families and the society itself.[1] Throughout history, and still prominent today, are forces relating to the charisma of exceptional individuals.[2] An overt example is Adolph Hitler and the Nazi movement. More subtle are the cultist movements and their leaders, such as James Jones, Charles Manson, and the Reverend Moon. There are many psychological factors that lead to the total acceptance of such cults—a great need for stimulus, recognition, contact, structure, dependency, and security; atypical associative disorders; and the turmoil of developmental changes in adolescents. Enhancing the charisma of the leader are characteristics of the cultist movement itself, such as use of deception and intensification of total dependency.[1] Sexual magnetism may be a factor in some cults, but in others celibacy is enforced in order to divert sexual energy for other purposes.[2] The number of people in such cults in the United States has been estimated as between one and five million, with about 85% from middle and upper class families.[3]

Freud stated that the personality of such charismatic individuals is occasionally more important than the idea they put forward.[4] Thus "We know that in the mass of mankind there is a powerful need for an authority who can be admired, before whom one bows down,

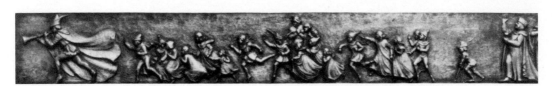

Pied Piper Phenomenon   The Pied Piper leading his flock of children.[12] (frieze by Robert Miller, 1937)

by whom one is ruled and perhaps even ill-treated . . . . It is a longing for the father felt by everyone from his childhood onwards, for the same father whom the hero of legend boasts he has overcome."

The Pied Piper was an enticer of both rats and children. He is a thirteenth century legend from German folklore that may have some historical basis. There are various forms of the legend. The one best known is that found in a 1842 poem by Robert Browning.[5] The city leaders of Hamelin accepted the offer from a mysterious stranger, dressed in particolored (pied) clothes, to rid the town of a plague of rats in exchange for a specified amount of money. When the stranger began to play his pipe, all the rats followed him into the river Weser and drowned. When the city leaders refused to pay him the agreed upon amount of money the Pied Piper began playing his pipe again, and all the children of the town followed him away, never to be seen again.

The equivalent to the Pied Piper in Greek mythology is Orpheus, who played a lyre with such perfection that no living creatures could resist the charm of his music.[6] Of interest is a strikingly similar folktale of Francheville on the Isle of Wight.[7] An additional element has epidemiological implications. When the inhabitants first tried to destroy the rats, they used poison, but the rotting carcasses caused fever, possibly the plague which is spread by rats. A result of the seduction of all children by the piper was the fall of Francheville when the French landed in 1377, presumably because it occurred before a new generation of young men could grow up for its defense.

A proposed historical basis for the legend is that many children had actually died during an epidemic of typhus in Hameln (Hamelin), and were buried in a common grave outside of the city.[8] Supportive is the association with a rat infestation and the reference to a mottled coat, which may represent macular skin lesions.

The phrase Pied Piper has been used for child health care units that relieve anxiety by enthralling them with the trappings of decor and with books related to fantasy. Thus, there is the Pied-Piper Dentist[9] and the Pied Piper of Baltimore Head Start School Program.[10] The Pied Piper has been lightheartedly considered as the first instance in which ultrasound was used to control rodent infestation.[11]

1. Zerin, M. F.: The Pied Piper phenomenon and the processing of victims: The transactional analysis perspective re-examined: *Transact. Anal. J.*, 13:172–177, 1983.
2. Newman, R. G.: Thoughts on superstars of charisma: Pipers in our midst: *Am. J. Orthopsychiatry*, 53:201–208, 1983.
3. Keiser, T. W. & Keiser, J. L.: *The Anatomy of Illusion. Religious Cults and Destructive Persuasion*: Springfield, Illinois, Charles C Thomas, 1987.
4. Freud, S.: "Moses and Monotheism": *S.E.*, Vol. 23, p. 109.
5. Browning, R.: *The Pied Piper of Hamelin*: illustrated by H. Jones, London, Oxford University Press, 1962.
6. Bulfinch, p. 234.
7. Boasc, pp. 112–113.
8. Dirckx, J. H.: The Pied Piper of Hamelin. A medical-historical interpretation: *Am. J. Dermatopathol.*, 2:39–45, 1980.
9. Smoller, E.: Pied-Piper dentist: *Med. Affairs U. Penn.*, 32:40, 1970.
10. Phillips, B. L.: The Pied Piper of Baltimore: *Am. J. Nursing*, 71:304–305, 1971.
11. Dunlop, J. M.: The Mother Goose syndrome—A lighthearted look at paediatric literature: *Public Health*, 88:89–96, 1974.
12. Rochester Public Library, Rochester, Minnesota.

Pinocchio Appearance

A hemangioma on the tip of the nose can be of considerable embarrassment to both a child and its parents.[1] The lesion usually lies over the lower nasal cartilages, dipping between the medial crura of the alar cartilages. Removal is by a bloodless procedure followed by reconstruction of the nose.

Le Adventures di Pinocchio is a children's story written in 1883 by Collodi,[2] the pen name of Corlo Lorenzini of Florence, Italy.[3] Pinocchio was lovingly carved by the lonely Geppetto. The nose was the most prominent feature of this puppet come to life. It grew longer and longer when he told lies, but returned to normal when he told the truth. It is a children's morality story, as are so many of its genre.

In this eponym, the hemangioma appears to be equivalent to the lie (both abnormal), and the surgery to the truth (both restoration to normal). The best known equivalent to Pinocchio's nose is that of Cyrano de Bergerac, a seventeenth century French cavalier and writer, who was immortalized by a play written by Edmond Rostand in 1897.[4]

1. Wynn, S. K.: Aesthetic reduction of "Pinocchio"-nose hemangioma: *Arch. Otolaryngol.*, 102:416–419, 1976.
2. Collodi, C.: *The Adventures of Pinocchio*: Chiesa translator, London, Collier Macmillan, 1969, p. 197.
3. Benét, p. 790.
4. Rostand, E.: *Cyrano de Bergerac. A Heroic Comedy in 5 Acts*: L. Untermyer translator, New York, Heritage Press, 1954.

Pinocchio Syndrome

(psychosomatic conditions)

Psychosomatic patients have several inadequate reactions to their environment.[1] They are unfamiliar with their emotions and have occasional bouts of destructivity or abrupt despair; they cannot related their inner experiences meaningfully to action; they panic with losses; and they fail in repeated attempts to establish contact with transitional objects. One psychotherapeutic approach is based on a fixed arrangement that the therapy group will stay together for two years.[2]

The eponym is named after Pinocchio, the living puppet,[3] because he exhibited some of the characteristics of psychosomatic patients,[1] although he also had some legitimate illnesses. When Pinocchio was hanged by the neck, a beautiful maiden with dark blue hair (the fairy) sent for three famous doctors—a crow, an owl, and a talking cricket. When he developed a fever he refused to take medicine. When he got an earache his ears grew long and hairy, and he was diagnosed by the Dormouse as having donkey fever. It has been suggested that the fairy represents the author's mother.[4]

In the nineteenth century, when Pinocchio was written, psychosomatic conditions were labeled as nervous disorders and considered to be imaginary illnesses and malingering.[5] A current definition of psychosomatic is "the inseparability and interdependence of psychosocial and biologic (physiologic, somatic) aspects of humankind."[6] Psychosomatic medicine is defined as the branch of medicine that recognizes the importance of mind-body relationships for all illnesses, and in which therapy and management are thereby based.[7] The relationship between health, disease, the body, and the mind was recognized long before the modern era by Hippocrates and Maimonides.[8] As the latter has been quoted from his *Hygiene of the Soul*, "The physician should notice accordingly that every sick person is depressed whereas every healthy person is cheerful. He should therefore remove the mental effects which cause the depression for in this way is health maintained."[8]

1. Sellschopp-Rüppell, A. & Rad, M. von: Pinocchio—A psychosomatic syndrome: *Psychother. Psychosom.*, 28:357–360, 1977.
2. Rad, M. von & Rüppell, A.: Combined inpatient and outpatient group psychotherapy: A therapeutic model for psychosomatics: *Psychother. Psychosom.*, 26:237–243, 1975.
3. Collodi, C.: *The Adventures of Pinocchio*: C. D. Ciesa, translator, London, Collier Macmillan, 1969.
4. Smith, R. D.: The cricket and the marionette: *South. Med. J.*, 75:59–60, 1982.
5. McMahon, C. E.: Nervous disease and malingering: The status of psychosomatic concepts in nineteenth century medicine: *Int. J. Psychosom.*, 31:15–19, 1984.
6. Lipowski, Z. L.: What does the word "Psychosomatic" really mean? A historical and semantic inquiry: *Psychosom. Med.*, 46:153–171, 1984.
7. Thomas, p. 1411.
8. Soffer, A.: Maimonides and psychosomatic medicine: *Arch. Int. Med.*, 146:653, 1986.

Playboy Bunny Sign

The ultrasonic image of the junction between the hepatic veins and the inferior vena cava serves as an anatomical landmark.[1] The inferior vena cava has the appearance of the head of a rabbit, the middle and lateral hepatic veins of long rabbitlike ears, and the right hepatic veins of the Playboy Bunny's pipe.

The Playboy Bunny is the trademark of the *Playboy* magazine,[2] and is the designation given to waitresses at Playboy Clubs who are costumed as rabbits. The connotation of "bunny" in this usage is that of a female who is libertarian in her relationships with the other sex.[3] It is not apparent why the radiological rabbitlike appearance was named after a lagomorphized human when it could just as well have been named after an anthropomorphized rabbit as, for example, Bugs Bunny.

1. Eisenberg, p. 453.
2. *Playboy*: Chicago, HMH Publications.
3. Partridge, p. 158.

Pollyanna Posture

(pollyannaism)

One pattern of the doctor-patient interaction is an unconscious collusion between the two, in which the patient and doctor behave toward each other in an overly optimistic fashion.[1] The physician exhibits his optimism by backslapping, insincere jokes, and unrealistic supportive remarks. The result may well be that the patient conceals his symptoms or complaints that need to be investigated. This is classified as one of three basic types of patient-doctor collusion which deny underlying anxiety about the disease.[1] The other two types are the needy child–omnipotent parent posture and the persecutor-victim posture. Another classification of doctor-patient relationships includes activity-passivity, guidance-cooperation, and mutual participation categories (see Pygmalion Complex).[2]

Pollyanna is the young, excessively optimistic, female heroine created by Eleanor Porter, an American author.[3] Pollyanna was struck by an automobile, which injured her back. The medical diagnosis was permanent paralysis. Her Aunt Polly was horrified, but Pollyanna's response was, "Why, Aunt Polly, there is something I can be glad about after all. I can be glad I've *had* my legs . . . !" But she did recover the use of her legs. Pollyanna was an expert at playing her favorite game, the "glad game," which was based on always looking at the best side of her numerous misfortunes.

An actual instance of the Pollyanna Posture has been described in the *Journal of the American Medical Association*, the patient referred to being Samuel Vaisrub, M.D., one of its former editors.[4] "Even when the cancer had long progressed and the various treatments had been abandoned, this knowledgeable but misguided physician cheerfully announced to family and friends that he would 'have Sam on his feet and back at the office in no time.' My father died two nights later, with my mother and me at his bedside." "Although knowing in advance that a loved one is terminally ill does not alleviate the survivors' subsequent grief, it does allow them to face the prospect of the death, aware, and to be prepared."

Examples of such fatuously optimistic behavior on the part of physicians can also be found in fictional works, although patient collusion is not necessarily a feature. The doctor in Tolstoy's *The Death of Ivan Ilyich* (1886) is "fresh, hearty stocky, cheerful, . . . with a look on his face that seems to say: 'Now, now . . . we're going to fix everything right away.' The doctor knows this expression is inappropriate here, but he has put it on once and for all and can't take if off."[5] The result of such pollyannaism was that "Ivan Ilyich suffered most of all from the lie which, for some reason, everyone accepted: that he was not dying but was simply ill. . . ." The withholding from the patient of a fatal diagnosis is strongly sanctioned, if not mandated in the Russian medical culture.[6] The description of Ivan Ilyich's fatal illness has been interpreted as carcinoma of the body of the pancreas.[7] Basic psychological phenomena are also evident in Tolstoy's *Childhood*.[8]

George Eliot featured Dr. Lydgate in her 1871–72 novel *Middlemarch*.[9] His relationship with patients was tempered by his idealism.[10] "I don't really like attending such people [the rich] so well as the poor. The cases are more monotonous, and one has to go through more fuss and listen more deferentially to nonsense."[9]

Another physician relationship is found in Stanislow Lem's science fiction tale *Return from the Stars*,[11] although under different circumstances. "What did arouse my antipathy were the ones who looked after us . . . Dr. Abs . . . treated me the way a doctor would an abnormal patient, pretending, and very well too, that he was dealing with someone quite ordinary. When that became impossible he would joke. I had had enough of his . . . joviality." This is another variant of the physician behavior, the facetious, jocose physician who makes inane, supposedly humorous comments at every opportunity.[12]

Anne Hudson Jones considers of value such "Literary models of the healer relationship [which] flesh out the dynamics of the human relationship . . . . By so doing, they demonstrate the many nuances of emotions that enter in any human exchange."[13]

Pollyannaish behavior toward patients has been called a mask of infallibility which is used to maintain professional control, the placebo effect of physicians, and a father-knows-best attitude.[14] It is an extreme of optimism which is satirized by Voltaire in *Candide*.[15] " 'What's optimism,' asked Cacambo. 'Alas,' said Candide, 'it's a mania for insisting that everything is all right when everything is going wrong' " (see Panglossian Paradigm). The opposite of the Pollyanna Posture is related to Pascal's wager. The physician gives a gloomy prediction for a seriously ill patient.[16] If the patient dies, the doctor has made an accurate prediction. If the patient survives, the doctor also receives credit—this time for achieving an impossible cure.

It has been suggested that the predominant emphasis on science during the entire continuum of medical education and training "can have a devastating impact where science is used to define . . . the physician-patient relationship. The patient is reduced 'either to an insentient automaton or to a bundle of appetites . . . ."[17]

Pollyanna has entered the vocabulary of our society as an excessively or blindly optimistic person.[18] The related noun, pollyannaism, is used in a more psychological sense, as, for example, for well-adjusted people who tend to be pollyannaish.[19] There are four further pollyanna eponyms oriented to positive and pleasant psychological aspects. The Pollyanna Principle states that people process pleasant information more efficiently and accurately than less pleasant information.[20] The Pollyanna Phenomenon refers to the fact that pollyannaistic individuals are more liable to change their judgment on a subject when more positive information is provided then negative.[21]

The Pollyanna Hypothesis asserts that there is a human tendency to use evaluatively positive words more frequently and more diversely than evaluatively negative words.[22] The Pollyanna Process has been applied to the transition from initial feelings of despair after an intestinal resection and colostomy to eventual positive feelings toward the stoma.[23]

Another psychological pollyannaish phenomenon is the fact that whereas normal individuals recall significantly more pleasant than unpleasant words, there is no such differential recall in schizophrenics.[24] A study of college students has demonstrated that positive thinking about past stressful events provides a temporary feeling of well being, whereas thinking negatively of the past decreases the feeling of well being for a much longer period of time.[25]

1. Twemlow, S. W.: Iatrogenic disease or doctor-patient collusion?: *Am. Fam. Physician*, 24:129–134, 1981.
2. Szasz, T. S. & Hollender, M. H.: A contribution to the philosophy of medicine. The basic models of the doctor-patient relationship: *Arch. Int. Med.*, 97:585–592, 1956.
3. Porter, E. H.: *Pollyanna*: New York, A. L. Burt, 1913.
4. Vaisrub, S.: Let's face facts: *J.A.M.A.*, 255:3166, 1986.
5. Tolstoy, L.: *The Death of Ivan Ilych*: L. Solotaroff translator, Toronto, Bantam Books, 1981.
6. Crawshaw, R.: Lying: in *In Search of the Modern Hippocrates*, Bulger, R. J., Ed., Iowa City, Iowa, University of Iowa Press, 1987, pp. 189–190.
7. Schein, C. J.: The Death of Ivan Ilych. An axiomatic hypothesis: *N.Y. State J. Med.*, 81:416, 1981.
8. Smyrniw, W.: Tolstoy's depiction of death in the context of recent studies of the "experience of dying": *Can. Slavonic Papers*, 21:367–379, 1979.
9. Eliot, G.: *Middlemarch*: New York, Penguin Books, 1976, p. 327.
10. White, M. C.: Dr. Lydgate: The literary characterization of the doctor at a historical turning point: *Asclepsio*, 37:321–341, 1985.
11. Lem, S.: *Return from the Stars*: B. Marszal & F. Simpson translators, New York, Harcourt Brace Jovanovich, 1980, p. 4.
12. Nicol, H. G.: Facetious doctors: *Br. Med. J.*, 289:28, 1984.
13. Jones, A. H.: The healer-patient family relationship in Vonda A. McIntyre's "Of Mist, and Grass, and Sand": *Perspect. Biol. Med.*, 26:274–280, 1983.
14. Katz, J.: *The Silent World of Doctor and Patient*: New York, Free Press, 1984, p. 198.
15. Voltaire: *Candide*: L. Bair translator, New York, Bantam Books, 1959, p. 73.
16. Haubrich, p. 179.
17. Herrick, C. R.: Cognitive dissonance and physician training: *Pharos*, 49:2–6, 1986.
18. Stein, p. 1114.
19. Scott, W. A. & Peterson, C.: Adjustment, pollyannaism, and attraction to close relationships: *J. Consult. Clin. Psychol.*, 43:872–880, 1975.
20. Matlin, M. W. & Gawron, V. J.: Individual differences in pollyannaism: *J. Personal. Assess.*, 43:411–412, 1979.
21. Lewicka, M.: Zjawisko Polyanny (the Pollyanna phenomenon): *Przegl. Psychol.*, 21:446–466, 1978.

22. Boucher, J. & Osgood, C. E.: The Pollyanna hypothesis: *J. Verb. Learn. Verb. Behav.*, 8:1–8, 1969.
23. Mullen, B. D.: The Pollyanna process: *Nursing Times*, 13:182–184, 1983.
24. Koh, D. et al.: Affective memory and schizophrenic anhedonia: *Schizophrenia Bull.*, 7:292–307, 1981.
25. Goodhart, D. E.: Some psychological effects associated with positive and negative thinking about stressful event outcomes: Was Pollyanna right?: *J. Personal. Social Psychol.*, 48:216–232, 1985.

Popeye Syndrome

(brachial entrapment syndrome)

In muscular, middle-aged men who do heavy work with their arms, rapid muscular fatigue of the forearm and hand may occur, with paresthesia or deadening of sensation in the fingers.[1] The flexors of the elbow (biceps and brachials), and the bellies of the flexors and extensors of the hand and fingers are confined in the rigid antecubital space of the elbow between bone and the lacertus fascia. If there is significant hypertrophy of these muscles, the brachial artery is compressed by their increase in mass on contracting to flex the elbow. This may be determined by palpation of the brachial artery, or by angiography.[2] Treatment is by division of the lacertus fascia, which permits return to usual activities.

The cartoon character, "Popeye the Sailor Man," first appeared on January 17, 1929, the creation of E. G. Segar.[3] He was one of the first "muscle bound" heroes of the comic strips, being preceded by only a few—such as Katrinka of "Toonervillle Folks."[4] After Segar's death in 1938, the strip was continued by a variety of individuals, with varying success. One of Popeye's major physical attributes is marked enlargement of the muscles of the forearm and elbow region, particularly after eating spinach. Justification for this syndrome is provided by one cartoon episode in which Popeye lost muscular control while lifting crates of spinach.[1]

Other medical references to Popeye are related to his use of spinach for strength and nutrition. The cartoon character did much to increase the consumption of spinach, a beneficial influence as it contains calcium and iron and is rich in vitamins A and C.[5] The recent decrease in the use of spinach, especially in less developed regions of the world, is considered unfortunate because it can easily be home grown, and is of significant nutritional value for infants.[6] There have been concerns, however, regarding its high nitrogen content which may result in vomiting, diarrhea, and methemoglobinemia in infants.[7]

Spinach has been used as a test of the influence of nutritional role models. Three groups of children were given an identical diet, including spinach. One group was shown a Popeye cartoon before eating, another group had a child model who ate his spinach with gusto and commented on its tastiness, and the third group had no attempted reinforcement.[8] The number of children who ate spinach increased in both of the first two test groups in comparison with the third group. The power of Popeye was no more effective than the peer role model in this study.

Comics may even have a detrimental effect on health. Shortly before and following the 1970s, some had indirect subtle themes and references which could develop positive attitudes toward drug abuse.[9] Some adult drug users have implicated comics and cartoons in general as influencing their behavior.[10] However, there have been no definitive studies to investigate such rationalizations. The image of Popeye should not be denigrated, as he has served as a positive role model in other areas.

1. Biemans, R. G. M.: The Popeye syndrome—Brachial artery entrapment as a result of muscular hypertrophy: *Neth. J. Surg.*, 36:103–106, 1984.
2. Biemans, R. G. M.: Brachial artery entrapment syndrome. Intermittent arterial compression as a result of muscular hypertrophy: *J. Cardiovasc. Surg.*, 18:367–371, 1977.
3. Segar, E. C.: *Thimble Theatre Starring: Popeye the Sailor*: New York, Nostalgia Press, 1971.
4. Blackbeard, B.: The First (Arf, Arf) Superhero of Them All: in *All in Color for a Dime*, D. Lupoff & D. Thompson, New Rochelle, New York, Arlington House, 1970, pp. 97–111.
5. Hunter, R.: Why Popeye took spinach: *Lancet*, 1:746–747, 1971.
6. Jelliffe, D. B.: Popeye's influence overseas?: *Lancet*, 1:1245, 1971.
7. Leading Article: Spinach—A risk to babies: *Br. Med. J.*, 1:250–1966.
8. Harris, M. B. & Baudin, H.: Models and vegeta-

ble eating: The power of Popeye: *Psychol. Rep.* 31:570, 1972.

9. Wertham, F.: *Seduction of the Innocent*: New York, Rinehart, 1954.

10. Siegal, R. K.: Seduction of the innocent. A clinical note on the effects of cartoons and comics on drug use: *J. Psychoact. Drugs*, 17:201–204, 1985.

Priapism

Priapism is a persistent, painful erection of the penis which is often unrelated to sexual activity.[1] It is usually idiopathic but can occur in patients with sickle cell anemia, chronic granulocytic leukemia, or spinal cord injury.[2] It may be due to clotting within the penile venous systems. Another unusual penile erection can occur during endoscopic manipulation.[3] Priapism has been attributed to tumors of the prostate and bladder,[4] and may occur with large doses of cantharides (spanish fly) (see Aphrodisiac).[5] Priapism has also occurred in one-third of all male patients taking a recently developed antidepressant, trazodone (Desyrel).[6]

Priapus was the son of Bacchus and Venus (Aphrodite).[7] Hera, who was jealous of Venus, caused Priapus to be born with an enormous penis.[8] His horror-stricken mother abandoned

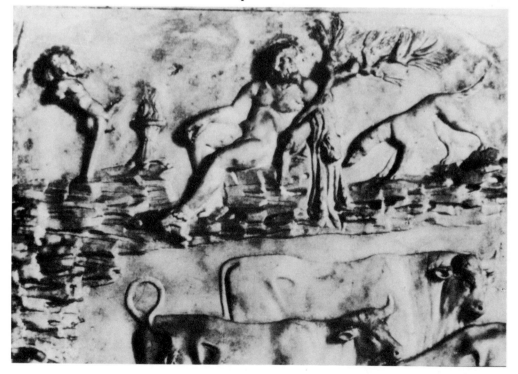

Priapism   Priapus (left), the god of fertility, with erect penis in a rustic scene.[14]

him and he was taken in by shepherds. Priapus was regarded as the god of fecundity of fields, flocks, raising of bees, culture of vines, and fishing. His phallic symbol was placed in gardens and orchards for their protection. The god Hermes was represented with an erect penis in an early Grecian herm (a stone pillar with the bust of a god).[9]

The term priapism has been used with the connotations of licentiousness, intentional indecency, prostitution, or whatever is low or base.[1] In Shakespeare's *Pericles*, Dionyza, the poisonous wife of the governor of Ephesus, is captured by pirates and sold to a brothel keeper.[10] Her performance there was less than satisfactory. "Fie, fie upon her! she is able to freeze/ the god Priapus, and undo a whole generation . . ."

The word priapus has been used for any penis or representation therefrom, but now more commonly means any penis of enormous size.[11] Priapism was a component of penis worship in the erotic literature of eighteenth and nineteenth century England, when it was also known as horn colick.[12] Phallic worship has also been a pervasive feature of many cultures, often expressed in fertility cults and seen as representations of the penis in figurines and amulets.[13] Lingam is the name given to the phallus that represents the god Siva in Hindu mythology.[9]

1. OED: VIII:1341–1342.
2. Braunwald, p. 218.
3. Moshe, O. B. & Vandendris, M.: The treatment of incoercible erection during endoscopic surgery: *J. Urol.*, 135:1272, 1986.
4. Thomas, G. & Schreiner, L. R.: *That's Incurable!*: Penguin Books, 1984, p. 96.
5. Howell, M. & Ford, P.: *The Beetle of Aphrodite and Other Medical Mysteries*: New York, Random House, 1985, p. 255.
6. *Physicians' Desk Reference*: 41st ed., Oradell, New Jersey, Medical Economics, 1987, p. 1266.
7. Bulfinch, p. 494.
8. Guirand 1964, p. 120.
9. Jung, p. 155.
10. Shakespeare, *Pericles, Prince of Tyre*: IV,vi.
11. Dickson, P.: *Words*: New York, Delacorte Press, 1982, p. 239.
12. Bloch, pp. 45, 265–266.
13. Knight, R. P.: *A Discourse on the Worship of Priapus* (1786): reprinted in *Sexual Symbolism. A History of Phallic Worship*, New York, Julian Press, 1957.

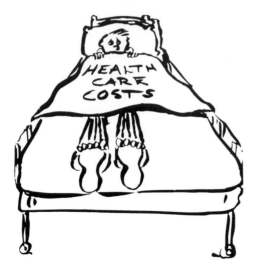

Procrustean Perspective Health care finances not enough to cover health care needs personified in its procrustean bed.[9] (Copyright 1987, *USA Today*. Reprinted with permission)

Procrustean Perspective

A review of the 1984 book *The Painful Prescription*[1] (by Aaron and Schwartz) has called it a Procrustean Perspective because of the impression given that some of Great Britain's health policies foster indifference to human needs.[2] The reviewer disagreed with the authors, indicating that British policies prioritize health care and American policies fail to make medical services functionally accessible to its 28 million uninsured. Furthermore, "Although the United States spends almost twice as large a percentage of its gross national product on health care as does Great Britain, the results as measured by generally accepted indexes of public health do not reflect increased value for the extra expenditure."[3] The authors of *The Painful Prescription* have objected to this review of their book on the basis that "we have presented compelling, direct evidence of widespread rationing of health care in Great Britain."

The Procrustean eponym is derived from Procrustes, a giant in Greek mythology.[4] He had an iron bedstead to which he tied all travelers who fell into his hands. If they were shorter than the bed, he stretched them until they fit, and if they were longer he cut off their limbs. Procrustes was killed by Theseus, who was to become king of Medea. The book accuses British socialized medicine of emulating Procrustes by cutting off health care because its cost does not fit the budget. The book review, then, would be equivalent to Theseus, in that it attempts to slay the monstrous accusation.

Comparisons of health care in Britain and the United States are becoming more numerous with the increasing concern about the American system. The Sidels have pointed out that the United States has higher morbidity, mortality, and disability rates than Britain, neglects health maintenance, and has little accountability.[5] Others deplore the redundancy, the excess capacity, and the inefficiency of American hospitals.[6]

The adjective procrustean is defined as "tending to produce conformity by violent and artificial means."[7] Thus, conscientious physicians know that they cannot fit all patients into specific disease categories without using "procrustean measures" to reduce the number of criteria that are traditionally required to make specific diagnoses, as described in the Cheshire Cat Syndrome.[8]

1. Aaron, H. J. & Schwartz, W. B.: *The Painful Prescription: Rationing Hospital Care*: Washington, D.C., Brookings Institute, 1984.
2. Miller, F. H. & Miller, G. A. H.: *The Painful Prescription*: A procrustean perspective?: *N. Engl. J. Med.*, 314:1383–1386, 1986.
3. Schwartz, W. B. & Aaron, H. J.: The Painful Prescription: *N. Engl. J. Med.*, 315:1169, 1968.
4. Bulfinch, p. 192.
5. Sidel, V. W. & Sidel, R.: *A Healthy State: An International Perspective on the Crisis in United States Medical Care*: New York, Pantheon, 1978.
6. Editorial: Rationing, justice and the American physician: *J.A.M.A.*, 255:1176–1177, 1986.
7. Stein, p. 1147.
8. Bywaters, E. G. L.: The Cheshire Cat syndrome: *Postgrad. Med. J.*, 44:19–22, 1968.
9. Harian, S.: Cartoon: *USA Today*, Feb. 24, 1987, p. 104.

Promethean Genes

It has been postulated that some genes provide a connection between heredity and culture, a gene-culture coevoluton.[1] The human mind absorbs the existing culture and creates new culture which in turn alters biological processes. "Cultural innovations acted as a new class of mutations that accelerated evolution and pushed the species forward to its present genetic position."[1]

In Greek mythology, Prometheus was one of the Titans, a gigantic race which inhabited the earth before man.[2] He and his brother, Epimetheus, were given the task by the gods to create man and give him and all other animals the facilities for preservation. Epimetheus gave many physical and mental gifts to animals, but had nothing left to provide for man's superiority over animals. With Minerva's aid, Prometheus, went up to heaven and lit his torch at the chariot of the sun. He then gave humans the gift of fire. Jupiter became enraged at this theft, and created woman as man's punishment for accepting Prometheus's gift. The first woman, Pandora, was endowed with many gifts including beauty, and Epimetheus was tricked into marrying her. Prometheus, however, was punished by being chained to Mount Caucasus where a vulture ate away his liver, which was renewed as fast as it was devoured. Because he

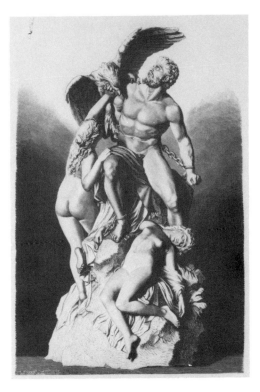

Promethean Genes The chained Prometheus with ocean nymphs and attacking eagle.[12]

refused to submit to his oppressor, Prometheus was condemned to experience pain forever. Finally, Hercules killed the vulture and set Prometheus free.

Presumably an effect of culture on genes would have a beneficial effect on humanity, as did the fire which was brought by Prometheus. The concept of Promethean Genes is a compromise between the rigid viewpoint that the environment has no influence on heredity, and Lysenko's teachings that the environment is predominant in inheritance.[3] The phrase, the Curse of Prometheus, has been used in the sense that he was punished for using foresight in obtaining fire for man; foresight being equated with the development of an immune system which can generate numerous random antigen-binding sites.[4] The curse is that this is placed under the surveillance of natural selection—resulting in a rather convoluted eponym.

Prometheus Bound is the name of a play by Aeschylus, written in the fourth century B.C.[5] Percy Shelley's major poem, *Prometheus Unbound*,[6] has been interpreted as a father-son conflict, as occurred between Jupiter and Prometheus, with resultant phallic assertiveness and fears of castration by the son.[7] In both the ancient and later versions, Prometheus is depicted as a heroic figure. Another poet, William Carlos Williams, has been called an "embattled Prometheus" because of the embittered, assertive, and rebellious nature of some of his essays.[8] The subtitle of Mary Shelley's *Frankenstein* is "A Modern Prometheus," presumably because he was given life by fire (in the form of electricity) as an innocent creature until goaded into destructive behavior.[9]

A more general use of Prometheus's name is as an adjective. Promethean is defined as anything that is life giving in a daringly original or creative fashion.[10] Thus, "test tube babies" might be called a promethean undertaking. In science fiction, Lem has given the name Prometheus to the space ship that made an audacious round trip from earth to Fomalhaut, twenty-three light years away.[11]

1. Lumsden, C. J. & Wilson, E. O.: *Promethean Fire. Reflections on the Origins of Mind.*: Cambridge, Massachusetts, Harvard University Press, 1983, pp. 56, 117–119, 181–183.

2. Bulfinch, pp. 19–28.
3. *Encyclopaedia Britannica*: VI:420.
4. Ohno, S. et al.: The curse of Prometheus is laid upon the immune system: *Prog. Allergy*, 22:8–39, 1981.
5. Aeschylus: *Prometheus Bound*: G. Murray translator, London, George Allen & Unwing, 1931.
6. Shelley, P. B.: *The Complete Poetical Works of Percy Bysshe Shelley*: Cambridge edition, Boston, Houghton Mifflin, 1901.
7. Waldoff, L.: The father-son conflict in Prometheus Unbound: *Psychoanal. Rev.*, 62:79–96, 1975.
8. Breslin, J. E. B.: *William Carlos Williams. An American Artist*: Chicago, University of Chicago Press, 1985, p. 16.
9. Shelley.
10. Espy, p. 33.
11. Lcm, S.: *Return From the Stars*: New York, Harcourt Brace Jovanovich, 1980, p. 28.
12. Brewer, 3:248.

Prometheus the Impostor

The eponym Prometheus the Impostor[1] has been used as the title of a detailed review of a book, *Betrayers of the Truth*,[2] which indicts the whole system of science because of some instances of fraudulent claims. The review does not deny deceit in science, but that human infallibility is unavoidable— ". . . we need not protect science against any tempting ideas, only against immoral scientific practices."[1] René Dubos has used the same theme in a more general context. " . . . as far as the unjustified promises about cancer are concerned, such promises are really a form of dishonesty . . . that's deemed justified because the goal is praiseworthy."[3]

Prometheus the Impostor could be considered as a metaphor for the scientist who can and does bring blessings to mankind, although occasionally the blessing may be fraudulent. The comparison is to Prometheus who benefited the human race by stealing fire from the sun. But, in doing so he was dishonest, having committed a crime against the gods, and so is the fraudulent scientist, at least against humanity. It has been pointed out that there were only four known instances of scientific fraud in 18,000 research projects funded in one year by the National Institutes of Health, and these were not related to crucial issues.[4]

In a more positive sense, Benjamin Franklin has been called the "modern Prometheus" because of his capture of the electricity of lightning descending from the heavens in his famous kite experiment of 1752.[5] Legislation that separates private practice from the National Health Service in Britain has been called a Promethean effort because it creates benefits without regard for the inevitable deficits caused by duplication of facilities.[6] Prometheus's risking the wrath of gods by stealing fire for the sake of humanity has been used as an example of the commitment needed for members of the National Health Service Corps.[7] The conflict for geriatrics between the enormous and expensive technology needed for medical therapy and the scarcity of sufficient economic sources to provide them at will has been called the confrontation of Prometheus and Malthus.[8] Attacks on medicine from many directions have been called new chains for Prometheus,[9] thus equating the punishment of Prometheus for benefiting man with the constraints placed upon health care delivery.

Similar to the Promethean myth was the explanation, in more primitive times, of why mankind appeared to be superior to other creatures and yet suffered and died.[10] His suffering of pain forever has been compared with man's exaggerated fear that when death comes it will be neither quick nor painless.[11] It has been this fear that led to Natural Death Acts which allow refusal by terminally ill patients of extraordinary therapeutic measures to prolong life. More philosophical is the use of the title *Prometheus Experiment* for a collection of poems by Bernard Strehler.[12] They relate to the desire for synthesis between the ideas of science, the perceptions of our emotions, and the need to know the meaning of existence.

1. Laor, N.: Occasional review: Prometheus the impostor: *Br. Med. J.*, 290:681–684, 1985.
2. Broad, W. & Wade, N.: *Betrayers of the Truth. Fraud and Deceit in the Halls of Science*: New York, Simon & Schuster, 1982.
3. Dubos, R. & Escande, J.-P.: *Quest. Reflections on Medicine, Science, and Humanity*: P. Ranum translator, New York, Harcourt Brace Jovanovich, 1979, p. 42.
4. Thomas, L.: "Falsity and Failure": in *Late Night Thoughts on Listening to Mahler's Ninth Symphony*: New York, Viking Press, 1983, pp. 108–113.

5. Roth, N.: Benjamin Franklin, the 'modern Prometheus': *Med. Instrum.*, 11:32–33, 1977.
6. Woodhouse, D. F.: Politics and Prometheus: *Lancet*, 1:1350, 1976.
7. Scutchfield, F. D.: Prometheus and Sisyphus: Medical Mythology: *Pharos*, 43:16–18, 1980.
8. Avorn, J.: Benefit and cost analysis in geriatric care. Turning age discrimination into health policy: *N. Engl. J. Med.*, 310:1294–1301, 1984.
9. Vaisrub, S.: New chains for Prometheus: *J.A.M.A.*, 229:1213–1214, 1974.
10. Bova, B.: "The Role of Science Fiction" in *Science Fiction Today and Tomorrow*, R. Bretnor, Ed., Baltimore, Penguin Books, 1974.
11. Dowben, C.: Prometheus revisited: Popular myths, medical realities, and legislative actions concerning death: *J. Health Politics Policy Law*, 5:250–276, 1980.
12. Strehler, B. L.: The Prometheus experiment: *Perspect. Biol. Med.*, 11:293–324, 1968.

Proteus

(protean)

Proteus is the name of a genus of gram-negative bacteria that are usually straight rods, but which can assume coccoid forms, filaments, and spheroblasts under certain conditions.[1] Characteristic of the genus is spontaneous swarming on solid surfaces of most strains. The four species of *Proteus* that are most pathogenic are *P. vulgaris*, *P. mirabilis*, *P. morganii*, and *P. rettgeri*.[2] They cause such infections as cellulitis, prostatitis, pyelonephritis, and septicemia.[2]

The bacillus is named after Proteus, the old man of the sea who tended Neptune's flocks of seals.[3] He had the gift of prophesy. At midday Proteus rose from the sea and slept in the shade of rocks. Anyone wishing to find out the future from him had to catch him at that time. To escape having to prophesize, he assumed every possible shape, including a wild boar, a tiger, or a raging fire. If he still could not escape, he resumed his real form, prophesized, and returned to the sea.

Like the Greek god, *Proteus* organisms can assume many shapes and can even foretell the future of infected patients—insofar as the result of testing cultures of *Proteus* organisms for susceptibility or resistance to antibiotics. In the vernacular as well as the medical, the adjective protean is applied to anything that can readily assume many shapes.[4] Richard Burton in his book of 1621 on melancholy posited that "Proteus himself is not so diverse [as melancholy]."[5]

A more modern text states that "The microscopic appearances of nephroblastoma are protean."[6]

1. Buchanan, R. E. & Gibbons, N. E., Eds.: *Bergey's Manual of Determinative Bacteriology*: 8th ed., Baltimore, Williams & Wilkins, 1974, p. 327.
2. Berkow, pp. 5, 99.
3. Bulfinch, p. 494.
4. Espy, p. 41.
5. Burton, R.: *The Anatomy of Melancholy. What It Is*: London, Thomas Tegg, 1845.
6. Bennington, J. L. & Beckwith, J. B.: *Tumors of the Kidney, Renal Pelvis and Ureter*: Washington, Armed Forces Inst. Pathol., 1975, p. 60.

Proteus Syndrome

The designation of the Proteus Syndrome was given to an apparently new syndrome described in four children in 1983 by Wiedemann and others.[1] Components are partial gigantism of hands, feet, and some digits; and the presence of skin nevi, keratotic areas, subcutaneous tumors, macrocephaly, and bony growths of the skull. Also present may be hemihypertrophy and accelerated growth. There have been similar cases reported before the specific designation of the syndrome.[2] Some of the abnormalities are present at birth and others develop during infancy and early childhood. None have had positive family histories. By 1975, thirteen reported cases were included under this designation, two of which also had pelvic lipomatosis.[3]

The name of the Greek god Proteus has been used for this syndrome because it presents a marked variability (polymorphous) from case-to-case, as did Proteus's appearance from time-to-time (see Proteus). Such variability has resulted in confusion with other soft tissue syndromes which involve skin, connective tissue, fat, and bone.[4] Although overgrowth of limbs may occur in neurofibromatosis, neurofibromata have not been found in patients with the Proteus Syndrome.[5]

A well-known patient of the nineteenth century exemplifies some of the difficulties in differentiating between similar syndromes. Joseph Merrick, the Elephant Man, was recently labeled as an example of neurofibromatosis.[6] However, it has now been suggested that he suffered from the Proteus Syndrome because there is no evidence that he had neurofibrous tumors, and because his soft tissue changes were very bizarre.[7] He had typical features of the Proteus Syndrome, such as macrocephaly, hyperostosis of the skull, thick skin and subcutaneous tissues, and lipomas. It is possible that these patients with soft tissue and bony overgrowths do not represent separate, distinct entities but are variable manifestations along a spectrum of change (see Quasimodo's Tumor).

1. Wiedemann, H. R. et al.: The Proteus syndrome: *Eur. J. Pediatr.*, 140:5–12, 1983.
2. Lezama, D. B. & Buyse, M. L.: The Proteus syndrome. The emergence of an entity: *J. Clin. Dysmorphol.*, 12:10–13, 1884.
3. Costa, T.: Proteus syndrome: Report of two cases with pelvic lipomatosis: *Pediatrics*, 76:984–989, 1985.
4. Riccardi, V. M.: Von Recklinghausen neurofibromatosis: *N. Engl. J. Med.*, 305:1617–1627, 1981.
5. Cohen, M. M., Jr. & Hayden, P. W.: A newly recognized hamartomatous syndrome: *Birth Defects Original Article Series*, 15:291–296, 1979.
6. Rai, G. S. & Coni, N. K.: The "Elephant Man" of Cambridge. A case report of neurofibromatosis: *J. Am. Geriatr. Soc.*, 29:129–130, 1981.
7. Tibbles, J. A. R. & Cohen, M. M., Jr.: The Proteus syndrome: The Elephant Man diagnosed: *Br. Med. J.*, 293:683–685, 1986.

Psyche

(psychology[1])

Psyche is a somewhat obsolete term for the subjective aspects of the mind and of the individual.[2] It is also used as the prefix for many related medical words. In Greek mythology, Psyche, the daughter of a king, was the personification of fervent emotion.[1] She had such wonderous beauty that crowds of people came from many countries to see and pay homage to her.[3] Venus (Aphrodite), the goddess of beauty, was so greatly offended that she asked her son, Cupid (Eros), to have Psyche develop a passion for a mean and lowly person. Cupid, however, erred and fell in love with Psyche himself. Henceforth Venus frowned upon Psyche, so that no one would ask for her in marriage. She became lonely and sick of the beauty which received flattery but did not arouse love.

Psyche's parents consulted the oracle of Apollo, who stated that Psyche was destined to be the bride of a monster, who awaited her on the top of a mountain. There she lived in a

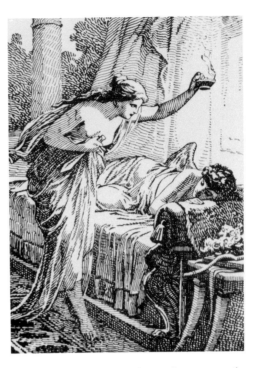

Psyche Psyche disobeying the warning not to see her husband.[8]

magnificent palace where she heard her husband's voice but never saw him, as he only came at night. One night she lighted a lamp above her sleeping husband, and found him to be Cupid. He vanished, and so did the palace. She was then subjected to many horrible ordeals by the angry Venus but overcame them. Finally, Cupid implored Zeus to help Psyche. Zeus consented and conferred immortality on Psyche. She and Cupid were finally united on Mount Olympus amid great rejoicing.

The Greek word for breath is psyche, derived from Cupid's beloved. It signifies life, the source of all vital activities of man and the soul or spirit—in distinction from his material aspects.[1] The phrase Psyche task is derived from the seemingly impossible tasks set for her as punishment by the jealous Venus,[4] and is similar to the eponym Sisyphean Task (see Sisyphean Reaction).

A Hans Christian Andersen story is named "Psyche" after the statue made by a struggling artist who was inspired by a lovely girl he had seen.[5] When she rejected him, his life was devastated, and he died unfulfilled. Centuries later, the statue was unearthed and considered to be a masterpiece, although the artist was not known. The moral is that "What belongs to heaven shines in its creator and, when he dies, his Psyche lives still."[5]

A derivative word from psyche is psychic, which has been given a confusing variety of meanings ranging from the human mind to the supernatural.[6] Dryer has listed the following applications of the word psychic—acupuncture, biofeedback, spiritism, meditation, prayer, laying on of hands, voodoo, satanic possession and the evil eye.[7]

1. OED: VII:1549–1552.
2. Stedman, p. 1163.
3. Bulfinch, pp. 100–112.
4. Weekley, p. 1163.
5. Andersen, H. C.: "Psyche": in *Hans Christian Andersen. The Complete Fairy Tales and Stories*, E. C. Haugaard translator, Garden City, New York, Doubleday, 1974, pp. 785–795.
6. Stein, p. 1160–1162.
7. Dryer, B. V.: *A Symbolic Triangle: Hippocrates, Psyche and Pandora*: Philadelphia, Society Health Human Values, 1978.
8. Gayley, p. 130.

Pygmalion Complex

The guidance-cooperation model of physician-patient relationships[1] includes several subsets, one of which involves the attempt by one person (the physician) to shape another person (the patient) to be more like one's ideal image for that person.[2] This approach may contribute to noncompliance of the patient because of differences in expectations or of insults to the self-esteem of the patient.

The related complex is named after Pygmalion, a Greek god who saw much to blame in women and resolved never to marry.[3] He was a sculptor and made an ivory statue of a woman more beautiful than any living. He fell so in love with his statue that he clothed it and gave it presents of beads and jewels. Pygmalion laid the statute on a couch and called it his wife. At a festival of Venus he asked the gods for a wife like his ivory statue. Venus heard him, and when he returned home the statue was alive. She was named Galatea and their union resulted in a son, Paphos, after whom the city sacred to Venus was named.

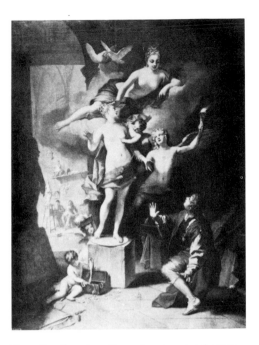

Pygmalion Complex Pygmalion observing the transformation of Galatea.[15]

The Pygmalion Complex refers to the making over of an individual to suit the likes of another. It does not seem quite appropriate as an eponym related to possible noncompliance because Galatea was very compliant. Not as compliant is Eliza of the 1913 play by George Bernard Shaw, *Pygmalion*,[4] in which Professor Henry Higgins, a teacher of phonetics, transformed a Cockney flower girl, Eliza Doolittle, into his concept of an elegant woman, only to have her fall in love with him. Unlike Pygmalion, he does not marry her. Shaw's altered myth was made into a very successful musical comedy, *My Fair Lady*, in 1957.[5] "What could possibly matter more than to take a human being and change her into a different human being . . . ?" The theme is not unique to Shaw. It is also found in an eighteenth century novel by Tobias Smollett, an English physician.[6] His novel, *The Adventures of Peregrine Pickle*, contains an episode in which a gypsy is taught to speak "proper" English.[7]

Named after Shaw's Eliza Doolittle is ELIZA, the acronym for a natural language computer program designed to function as a nondirective psychological therapist.[8] As occurs with the works of well-known authors, Pygmalion has been the basis for a psychoanalytic analysis of Shaw's childhood.[9]

Pygmalion in the Classroom[10] is the title of a book which applies to education the well-known psychological principle that people are affected by the expectations which others hold about them.[11] Studies of such expectations in the classroom have demonstrated that achievement expectations relate to achievement outcomes, including sex-related expectations for subjects such as mathematics.[12] Galactea, Pygmalion's beautiful statue, and Golem, the mechanical monster of Hasadic myth, have been evoked as positive and negative effects, respectively, of biased and unbiased expectations of their teachers on student outcomes.[13]

The eponym Pygmalionism has been applied to a psychotherapist who treats patients as children because he or she assumes that they know little or nothing.[14] Pygmalionism is also the name given to a fetish in which the sex object is a dressmaker's mannequin, the equivalent of Pygmalion's statue.

1. Szasz, T. S. & Hollender, M. H.: A contribution to the philosophy of medicine. The basic models of the doctor-patient relationship: *Arch. Int. Med.*, 97:585–592, 1956.
2. Stone, G. C.: Patient compliance and the role of the expert: *J. Social Issues*, 35:34–39, 1979.
3. Bulfinch, pp. 79–80.
4. Shaw, G. B.: *Pygmalion*: in *Pygmalion and Other Plays*: New York, Dodd, Mead, 1967, pp. 3–120.
5. Lerner, A. J. & Loewe, F.: *My Fair Lady*: New York, Coward-McCann, 1956.
6. Mannion, R. A.: Tobias George Smollett, 1721–1771: *J. Indiana State Med. Assoc.*, 71:706–709, 1978.
7. Smollett, T.: *The Adventures of Peregrine Pickle. In Which are Included, Memoirs of a Lady of Quality*: London, D. Wilson, 1751.
8. Jones, A. H.: Psychiatrists on Broadway, 1974–1982: *Lit. Med.*, 4:128–140, 1985.
9. Weissman, P.: Shaw's childhood and *Pygmalion*: *Psychoanal. Study Child.*, 13:541–561, 1958.
10. Rosenthal, R. & Jacobson, L.: *Pygmalion in the Classroom*: New York, Holt, Rinehart & Winston, 1968.
11. Zanna, M. P., Sheras, P. L. & Cooper, J.: Pygmalion and Galatea: The interactive effect of teacher and student expectancies: *J. Exp. Social Psychol.*, 11:279–287, 1977.
12. Smead, V. S.: Pygmalion vs. Galatea: Expectations of eighth grade girls and boys and their significant others as they relate to achievement

in mathematics class: *Dissert. Abstr.*, 37:7051–A, May, 1977.

13. Babad, E.Y. et al.: Pygmalion, Galatea, and the Golem: Investigations of biased and unbiased teachers: *J. Ed. Psychol.*, 74:459–474, 1982.

14. Campbell, p. 526.

15. Brewer, 3:262.

Q

Quasimodo Syndrome

A study of five patients who were hunchbacked as a result of kyphoscoliosis revealed three with complaints of disturbed sleep. They also had hypopnea and apnea associated with oxygen desaturation.[1] It is postulated that the respiratory abnormalities that occur in kyphoscoliotic patients while awake are increased in REM sleep during which the intercostal and accessory respiratory muscles are inhibited.

The source of the eponym is Victor Hugo's *The Hunchback of Notre Dame*,[2] published in 1830. One of Hugo's best known creations is its antihereo, Quasimodo. He was a deformed bellringer who was devoted to Esmeralda, a beautiful gypsy girl. Quasimodo hid Esmeralda in the belfry of Notre Dame, in order to save her from being burnt as a witch. She had been denounced as a witch by the archdeacon, Claude Frollo, whose passion for her she had rejected. Esmeralda was finally found and executed. Quasimodo then killed Frollo by throwing him from the heights of Notre Dame.

The character Quasimodo only resembles the syndrome in respect to having a hunchback; respiratory difficulties are not described. This did not, however, prevent the coiners of the syndrome from suggesting that Hugo may have described Quasimodo as a hunchback in order to explain his gentle yet heroic personality and behavior—on the basis of the long-term action of sleep-related hypoxemia on brain function.[1] This presupposes that Hugo had such knowledge in the nineteenth century.

1. Guilleminault, C. et al.: Severe kyphoscoliosis, breathing, and sleep. The "Quasimodo" syndrome during sleep: *Chest*, 79:626–630, 1981.
2. Hugo, V. W.: *The Hunchback of Notre Dame*: New York, Dodd, Mead, 1947.

Quasimodo's Tumor

(facial hamartoma)

Facial deformities can be caused by tumors of the skin, such as lymphangiomas and neurofibromas.[1] These two entities have some gross and microscopic similarities that could warrant their designation as mixed hamartomas.[2] Such lesions can produce extensive and grotesque disfigurements of the face and other body parts, as was described by Victor Hugo for Quasimodo, the grotesque yet gentle hunchback of Notre Dame. " . . . the right [eye] was completely overwhelmed and buried by an enormous wen; . . . [the] horny lip, over which one of those teeth projected, like the tusk of an elephant; . . . [the] forked chin; and, above all, the expression overlying the whole—an indefinable mixture of malice, bewilderment, and melancholy."[3]

Neurofibromatosis has been suggested as being depicted by Quasimodo's deformities, including his tetrahedral nose, horny lip, an enormous hump, warped thighs, broad feet, and monstrous hands.[4] Neurofibromatosis is an autosomal dominant disorder in which there is considerable variation in manifestations and complications, including peripheral and central neurofibromas,[5] The grotesque appearance of the nonfictional Elephant Man, John (Joseph) Merrick,[6,7] has been attributed to neurofibromatosis,[8,9] along with a related disorder, fibrous dysplasia (see Proteus Syndrome).[10] In either instance, the real or the fictional, there can exist behind the grotesque exterior an inner warm and intelligent being,[11] who responds to consideration and kindness.[12] Both Hugo's Quasimodo and Doctor Treves' patient, Merrick, died as a consequence of socialization.[13]

A related physical deviation is that of the elephant-headed Hindu god, Ganesa, son of Siva and Parvati.[14] In literature, however, it is malevolent characters who are depicted more commonly as having physical deformities.[15] Quasimodo is a noteworthy exception because

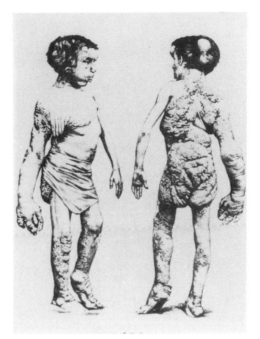

Quasimodo's Tumor Joseph Merrick, the Elephant Man, in 1884, at the age of 24.[6, pl. 20]

his intentions were noble in spite of his monstrous deformities.

The Quasimodo Complex has been defined as "emotional conflict, personality disorder, or social maladaption developing as a result of disfigurement."[16] Theatrical presentations based on severely deformed individuals, such as Quasimodo and Merrick, have been considered as beneficial because they engender mutual understanding between the sufferer and the nonsufferer, including physicians.[13]

1. Crikelair, G. F. & Cosman, B.: Histologically benign, clinically malignant lesions of the head and neck: *Plastic Reconstr. Surg.*, 42:343–354, 1968.
2. McDowell, F.: Facial hamartoma, or Quasimodo's Tumor: *Plastic Reconstr. Surg.*, 42:369–370, 1968.
3. Hugo, V. W.: *The Hunchback of Notre Dame*: New York, Dodd, Mead, 1947, pp. 48–49.
4. Cox, J.: Quest for Quasimodo: *Br. Med. J.*, 291:1801–1803, 1985.
5. Huson, S. M.: The different forms of neurofibromatosis: *Br. Med. J.*, 249:1113–1114, 1987.
6. Treves, F.: A case of congenital deformity: *Trans. Pathol. Soc. Lond.*, 26:492–498, 1884–1885.
7. Howell, M. & Ford, P.: *The True History of the Elephant Man*: Harmondswork, Middlesex, England, Penguin Books, 1980.
8. Zapatka, F.: The Elephant Man: *Plastic Reconstr. Surg.*, 69:563–564, 1982.
9. Rai, G. S. & Coni, N. K.: The "Elephant Man" of Cambridge. A case report of neurofibromatosis: *J. Am. Geriatr. Soc.*, 29:129–130, 1981.
10. Bean, W. B. et al.: A nonletter from the editor and a case for all seasons: *Semin. Roentgen.*, 17:153–162, 1982.
11. Karp, L. E.: The Elephant Man: *Am. J. Med. Genet.*, 10:1–3, 1981.
12. Waldron, G.: Sir Frederick Treves and the Elephant Man: *Lancet*, 2:42, 1980.
13. Belli, A.: Mortality and medicine on the modern stage: *Pharos*, 47:11–16, 1984.
14. *Encyclopaedia Britannica*: IV:407.
15. Thurer, S.: Disability and monstrosity: A look at literary distortions of handicapping conditions: *Rehab. Lit.* 41:12–15, 1980.
16. Campbell, p. 123.

Queen of Hell Syndrome

In some instances, the love between mother and child may result in severe depression in the mother.[1] Characteristic backgrounds of these women include periods of sexual acting out alternating with living as a docile daughter with their mothers; being very close to indulgent mothers during childhood; isolation from childhood peers; first child born when 16 to 18 years of age; and erratic work history.

The derivation of the eponym is from Greek mythology. The Queen of Hell Syndrome is based on the same mother-daughter relationship as the Persephone Syndrome.[2] The orientation of the latter, however, is on the separation of immigrant Greek wives (Persephone) from their mothers (Ceres) who remain in the homeland. In the Queen of Hell Syndrome, the relationship to the myth is Persephone's being forced into an adult role as a result of her abduction by Hades while still an adolescent. Ceres found her daughter and reached a compromise. Persephone would be the Queen of Hell (during the winter), and the obedient daughter of Ceres (during spring and summer). It is such a duality of roles that leads to the psychological abnormalities, and provides a fairly good "fit" with the eponym.

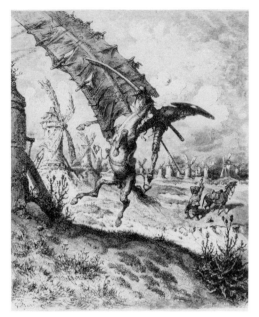

(A)

1. Crockett, M. S.: The Queen of Hell syndrome: Social isolation, teenage pregnancy, and depression: *Health Care Women Int.*, 5:125–143, 1984.
2. Dundas, N. & Nikelly, G.: The Persephone syndrome. A study of conflict in the adaptive process of married Greek female immigrants in the U.S.A.: *Social Psychiatry*, 7:211–216, 1972.

Quixotic Medicine

(quixotism[1])

Physicians and the medical establishment before the twentieth century had little in the way of specific cures for disease. They exhibited a relatively high degree of quackery, and were often more interested in their income than in patient welfare.[2] Fault finders with the traditional system were called traitors and heretics, as was Cervantes, the creator of the deluded knight errant, Don Quixote. Quixote was so crazed by the constant reading of romances of chivalry that he believed that he was called upon to right all the wrongs of the world.[3] He imagined evil everywhere, mistaking windmills for giants, and flocks of sheep for armies.

The justification for the eponym Quixotic Medicine is that Cervantes fought against the evils of corruption in Spain in the seventeenth century. The eponym relates to the ignorance and corruption of medical practitioners of the

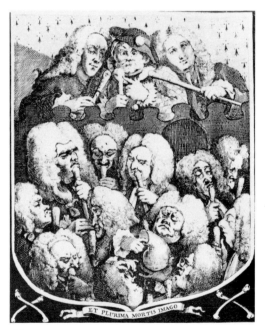

(B)

Quixotic Medicine A. Don Quixote tilting at the monstrous windmills.[11] (by Gustav Doré, 1863) (by permission, Dover Pubns., Inc.) **B.** The Company of Undertakers–a 1736 satire of quack physicians.[12] (by William Hogarth, 1737) (by permission, Dover Pubns., Inc.)

time rather than only to the behavior of Don Quixote, who tilted at supposed evil windmills. Thus, Quixotic Medicine is a mixed eponym, referring to both the corrupt medicine of the seventeenth century and the ill-used fault finders who "Cassandra-like . . . prophesy evil to mocking audiences."[2]

It was not only those who found fault with traditional medicine who were dealt with harshly, but also those who pioneered new concepts, such as Jenner, Semmelweis, Pasteur, and Bernard.[4] *The Adventures of Don Quixote de la Mancha*[3] has also been interpreted as "an ironic story of an idealist frustrated and mocked in a materialistic world."[5] It is possibly in this sense that Norman Cousins refers to "the underlying resentments that are sometimes part of the physician's quixotic attitudes towards his patients."[6] More generally, the label of quixotic is applied to someone who is idealistic without regard to practicality.[7] The great Spanish neurological anatomist Santiago Ramón y Cajal (1852–1934) has been called the Don Quixote of the microscope because of his unorthodox, rebellious, and imaginative behavior, both scientifically and personally.[8]

Knight errantry, as satirized by Cervantes, had many risks, not the least of which were severe wounds.[9] Quixote considered skill "in physic, especially in the botanical part of it" to be necessary for such knights. In fact he had the formula for an elixir "one drop of which would heal all wounds as perfect as if they had never been made." More related to the eponym, Quixotic Medicine, are statements by Quixote's squire, Sancho. "A doctor gives his advice by the pulse of your pocket." " . . . she [a peasant] was killed by a damned doctor who gave her a purge when she was a child." Thomas Sydenham, the great seventeenth century English clinician, was asked what to read to learn medicine; he replied, Don Quixote, probably referring more to the humanistic orientation of the book than to its medical content (see Don Quixote Syndrome).[10]

1. OED: VIII:75.
2. Kahn, R. G. & Kahn, M.: Quixotic medicine: *Med. Life*, 33:170–194, 1926.
3. Cervantes, M.: *The Adventures of Don Quixote de la Mancha*: New York, Dodd, Mead, 1971.

4. Radner, D. B.: The intolerance of great men: *Med. Hist.*, 5(ns):561–565, 1932.
5. Benét, pp. 280–281.
6. Cousins, N., Ed.: *The Physician in Literature*: Philadelphia, W. B. Saunders, 1982, p. xvii.
7. Editors of the American Heritage Dictionaries, pp. 197–198.
8. Williams, H.: *Don Quixote of the Microscope*: London, Cope, 1954.
9. Head, J. R.: Medical allusions in Don Quixote: *Ann. Med. Hist.*, 6:169–179, 1934.
10. Literature and medicine: *MD*, Aug., 1962, pp. 115–119.
11. Doré, G.: *Doré's Illustrations of Don Quixote*: New York, Dover, 1982, p. 11.
12. Hogarth, W.: "The Company of Undertakers": in Shesgreen, S., *Engravings by Hogarth*, New York, Dover, 1973, plate 40.

R

Raggedy Ann Syndrome

(chronic fatigue syndrome, chronic mononucleosislike syndrome)

A state of chronic debilitating fatigue has been recognized for about fifty years under a large variety of names.[1] It became a focus of interest when approximately ninety patients were studied and reported to the Centers for Disease Control by Peterson and Cheney.[2] These cases had occurred in Incline Village on the North Shore of Lake Tahoe from November 1984 through August 1985. Approximately 75% have occurred in women.[3] Age range is from twenty to fifty years. Excessive and at times overwhelming and disabling fatigue is the primary symptom of this disorder. It is often accompanied by muscle pains, short-term memory loss, difficulty in concentration, and in some patients, panic attacks, balance disorders, and apraxia. The fatigue is associated with lymphadenopathy, pharyngitis, and splenomegaly or hepatomegaly. In some patients, 2 to 4 mm multifocal defects in subcortical white matter may be seen with magnetic resonance imaging. Disabling daytime sleepiness in patients with similar symptoms has been given the awkward designation of idiopathic central nervous system hypersomnia,[4] probably an unnecessary term.

Because of the chronicity of the fatigue, and because it often follows acute episodes of infectious mononucleosis, patients with such complaints were tested for Epstein-Barr virus (EBV) antigen.[1] Elevated blood levels have been found in many. But this does not necessarily implicate a chronic EBV condition because such infection is almost universal.[5] Although EBV-specific antigens were higher in patients than in controls the differences were not statistically significant.[6] These patients may demonstrate some humoral and cellular responses that occur with EBV infection, but the association with the chronic fatigue syndrome may be coincidental rather than causal.[7] It has been postulated that a variant of the EBV is the basis for this illness.[8] In the past, most of these patients were considered to be suffering from a psychoneurotic disorder (see Oblomov Syndrome).[9]

The eponym Raggedy Ann Syndrome was used in a brief report[10] of a lengthy account of the Incline Village epidemic of the chronic fatigue syndrome. The latter was published in the journal *Hippocrates* in July, 1987.[11] It was titled "Raggedy Ann Town," derived from the statement of a female victim that "the overwhelming fatigue made her feel like a Raggedy Ann without stuffing." Raggedy Ann was created in 1917 as a character by Johnny Gruelle, an American newspaper cartoonist, for a series of children's books about Raggedy Ann's adventures.[12] In order to attract attention to the books, a Raggedy Ann doll was made and placed by the book display in a store window.[13] It has shoe-button eyes, a smile, and carrot-colored yarn hair. After 70 years, both the Raggedy Ann books and dolls are still popular. The equating of marked enervating fatigue with a stitched rag doll would appear to be appropriate, especially without its stuffing. The literary character is, however, described as having many adventures, some of which are quite energetic.

The chronic fatigue syndrome has also been called the "yuppie" flu, or plague, the acronym referring to young urban professionals because of an apparent propensity for such individuals.[11] One example is evident in a letter received by one of the authors from a friend.

I have, for me, sad news to impart. As of July 1st, 1987 my practice of medicine will be taken over by Dr. _____. Some time ago I developed a form of chronic mononucleosis. This is a rather newly described illness that has many manifestations. In me, the chief symptom is fatigue. I no longer have sufficient energy to take care of an expanding practice, the reading of 8 to 9 medical journals regularly, serving four rather widely spread hospitals, keeping up with the research groups I belong to, and going to two or more conventions a year.[14]

1. Holmes, G. P. et al.: A cluster of patients with a chronic mononucleosis-like syndrome. Is Epstein-Barr virus the cause? *J.A.M.A.*, 257:2297–2302, 1987.
2. Chronic fatigue possibly related to Epstein-Barr virus—Nevada: *MMWR*, 35:350–352, 1986.
3. Dwyer, B.: Chronic fatigue: A new immunosuppressive virus: *Psychiatr. Times*, 4:1, 21–22, 1987.
4. Guilleminault, C., & Mondini, S.: Mononucleosis and chronic daytime sleepiness: *Arch. Int. Med.*, 146:1333–1335, 1986.
5. Buchwald, D. et al.: Frequency of 'chronic active Epstein-Barr virus infection' on a general medical practice: *J.A.M.A.*, 257:2303–2307, 1987.
6. Merlin, T. L.: Chronic mononucleosis: Pitfalls in the laboratory diagnosis: *Human Pathol.*, 17:2–8, 1986.
7. Editorial: Enervating illness and Epstein-Barr virus: *Lancet*, 2:141–142, 1986.
8. Jones, J. F. et al.: Evidence for active Epstein-Barr virus infection in patients with persistent unexplained illness: Elevated early antigen antibodies: *Ann. Intern. Med.*, 102:1–7, 1985.
9. Straus, S. E.: EB or not EB—That is the question: *J.A.M.A.*, 257:2335–2336, 1987.
10. Donahue, D.: Magazines: *USA Today*, 7D, July 3, 1987.
11. Boly, W.: Raggedy Ann town: *Hippocrates*, 1:30–40, 1987.
12. Gruelle, J.: *The Raggedy Ann & Andy Storybook*: New York, Grosset & Dunlap, 1980.
13. Meyers, W. D.: "The Love Package": *McCall's*, 102:36–37, Dec., 1974.
14. Personal Communication to AER, 1987.

Rapunzel Syndrome

The Rapunzel Syndrome has been applied to long strands of hair which extend into the intestine and cause obstruction.[1] Such masses of hair are swallowed and can form large clumps in the stomach or intestine, which are called trichobezoars. Over two hundred cases of foreign material impacted in the stomach or intestine have been reported. Swallowing of hair in particular is usually found in young girls who are mentally defective or have psychiatric problems. Related is the pulling out of the hair (trichotillomania), which may be a reaction to serious family problems.[2]

The Rapunzel Syndrome is based upon a Grimm fairy tale. It begins with a man stealing some rampion (edible white tuber) from a witch's garden for his wife, who was barren.[3] He was caught by the witch, who said she would not punish him but would cause them to have a female child on the condition that the girl would be given to her. This occurred, and the witch claimed the beautiful Rapunzel, whom she shut up in a tower in a forest at the age of twelve. When the witch wished to visit Rapunzel she would cry out, "Rapunzel, Rapunzel! Let down thine hair!" The girl then unfastened her beautiful golden hair, twenty ells in length (about 75 feet), which the witch would then climb. A king's son heard the call on passing by and repeated it the next day. He climbed up the hair and fell in love with Rapunzel. When the witch found out, she cut off Rapunzel's hair and hid her in a desert. Then the witch fastened the cut hair to the tower. When the king's son climbed up and saw the witch he jumped from the tower, but fell on thorns, which put out his eyes. He wandered many years until he chanced on Rapunzel, and her tears restored his sight. "They lived long and happily."

The cutting of Rapunzel's hair has been considered as symbolic of patients who report thoughts of cutting their own hair.[4] On a psychiatric level, it represents castration, loss of the mother, and reparation. Elements of the Rapunzel story may represent a symbiotic mother-daughter relationship.[5] Another psychiatric interpretation is that of borderline personality. "Rapunzel . . . who might pass for normal except for her own recognition that, inside the false self represented by the tower in the woods, there was a person who felt essentially fragmented and who craved the completion of a self-object in the form of the rescuing prince."[6]

The eponym Rapunzel Syndrome is derived only from the fact that both the girl and some trichobezoars have long hairs. Rapunzel may have had a psychiatric disorder, but there is no indication that she ever swallowed her hair. It may occur with hair-biting, which is the equivalent of biting fingernails in nervous girls,[7] as Rapunzel may well have been, given her rather unique living conditions.

The generic term bezoar is derived from the arabic bazahr, meaning protection against poi-

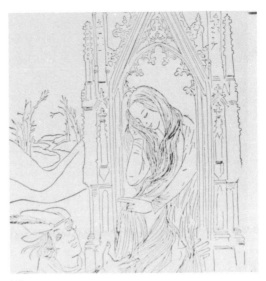

(A)

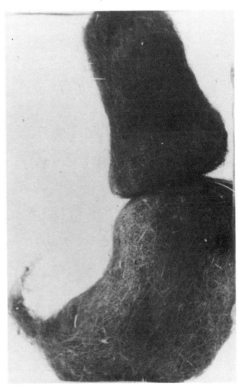

(B)

Rapunzel Syndrome **A.** The prince using Rapunzel's hair to reach her tower prison.[3, p. 71] **B.** Trichobezoar (hair mass) that completely filled a stomach.[13] (by permission A. Rodin)

259

son.[8] Thus, the bezoar-stone, an intestinal calculus found in some animals, was thought to have medicinal powers.[9] Bezoars may be composed not only of hair, but also of vegetable and fruit fibers (phytobezoar).[10] They may also be formed by tar, shellac, resin, string, wood, and rubber bands, or even gum.[11] A drug used for the treatment of acute duodenal ulcers may also be the culprit. Sulfcrate combines with hydrogen ions to form an ulcer-adherent complex that protects the ulcer against pesin and bile salts, but may become so excessive that it forms a large mass, a sulfcrate bezoar.[12]

1. Vaughan, E. D. Jr. et al.: The Rapunzel syndrome: An unusual complication of intestinal bezoar: *Surgery*, 63:339–343, 1968.
2. Kolb, p. 695.
3. Grimm, J. & Grimm, W.: "Rapunzel": in *Grimm's Fairy Tales*, Garden City, New York, Junior Deluxe Editions, n.d. pp. 69–74.
4. Andersen, J. J.: Rapunzel: The symbolism of the cutting of hair: *J. Am. Psychoanal. Assoc.*, 28:69–88, 1980.
5. Weimer, S. R.: Using fairy tales in psychotherapy. "Rapunzel": *Bull. Menninger Clin.*, 42:25–34, 1978.
6. Lonie, I.: From Humpty-Dumpty to Rapunzel: *Aust. N.Z. J. Psychiatry*, 19:372–381, 1985.
7. Gonzalez-Crussi, F.: Three forms of sudden death: New York, Harper & Row, 1986, pp. 91–93.
8. Thomas, p. 1772.
9. Weekley, p. 147.
10. Deslypere, J. P. et al.: An unusual case of trichobezoar: The Rapunzel syndrome: *Am. J. Gastroenterol.*, 77:467–470, 1982.
11. Ikard, R. W.: Bubble gum bezoar: *Surg. Rounds*, Feb., 1985, pp. 104–105.
12. Barnhart, E. R. pub.: *Physicians' Desk Reference*: 41st ed., Oradell, New Jersey, *Med. Econom.*, 1987, p. 1173.
13. Rodin, A. E.: *Oslerian Pathology*: Lawrence, Kansas, Coronado, 1981, p. 191.

Red Queen Hypothesis

"A change in the realized absolute fitness of one species is balanced by an equal and opposite net change in the realized absolute fitness of all interacting species considered together."[1] This relates to the ability of organisms to control the available trophic (nutritional) energy on which fitness depends.[2] Thus, evolution is depicted as keeping a balanced ecosystem even with the passage of time.

This hypothesis has been named after the Red Queen in Lewis Carroll's *Through the Look-*

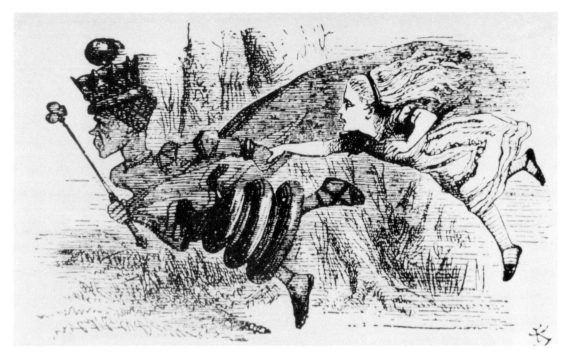

Red Queen Hypothesis   Alice and the Red Queen running as fast as they can to keep in the same place. (by John Tenniel) (Dodgson)

ing Glass,[3] whose country was "marked out just like a large chess board." Alice was standing in the second square and the Red Queen told her she could be the White Queen's pawn, and then become the Queen when she got to the eighth square. They then began to run very fast; but Alice noticed "that the trees never changed their places at all: however fast they went, they never seemed to pass anything. I wonder if all the things move along with us." The Red Queen said, "Now, *here*, you see, it takes all the running *you* can do, to keep in the same place. If you want to get somewhere else, you must run twice as fast as that."

The Red Queen eponym appears to be so named because, like the Red Queen, the hypothesis is that of a nonprogressive evolution in terms of maintaining a balanced, stable ecosystem, irrespective of the flight of time. Questioned has been the assumption implicit in the hypothesis that there is an all-pervading competition in nature at the expense of mutuality of coexistence,[4] and that it imparts a bias toward a linearity of extinction rate.[5]

Other studies, published under the title of

"Homage to the Red Queen,"[6] support the hypothesis that natural selection works in favor of a balance of nature. Coevolution of two species tends to enhance dynamic stability, although artificial enrichment erodes the stability. Events in the Red Queen's kingdom have also been applied to interferon research which is forced by decreased funding to run just to stay even.[7]

1. Van Allen, L.: Energy and evolution: *Evol. Theory*, 1:179–229, 1976.
2. Van Allen, L.: The Red Queen lives: *Nature*, 260:575, 1976.
3. Carroll, pp. 207–210.
4. Castrodeza, C.: Non-progressive evolution, the Red Queen hypothesis, and the balance of nature: *Acta Biotheoret.*, 28:11–18, 1979.
5. Hanam, A.: The Red Queen dethroned: *Nature*, 259:12–13, 1976.
6. Rosenzweig, M. L. & Schaffer, W. M.: Homage to the Red Queen. II. Coevolutionary response to enrichment of exploitation ecosystems: *Theoret. Pop. Biol.*, 14:158–163, 1978.
7. Friedman, R. M.: Interferon research in the Red Queen's kingdom: *Arch. Pathol.*, 98:73–75, 1974.

Rhesus Factor

(Rh factor)

The Rh factor is a blood antigen which is present in 85% of whites.[1] If an Rh-negative female is impregnated by an Rh-positive male, an Rh-positive fetus may be conceived. Rh incompatibility then occurs when the Rh-positive fetal red cells enter the material circulation, producing antibodies to them. When these Rh antibodies return to the fetus and destroy its red blood cells the resultant anemia constitutes erythroblastosis fetalis. This human blood group is now characterized by a complex of over thirty antigens and antibodies. The Rh factor is named after the rhesus monkey, which in turn was so named after a king of Greek mythology.[2]

Rhesus was the mythical king of Thrace, who came to the aid of the Trojans with a large army.[3] He was told by an oracle that Troy would be safe should his horses drink from the River Xanthus and feed upon the grass of the Trojan plains. Rhesus was, however, slain by Odysseus and Diomedes before this was done. Thrace was the name given by the ancient Greeks to that part of the Balkans between the Danube and the Aegean Sea.[4]

It was through experiments with the rhesus monkey that the Rh factor was first discovered in 1940. This species (*Macaca mulatta*) is one of the macaques found in India. It is widely used in research because of its high intelligence and motivation,[5] and as a popular performing animal in traveling menageries, annual fairs, and circuses.[6] Uncertain is why this species was named after King Rhesus, although Espy suggests (tongue-in-cheek no doubt) that it was because the Greeks made a "monkey" out of him.[7]

1. Wintrobe, M. M. et al.: *Clinical Hematology*: 8th ed., Philadelphia, Lea & Fibiger, 1981, p. 463.
2. OED: VIII:626.
3. Guirand 1964, p. 46.
4. *Encyclopaedia Britannica*: IX:976–977.
5. Bourne, G. H.: *Primate Odyssey*: New York, G. P. Putman & Sons, 1962, pp. 116, 126.
6. Berger, G.: *The Monkeys and Apes*: New York, Arco, 1985, p. 125.
7. Espy, p. 291.

Rip Van Winkle Syndrome

(hypersomnia)

Long-term hypersomnia of uncertain cause is quite rare.[1] It usually begins at puberty or later and then lasts for life. It may be familial. Unlike narcolepsy, hypersomnia is not irresistible, sleep usually lasts from several hours to several days, and it does not have sleep-onset REM periods.[2] Hypersomnia occurs on a periodic basis in the Klein-Levin Syndrome and the Pickwickian Syndrome. It may also be a symptom of depression, or represent an escape from everyday life. Pathological somnolence has been reported in patients with upper brain stem infarctions due to strokes.[3]

Rip Van Winkle[4] was the creation of Washington Irving in 1819. The main character is a henpecked husband who met dwarfs playing ninepins in the Catskill mountains before the Revolutionary War. He drank from their keg and fell asleep for twenty years. When he awoke he discovered that his wife was dead, his daughter married, and King George's picture replaced by that of George Washington. This folktale was used by Irving to contrast the new and old societies.[5] Oliver Wendell Holmes wrote a lengthy poem in 1870 on the same theme, *Rip Van Winkle, M.D.*, the theme being a satire of

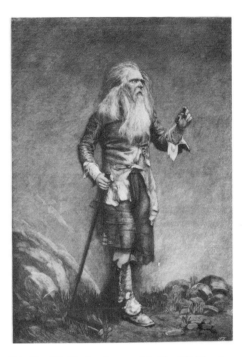

Rip Van Winkle Syndrome Rip Van Winkle after 20 years of sleep (portrayed by Jefferson).[10]

physicians who practice old-fashioned medicine.[6] Doctor Van Winkle slept for thirty years and awoke out of date, still using blood letting, leaches, and tartrate. This is evident in his description of treatment of the ailing Deacon.

Fever—that's certain—pleurisy, perhaps.
A quart of blood will ease the pain, no doubt,
Ten leaches next will help to suck it out,
Then clap a blister on the painful part—
But first two grains of *Antimonium Tart.*
Last with a dose of cleansing caromel
Unload the portal system—(that sounds well!)

The Rip Van Winkle experience has also been applied to a psychiatric syndrome of alienation.[7] In more common usage, an individual who is out of touch with the times is called a Rip Van Winkle.[8]

Related to the Rip Van Winkle theme is a still more extravagant example of hypersomnia, the myth of the Seven Sleepers of Epheus. They were Christian holy men who were sealed in a cave by an emperor. When the cave was opened 362 years later, they arose saying that they had been asleep for only one night.[9] The protector against insomnia and the patron saint of nightwatchmen is St. Pedro of Alcantara, who slept for only one-and-one-half hours each twenty-four hours.[9]

1. Cutler, E. A. & Marshall, J. R.: Rip Van Winkle Syndrome in Childhood: Familial Long-Term Hypersomnia: Original Articles Series, Annual Review of Birth Defects Symposium, March of Dimes Foundation, New York, Alan R. Liss, 14 (6B):367–368, 1978.
2. Freedman, p. 125.
3. Prendes, J. -L. & Rosenberg, S. J.: Rip Van Winkle syndrome: Confusion and irresistible somnolence after stroke: *South. Med. J.*, 79:1162–1164, 1986.
4. Irving, W.: *Rip Van Winkle*: Philadelphia, J. B. Lippincott, n.d.
5. Benét, p. 861.
6. Holmes, O. W.: "Rip Van Winkle, M.D.": in *The Poetical Works of Oliver Wendell Holmes*, Cambridge Edition revised, Boston, Houghton Mifflin, 1975, pp. 63–68.
7. Vaisrub, p. 22.
8. Espy, p. 340.
9. Murphy.
10. Brewer, 4:186.

Robin Hood Syndrome

(inverse cerebral steal)

When there is a decrease of circulating carbon dioxide in the blood (hypocarbia, hypocapnia) there is vasoconstriction of arterioles in normal areas of the brain with consequent increased flow to parts of the brain which have been damaged by acute cerebrovascular disease or tumors.[1] This has been called the inverse cerebral steal. The opposite of this happens in intracerebral steal in which increased carbon dioxide (hypercarbia) results in dilation of vessels in the normal brain, with consequent decreased blood flow to diseased areas of the brain (see Humpty Dumpty Phenomenon).[2]

Benevolent stealing, as occurs in the inverse cerebral steal, is symbolized by Robin Hood, an English legend dating from about the twelfth to fourteenth centuries.[3] It may have originated with Robert Hode, who fled the king's justices in York in 1225. According to ballads written on his adventures, Robin Hood was an outlawed earl who lived in Sherwood Forest in Nottinghamshire. He is now a folk hero who gave to the poor what he robbed from the rich. His main protagonist was the Sheriff of Nottingham.

Like Robin Hood, decrease in blood carbon dioxide robs blood from the rich (normal) brain tissue by causing its blood vessels to constrict, and thus diverts the richness of blood flow to the poor (abnormal) brain tissue. A false aneurysm of the right subclavian artery in a boy has been referred to as the Robin Hood Legacy because it was the result of an arrow wound inflicted in Old Sherwood Forest, Robin Hood's location.[4]

1. Lassen, N. A. & Pálvolgyi, R.: Cerebral steal during hypercapnia and the inverse reaction during hypocapnia observed by the ^{133}Xenon technique in man: *Scand. J. Lab. Clin. Invest.*, 22 (suppl. 102): 206, 1968.
2. Wollman, H.: The Humpty Dumpty phenomenon: *J. Anesthol.*, 33:379–381, 1970.
3. Holt, J. C.: *Robin Hood*: London, Thames & Hudson, 1982.
4. Earnshaw, J. J., Wenham, P. W. & Hopkinson, B. R.: Robin Hood's legacy: *Br. Med. J.*, 291:1766, 1985.

Romeo Error

Individuals may spontaneously revive even a few days after being wrongly certified as dead.[1] This was especially true before the development of electrocardiograms and electroencephalograms. Absence of electrical activity may, however, occur when absolute death is not present.

The eponym is named after Shakespeare's Romeo Montague, who fell in love with Juliet Capulet, a member of his family's enemy clan.[2] They were secretly married after Romeo killed Tybalt, the nephew of Lady Capulet, in a fight. Romeo then escaped to Mantua, where he heard that Juliet was dead, although actually she had only taken a potion to make her appear dead. Romeo went to her tomb and then poisoned himself to die at her side while lamenting.

Arms, take your last embrace! and, lips, you,
The doors of breath, seal with a righteous kiss
A dateless bargain to engrossing death! . . .
Here's to my love!
                                        [Drinks.
                    O true Apothecary!
Thy drugs are quick. Thus with a kiss I die.
                                        [Dies.

When Juliet awoke and found Romeo dead, she stabbed herself with his dagger. Perhaps the eponym should have been named after Juliet, who awoke after apparent death, although it was Romeo's error that led to their actual deaths.

There are many reports throughout history of supposedly dead individuals reviving spontaneously, some of whom had been buried, some during lying-in-state, and some on the dissecting table.[1] The death of Juliet was, however, only feigned, unlike the eponym, which indicates a nonpurposeful appearance resembling death. In the Lazarus complex death was contravened as a biblical miracle. Another biblical occurrence is the Elisha Method, the earliest example of resuscitation by mouth-to-mouth respiration.

The romantic tragedy of Romeo and Juliet has been psychoanalyzed as representing "the phenomenon of self-absorbed parents unable to respond to their children's strivings for greater selfhood."[3]

1. Watson, L.: *The Romeo Error. A Matter of Life and Death*: Garden City, New York, Doubleday, 1975.
2. Shakespeare, *Romeo and Juliet*: V, iii.
3. Muslin, H. L.: Romeo and Juliet: The tragic self in adolescence: *Adoles. Psychiatry*, 10:106–117, 1982.

Rumpelstiltskin Complex

Rejection of a child by parents may be overt or subtle. The latter appears in the form of praise, support, loyalty, or admiration.[1] An exaggerated overevaluation of their child's abilities can lead to serious psychological damage to a child's self-image. The results are frustrations and distortions of the parent-child relationship. Such distorted appreciation of one's child arises from an abnormal need for aggrandization, fulfilled by attributing to the child accomplishments which the parents themselves do not have.

The source of the eponym is the Grimm brothers' fairy tale *Rumpelstiltskin*.[2] A poor miller was so proud of his beautiful daughter that he bragged to the king that she could spin straw into gold. The king commanded that she be brought to court and do so. To comply, the girl made a pact with a dwarf to help her in return for giving up her first born to him. The king was so impressed by her apparent skill that he married her. A year later a child was born to them, and the dwarf came to claim the child. Because he had pity on the weeping mother, the dwarf offered to cancel the contract if she could tell him his name within a three-day period. She sent a messenger throughout the land for all the names he could find. On the third day the messenger encountered a comical little man singing a song which included his name, Rumpelstiltskin. The dwarf was so distressed when the queen told him his name that he stamped his left foot in such a fury that he split in two.

The child in the Rumpelstiltskin Complex is the beautiful daughter and the parent is the miller who greatly exaggerated her spinning skills. The fairy story can be criticized as highlighting materialistic values, such as the desire for gold, the absence in pride of workmanship, and the reliance on magical, mechanistic solutions.[1] The Rumpelstiltskin theme has also been interpreted as symbolic of "the facade of the innocent, virginal girl who achieves the trappings of womanhood and motherhood at the expense of those around her and who are indeed party to her efforts . . . . It conveys man's fear of woman's power. . . ."[3]

Also related to psychiatry is the so-called Principle of Rumpelstiltskin, which states that using the right word for the patient's disease is therapeutic in itself.[4] It conveys to the patient that someone of considerable status understands the condition and thus allays anxiety even if the words may have little meaning.

1. Katz, L.: The Rumpelstiltskin complex: *Contemp. Psychoanal.*, 10:117–124, 1974.
2. Grimm, J. & Grimm, W.: "Rumpelstiltskin": in *Grimm's Fairy Tales*. illustrated by L. Weisgard, Garden City, New York, Junior Deluxe Editions, pp. 232–237, n.d.
3. Rinsley, D. B. & Bergmann, E.: Enchantment and alchemy. The story of Rumpelstiltskin: *Bull. Menninger Clin.*, 47:1–14, 1983.
4. Torrey, E. F.: What western psychotherapists can learn from witch doctors: *Am. J. Orthopsychiatry*, 42:69–76, 1972.

Rumpelstiltskin Organization

Development of health care organizations may be caught in a complex of conflicting needs, resources, and expectations.[1] These problems are related to limited resources, discrepancies between supply and demand, fearful staff, a charismatic director, and demanding government and community agencies. When the facility finally opens the leader has become doubting and fearful of failure, and is fired.

The eponym Rumpelstiltskin Organization has been applied to such a situation. It was used to describe an unnamed psychoeducational facility for emotionally disturbed children and adolescents.[1] Midlevel administrators (the poor miller) are trying to create a new organization in the face of increasing demands for service, limited resources, and a cumbersome bureaucracy. The medical director (Rumpelstiltskin) has a powerful presence and a captivating dream of an ideal organization, but demands total control. The key staff group (the miller's beautiful daughter) is privately doubtful and fearful about its ability to accomplish the task. The consumers, community agencies, and government regulatory agencies (the king), expect many wonderful things (spun gold) from the organization.

This application of the Rumpelstiltskin fairy story is clever and imaginative, but somewhat strained.

1. Smith, K. K. & Simmons, V. M.: A Rumpelstiltskin organization: Metaphors on metaphors in field research: *Admin. Sci., Q.*, 28:377–392, 1983.

S

Saint Anthony's Fire

(ergotism, erysipelas)

Saint Anthony's Fire has been used as an eponym for two diseases, ergotism and erysipelas, each of different etiology, pathogenesis, and manifestations except for burning sensations which they have in common. Erysipelas is an acute infection of the skin and subcutaneous tissues caused by Group A streptococci, although rarely staphylococci and pneumococci may be responsible.[1] The commonest site is the face, with occasional involvement of wounds and surgical incisions. It occurs most frequently at the two extremes of age. There is abrupt onset with fever, headache, and vomiting, followed by itching and spreading redness of the skin. Positive cultures for Group A streptococci can also be obtained from the respiratory tract or blood stream.

Ergotism is a completely different entity, caused by ergot, the product of a fungus (*Claviceps purpurea*) that grows upon grains, especially rye.[2] The spores are carried by insects or the wind to the ovaries of young rye. The ovaries are then consumed by a dense tissue. The latter forms into a purple curved body, the sclerotium, which is a major source of commercial ergot alkaloids. Ergot, when ingested by the human, causes peripheral vasoconstriction, depression of vasomotor centers, peripheral adrenergic blockade, and stimulation of uterine contractions.

Ergot poisoning may occur after eating infected rye or by overdose when used as a drug

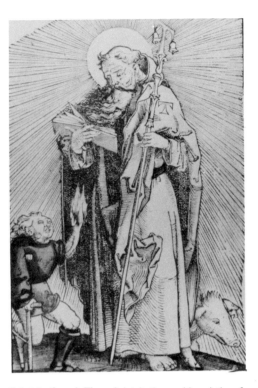

Saint Anthony's Fire   Saint Anthony with a victim of ergotism, represented by his flaming hand.[16] (woodcut by Johannes Wechtlin, 1540) (by permission, Dover Pubns., Inc.)

to cause abortion.[3] Acute poisoning is uncommon and causes vomiting, diarrhea, thirst, itching, and unconsciousness. In chronic poisoning, the effects are due to decreased circulation in the extremities caused by vasoconstriction and thrombosis with consequent coldness, muscle pain on walking, and eventually gangrene with loss of toes and sometimes fingers.

Saint Anthony (A.D. 251–356) was born in Upper Egypt.[4] At the age of twenty he gave away the estate he had inherited and lived as a hermit until the age of 54, when he founded his first monastery. Constantine the Great sought him out for prayers. He is noted for his ascetic religious life. In A.D. 561 his bones were reputed to have been discovered and eventually sent to Vienne, France, where they miraculously cured cases of ergotism. The dead holy man as a healing cult-figure has been more commonly found in Western religions than in Eastern ones.[5]

In the tenth century ergotism was also labeled St. Mary's Sickness, or Our Lady's Sickness, because many of the afflicted went to Notre Dame Cathedral in Paris where they were healed.[6] St. Geneviéve also was invoked as a protector against this burning evil.

Historically, the eponym Saint Anthony's Fire has been more appropriately used for ergotism,[7] in part because his confrontation with the demons of hell provides a link with the burning symptoms of the syndrome.[8] Ergot poisoning was confused with erysipelas in the middle ages owing to similarity of such symptoms.[9] The disease was also called ignis sacer, the holy fire.[10] A woodcut portrait of Saint Anthony from the sixteenth century includes the figure of a man on crutches with flames arising from his left hand and a wooden peg leg, suggesting loss of the leg, possibly due to gangrene,[11] Saint Anthony is also the patron saint of butchers and brushmakers.

A plague in Athens from 430 to 427 B.C. has been attributed, among many other diseases, to ergotism. It has also been called the Thucydides syndrome on the basis of a description by Thucydides, who survived the epidemic.[12] Influenza has been suggested as the cause, although this has been contested on the basis of inappropriate symptomatology.[13] A possible "plague" of St. Anthony's Fire occurred in 1951 in the small French village of Pont-Saint-Espirit.[14] Hundreds of people and animals went berserk. Symptoms included nausea, chills, hallucinations and convulsions, and many died. Ergot in bread bought from the one village baker was indited, although only minute amounts of ergot were found on analyses. This was before the discovery that the mold, ergot, when baked with dough produces lysergic acid diethylamide (LSD) a possible cause of this epidemic. The beneficial therapeutic effects of ergot in obstetrics dates back to the early nineteenth century.[15]

1. Bisno, A. L.: Streptococcal skin infections: in *Harrison's Principles of Internal Medicine*, R. G. Petersdorf et al., Eds., New York, McGraw-Hill, 1983, p. 932.
2. Rall, T. W. & Schleifer, L. S.: Ergot and the ergot alkaloids: in *Goodman & Gilman's The Pharmacologic Basis of Therapeutics*, A. G. Gilman et al., Eds., 7th ed., New York, Macmillan, 1985, pp. 931–940.
3. Haddad, L. M. & Winchester, J. F.: *Clinical Management of Poisoning and Drug Overdose*: Philadelphia, W. B. Saunders, 1983, pp. 880–881.
4. Thurston, pp. 104–109.
5. Petersen, J. M.: Dead or alive? The holy man as a healer in east and west in the late sixth century: *J. Med. Hist.*, 9:91–98, 1983.
6. Backman, E. L.: *Religious Dances in the Christian Church and in Popular Medicine*: London, George Allen & Unwin, 1952, pp. 295–297.
7. Barger, G.: *Ergot and Ergotism*: London, Gurney & Jackson, 1931.
8. Dixon, L. S.: Bosch's "St. Anthony's triptych" — An apothecary's apothesis: *Art J.*, 44:119–131, 1984.
9. Dotz, W.: St. Anthony's fire: *Am. J. Dermatopathol.*, 2:249–253, 1980.
10. Bargman, G. J. & Gardner, L. I.: Ignis sacer: *Lancet*, 1:197–108, 1969.
11. Wechtlin, J.: Colored Woodcut (1540) in *Medicine and the Artist*, C. Zigrosser, 3rd ed., New York, Dover, 1970, p. 84.
12. Langmuir, A. D. et al.: The Thucydides syndrome. A new hypothesis for the cause of the plague of Athens: *N. Engl. J. Med.*, 313:1027–1030, 1985.
13. Holladay, A. J.: The Thucydides syndrome: Another view: *N. Engl. J. Med.*, 315:1170–1172, 1986.
14. Fuller, J. G.: *The Day of St. Anthony's Fire*: New York, Macmillan, 1968.
15. Moir, J. C.: Ergot: From St. Anthony's fire to the isolation of its active principle, ergometrine (ergonovine): *Am. J. Obstet. Gynecol.*, 120:291–296, 1974.

16. Zigrosser, C.: *Medicine and the Artist*: 3rd ed., New York, Dover, 1970, p. 84.

Saint Main's Evil

(scabies)

Scabies is caused by the tick mite, *Sarcoptes scabiei*.[1] Clinical manifestations include superficial burrows in the skin, intense pruritus, and secondary infection. St. Main (Méen, Mewan) was a sixth century monk who lived in Britain and founded a monastery at Gael.[2] He is reported to have caused a fountain to flow with waters that had curative powers. St. Main is also reputed to have cured many patients with skin diseases. It is not known why his name was applied more specifically to scabies, although this infestation was undoubtedly quite prevalent in the unhygienic middle ages.[3] A herb, scabious, which was thought to be effective for scabies also has been called l'herbe de St. Main.

1. Berkow, pp. 2044–2045.
2. Delaney, J. J.: *Dictionary of Saints*: Garden City, New York, Doubleday, 1980, p. 402.
3. Murphy.

Saint Paul's Evil

(epilepsy)

Epilepsy was called Saint Paul's Evil in Ireland, based on the belief that he was a convulsive.[1] St. Paul was born of Jewish parents in the first century, and was named Saul.[2] He became a very influential preacher of the gospel, and was finally beheaded during the prosecution of Christians by Emperor Nero. There are several patron saints of epilepsy: St. Lupus, St. Thomas, St. Malhurn, St. Valentine,[1] and St. Giles.[3] The latter also has been associated with the "curing" of insanity, sterility, and demoniac possession. A description of epilepsy is given in the New Testament. "Teacher [Jesus], I have brought You my son, who has a dumb spirit; whenever it gets hold of him, it throws him down—he foams at the mouth, he grinds his teeth, and becomes rigid." Christ cured the boy by ordering the "Dumb and deaf spirit" to come out of him.[4]

An obsolete term for epilepsy is Hercules Morbus, supposedly because of the Herculean strength and violence during epileptic fits.[5] Hercules was the Roman name for Heracles of Greek mythology.[6] His exceptional strength enabled him to win immortality by completing the twelve tasks set on him by his cousin Eurystheus. More modern epileptic eponyms are Dark Warrior Epilepsy and Astro-Fighter Epilepsy, both referring to seizures caused by the flashing lights of video games.[7]

Literature contains descriptions of epileptics, not the least of whom is Prince Myshkin, the leading character in Dostoevski's 1868 novel, *The Idiot*.[8] The prince was called the idiot because of his gentle, childlike nature and his refusal to take offense at anything. The description of one of his epileptic attacks is as accurate as and more dramatic and humane than that found in clinical texts.

...when suddenly in the midst of sadness, spiritual darkness and oppression, there seemed at moments a flash of light in his brain, and with extraordinary impetus all his vital forces suddenly began working at their highest tension. The sense of life, the consciousness of self, were multiplied ten times at these moments which passed like a flash of lighting . . . . But these moments, these flashes, were only the prelude of that final second . . . with which the fit began. . . . At the moment the face is horribly distorted, especially the eyes. The whole body and the features of the face work with convulsive jerks and contortions. A terrible, indescribable scream that is unlike anything else breaks from the sufferer. In that scream everything human seems obliterated. . . .

This could only have been written by a superb, sensitive writer, who was also an epileptic.

1. Murphy.
2. Delaney, J. J.: *Dictionary of Saints*: Garden City, New York, Doubleday, 1980, pp. 448–449.
3. Ohry, A. & Ohry-Kossoy, K.: St. Giles, St. Francis et al.: Medical patron saints: *Adler Museum Bull.*, 18:18–22, 1986.
4. NT: Mark 9:17–18.
5. Campbell, p. 279.
6. Schmidt, pp. 125–130.
7. Gordon, R.: *Great Medical Disasters*: New York, Dorset Press, 1986, p. 107.
8. Dostoievski, F. M.: *The Idiot*: C. Garnett translator, New York, Modern Library, 1935, pp. 213, 222.

Saint Vitus Dance

(chorea, chorea minor, dancing mania, danse de St. Guy, Sydenham's chorea)

Chorea is a delayed central nervous system manifestation of rheumatic disease.[1] It is

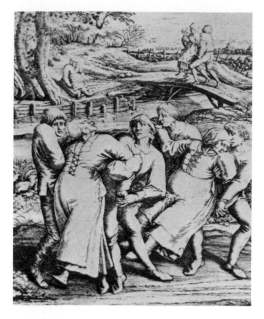

Saint Vitus' Dance   Saint Vitus dancers.[9] (by Peter Breughel the Elder)

characterized by sudden, aimless, irregular movements, muscle weakness, speech disturbance, and emotional instability. Its presumed association with St. Vitus began in the fourteenth century. In Aachen, Germany, about 1374, large crowds of men and women appeared in the streets, holding hands in circles to dance for many hours.[2] Such behavior spread throughout Germany. When it appeared in Strassburg in 1418, sufferers were sent to the Chapel of St. Vitus where they were cured by religious observances conducted by priests. In another version, it was a seventeenth century custom for young people to dance around a statue of St. Vitus in order to ensure good health.[3] In Germany, such dancing often became frenzied.

St. Vitus was an early Christian (c. A.D. 300), who lived in the Roman province of Lucania in southern Italy.[4] According to legend, he was baptized secretly at about the age of ten, and produced so many miracles and conversions that he was unfavorably noticed by Valerian, the administrator of Sicily. He escaped to Rome where he cured the son of the Emperor Diocletian by expelling what were thought to be the evil spirits which possessed him. St. Vitus was accused of sorcery and thrown into a cauldron filled with molten lead. He was saved by an angel, and then lived peacefully until his death. The reputed relics of St. Vitus reached Saxony in 836. A great devotion to him developed in Germany, where he was considered the protector from nervous diseases and hydrophobia. St. Vitus is also the patron saint of actors and dancers. He is invoked against all injuries that beasts do to men (bites of mad dogs and snakes).

Unlike the chorea of rheumatic fever, described by Sydenham in 1686, the dancing mania of the fourteenth century was undoubtedly a form of mass hysteria. The St. Vitus designation was given to chorea by Paracelsus.[2] A related dancing hysteria in medieval Italy was tarantualism, so named because it was thought to be caused by a bite of the tarantula, a very large spider that has a painful but nonpoisonous bite. An earlier name for tarantualism, St. John's Disease,[5] may have originated from the dance of Salome, which lead to the death of St. John the Baptist.[6] Freud considered the movements of victims of St. Vitus Dance to be symbolic of the sexual act.[7] He suggested that repression of sexual overstimulation as children was expressed by the dance mania.

In pre-Christian times and in the early church, dancing was used to influence invisible powers. It was considered to be an imitation of the dance of the Angels. There were also dances for the dead, to obtain their help in driving out illness. Among these dancers were "choreomaniacs" who engaged in dancing epidemics.[8] These latter may have been related to ergotism and tarantualism.

1. Braunwald, pp. 86–87.
2. Major, R. H.: *A History of Medicine*: vol. 1, Springfield, Illinois, Charles C Thomas, 1954, pp. 346–348.
3. Boycott, pp. 105–106.
4. Thurston, pp. 545–546.
5. Murphy.
6. NT: Mark 6:14–29.
7. Freeman, L. & Strean, H. S.: *Freud and Women*: New York, Frederick Ungar, 1981, p. 211.
8. Backman, E. L.: *Religious Dances in the Christian Church and in Popular Medicine*: London, George Allen & Unwin, 1952.
9. Sigerist, H. E.: *Civilization and Disease*: Itheca, New York, Chicago, University of Chicago Press, 1962, p. 196.

Sapphism

(lesbianism, tribadism)

Lesbianism and sapphism are designations for homosexual practices between women. Related is tribadism (derived from the Greek word tribein, rub), which indicates sexual pleasure by rubbing the external genitalia against that of another woman.[1] Confirmed lesbians often have histories of exposure to severe abusiveness and alcoholism, lack of gratifying relationships, and tendencies to depression and suicide.[2] Freud proposed that homosexuality in both sexes may be related to a very strong mother fixation.[3]

Sappho was an ancient Greek poetess, who lived on the island of Lesbos,[4] where it is implied that women carried out homosexual practices.[5] However, she fell in love with a beautiful youth, Phaon, who ferried a boat between Lesbos and Chios.[4] When her love was not returned she threw herself from the promontory of Leucadia into the sea because of a superstition that those who leaped from there would be cured of their love if not destroyed.

Books on Greek mythology appear to be somewhat reticent about discussing lesbian practices; but modern etymologies indicate "eccentric loving" on Sappho's part.[6] A modern book of photographs depicting lesbian love includes Sappho's name in its title.[7] More appropriately, Sappho has been called the Tenth Muse, the muse of poetry who used the four-lined verse form called sapphics.[8]

1. Stedman, pp. 776, 1253, 1480.
2. Kolb, p. 528.
3. Freeman, L. & Strean, H. S.: *Freud and Women*: New York, Frederick Ungar, 1981, p. 191.
4. Bulfinch, p. 253.
5. Espy, p. 225.
6. Partridge, E.: *Origins. A Short Etymological Dictionary of Modern English*: New York, Greenwich House, 1983, p. 349.
7. Smith, J. F.: *The Art of Loving Women: The Poetry of Sappho*: New York, Chelsea House, 1975.
8. Hendrickson, p. 181.

Saturnism

(plumbism, saturnine curse.)

The risk of lead poisoning increases considerably when its concentration in the blood rises to greater than 50 μ/dl.[1] Higher levels are found in urban than rural environments,[2] especially in slum areas (lead belts) where lead-rich flakes of paint may be ingested by children.[3] Not only lead workers have high blood levels, but also their children, who are exposed to lead dust which is carried home.[4] Those who work with leaded glass as a hobby are also at risk, unless precautions are taken.[5] Environmental pollution with lead has been a concern since the introduction of leaded gasoline in 1923.[6]

In adults, the effect of excessive lead can result in a chronic syndrome of headache, metallic taste, anorexia, colicky abdominal pain, and anemia.[1] It may also be manifested as chronic renal failure.[7] Lead poisoning presents more acutely in young children as an acute encephalopathy with forceful vomiting, intractable seizures, and finally coma. Subclinical lead poisoning may result in hyperactivity in children.[8] In a prospective study of 249 children from birth to two years of age, high prenatal exposure to lead (determined by umbilical cord levels) resulted in significantly lower cognitive development than in the control group.[9]

Saturn (Saturnus) was a god of ancient Roman mythology, although some have related him to the Greek Cronus, who was the father of Zeus.[10] He was the introducer of agriculture, and his wife, Ops (Rhea), the goddess of sowing and harvest. Cronus and Rhea, in Greek mythology, were Titans, the children of heaven and earth.[11] The eponym Saturnism was evidently derived from the designation of Saturn as the god of riches of the earth, including lead.[12]

Exposure to lead has not been restricted to our present civilization. Lead artifacts, and lead-lined water systems were used extensively by the Romans.[13] The first clinical account of lead poisoning has been accredited to Nicander in the second century B.C.[14] Although proposed, it is unlikely that Hippocrates described such a condition (see Bellman's Fallacy).[15] It has been postulated that gout among Roman aristocrats was actually caused by lead poisoning,[16] and thus may have contributed to the fall of Rome.[17] Lead also has been suggested as the cause of the decline of the British Empire during the eighteenth century and well into the nineteenth.[18] The "idiocy of the ruling classes" could have been in part due to lead poisoning rather than porphyria. Lead is now considered by some to be responsible for the variety of gout which is caused by blocking of the urinary excretion of uric acid.[19]

Saturnism has been reported from treatment with an Asian Indian lead-containing folk remedy.[20] Chronic plumbism has also been attributed to the addition of lead to wine for sweetening and preservation, which was carried out from the days of the Roman Empire to the nineteenth century.[21] This has been suggested as the cause of the psychiatric symptoms of George III rather than the more popular diagnosis of porphyria (see Lycanthropy).[22] The eccentricities in the paintings of Goya (1746–1828) have been attributed to exposure to lead in his paint.[23] Such an association was recognized by Ramazzini in 1713.[24] No wonder that lead poisoning has been called the Saturnine Curse.[25]

Saccharum saturni was another name for cerusa acetate, composed of lead acetate, or sugar of lead, and prepared by dissolving lead monoxide in vinegar.[26] It was used in the eighteenth and nineteenth centuries as an ointment for inflammatory diseases of the eye, skin cancers, sweating, and leukorrhea because of its cooling and desiccating properties.

In more common usage, the adjective saturnine is used for a person of sluggish, cold, and gloomy temperament, so used because lead is a heavy and sluggish metal.[27]

1. Berkow, pp. 1879–1880.
2. Cohen, C. J. et al.: Epidemiology of lead poisoning. A comparison between urban and rural children: *J.A.M.A.*, 226:1430–1433, 1973.
3. Fine, P. R. et al.: Pediatric blood lead levels. A study in 14 Illinois cities of intermediate population: *J.A.M.A.*, 221:1475–1479, 1972.
4. Baker, E. L. et al.: Lead poisoning in children of lead workers: *N. Engl. J. Med.*, 296:260–261, 1977.
5. Feldman, R. G. & Sedman, T.: Hobbyists working with lead: *N. Engl. J. Med.*, 292:929, 1975.
6. Rosner, D. & Markowitz, G.: A 'gift of God'?: The Public Health controversy over leaded gasoline during the 1920s: *Am. J. Public Health*, 75:344–352, 1985.
7. Craswell, P. W. et al.: Chronic renal failure with gout. A marker of chronic lead poisoning: *Kidney Int.*, 26:319–323, 1984.
8. Waldron, H. A.: Subclinical lead poisoning: A preventable disease: *Prevent. Med.*, 4:135–153, 1975.
9. Bellinger, D. et al.: Longitudinal analyses of prenatal and postnatal lead exposure and early cognitive development: *N. Engl. J. Med.*, 316:1037–1043, 1987.
10. Gayley, pp. 59–60.
11. Bulfinch, p. 6.
12. Vaisrub, p. 110.
13. Woolley, D. E.: A perspective of lead poisoning in antiquity and the present: *Neurotoxicology*, 5:353–362, 1984.
14. Waldron, H. A.: Lead poisoning in the ancient world: *Med. Hist.*, 17:391–399, 1973.
15. Waldron, H. A.: Hippocrates and lead: *Lancet*, 2:626, 1973.
16. Nriagu, J. O.: Saturnine gout among roman aristocrats. Did lead poisoning contribute to the fall of the empire?: *N. Engl. J. Med.*, 308:660–663, 1983.
17. Phillips, C. R.: Old wine in new bottles: Nriagu on the fall of Rome: *Class. Wld.*, 78:29–33, 1984.
18. Emsley, J.: When the Empire struck lead: *New Scientist*, 112:64–67, 1986/87.

19. Wedeen, R. P.: Irregular gout: Humoral or saturnine malady: *Bull. N.Y. Acad. Med.*, 60:969–979, 1984.
20. Pontifex, A. H. & Garg, A. K.: Lead poisoning from an Asian Indian folk remedy: *Can. Med. Assoc. J.*, 133:1227–1228, 1985.
21. Wedeen, R. P.: *Poison in the Pot. The Legacy of Lead*: Carbondale, Illinois, Southern Illinois University Press, 1984.
22. Macalpine, I. & Hunter, R.: *George III and the Mad Business*: London, Allen Lane Penguin Press, 1969.
23. Niederland, W. G.: Goya's illness. A case of lead encephalopathy?: *N.Y. State J. Med.*, 72:413–418, 1972.
24. Ramazzini, B.: *De Morbis Artificum (Diseases of Workers)*: W. C. Wright translator, New York, Hafner Publications, 1964, pp. 67–69.
25. Green, D. W.: The saturnine curse: A history of lead poisoning: *South. Med. J.*, 78:48–51, 1985.
26. Risse, G. B: *Hospital Life in Enlightenment Scotland. Care and Teaching at the Royal Infirmary of Edinburgh*: Cambridge, Cambridge University Press, 1986, pp. 371–372.
27. Haubrich, p. 218.

Satyriasis

(Don Juan syndrome, male hypersexuality, satyress[1])

Synonymous eponyms for male hypersexuality are satyriasis[2] and the Don Juan Syndrome.[3] There is often no organic cause;[4] but there may be an association with alcoholism.[5] Satyrs were Greek deities of the woods and fields. They attended Bacchus, the god of grape growing and of wine, along with the Nymphs who were the goddesses of nature.[6] Satyrs are described as being covered with bristly hair, and as having short horns and beards, with feet and legs like those of goats. Descriptions of their appearance are somewhat similar to that of Pan, the god of fields and fertility, but who was smaller in size (see Panic Terror). Satyrs roamed the countryside to satisfy their sexual appetites.[7]

The eponyms satyriasis and nymphomania represent the male and female counterparts of hypersexuality. They are both derived from the deities of nature and attendants of Bacchus. The name satyr has been used in the nonsexual sense of someone evil and dissipated by Oscar Wilde in characterizing the degenerate Dorian Gray.[8] Called satyr ears are the rounded ears found in a congenital syndrome of imperforate anus, abnormalities of hands and feet, and

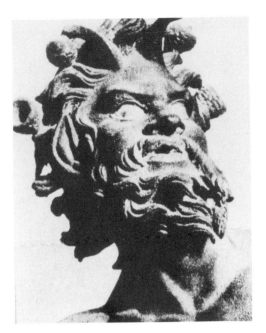

Satyriasis   Head of a satyr.[7, p. 114]

sensorineural deafness.[9] There is also a species of chimpanzee that is named *Pan satyrus*.[10]

1. OED: IX:127–128.
2. Moore, S. L. & May, M.: Satyriasis from a contemporary perspective: A review of male hypersexuality: *Rev. Male Hypersex.*, 4:83–93, 1982.
3. Freedman, p. 1507.
4. Moore, S. L.: Satyriasis: A case study: *J. Clin. Psychiatry*, 41:279–281, 1980.
5. deVito, R. A. & Marozas, R. J.: The alcoholic satyr: *Sex. Disabil.*, 4:234–245, 1981.
6. Gayley, pp. 44, 46.
7. Guirand 1968, p. 247.
8. Wilde, O.: *The Picture of Dorian Gray*: Harmondsworth, England, Penguin, 1985, p. 174.
9. Walpole, I. R. & Hockey, A.: Syndrome of imperforate anus, abnormalities of hands and feet, satyr ears, and gensorineural deafness: *J. Pediatr.*, 100:250–252, 1982.
10. McConnell, S. et al.: Monkeypox: Experimental infection in chimpanzee *(Pan satyrus)* and immunization with vaccina virus: *Am. J. Vet. Res.*, 29:1675–1680, 1968.

Serendipity

Serendipity is a noun defined as the faculty of making happy and unexpected discoveries by accident.[1] A prime example is that of Alexander Fleming, professor of bacteriology at St. Mary's Hospital, London.[2] In 1929, he noticed that an agar plate inoculated with staphylococci showed degeneration of bacterial colonies immediately around a contaminating mold. From this chance observation came the leap of educated intuition—the mold contained some substance that destroyed bacteria. Other historical examples are Wholer's discovery of urea, Galvani's of muscle stimulation by electricity, and Roentgen's of x-rays.[3] As outstanding was Jenner's realization that cowpox and smallpox are related;[4] and Laënnec's that there is a relationship between sounding barrels for depth and listening to thoracic sounds.[5]

Some more modern examples of serendipity are the observations that the tremor and rigidity of Parkinsonism disappears after an accidental tearing of the anterior choroidal artery;[6] that disulfiram (Antabuse) has a hypersensitizing effect for alcohol;[7] that organic mercurials have a diuretic action;[8] that narrowing of the main renal artery is a cause of hypertension;[9] that cutting of the spinothalamic tracts in the spinal cord can relieve intractable pain;[10] and many others.[11]

The eponym serendipity was coined by Horace Walpole, the fourth Earl of Oxford, in a letter to a friend dated January 28, 1754.[12] It is derived from the legend of the *Three Princes of Serendip*, Serendip being the ancient name for Ceylon, now Sri Lanka. "I once read a silly fairy tale, called 'The Three Princes of Serendip.' As their Highnesses traveled, they were always making discoveries, by accidents and sagacity, of things which they were not in quest of. . . ." When the Princes were sent out into the world by their father, the king, to further their education, they came upon the tracks of the large animal.[13] They deduced that it was a camel and lame because of the hoof prints; and that it was blind in one eye because the grass had been eaten on one side of the road, even though not as good as on the other side. When a stranger came looking for his lost animal, the princes described the camel's features so accurately that they were accused of stealing the animal. They were released, however, when they explained their observations to a judge.

The legend of the missing camel is stated to have first appeared in the Babylonian Talmud and in the lore of various oriental cultures.[14] The adventures of the three princes were compiled in a book in 1557 by Christoforo Armeno, an Italian, and translated into French in 1719.[15] In 1748, six years before Walpole's invention of the term serendipity, Voltaire used the same theme for "Zadig" who described accurately the features of the queen's lost animals by studying their tracks.[16] In a more recent book, Eco's *The Name of the Rose*, Brother William came across animal tracks from which he derived considerable information.[17]

According to Walpole's original definition, a serendipitous occurrence has three components—an accidental encounter while looking for something else, a valuable or agreeable finding, and determination of the significance by logical deduction. The dictionary definition omits the latter component, which is the vital one in relation to medical science. Related components of serendipity are acute observation, curiosity, opportunism, and receptivity.[18] Consistent with serendipity is Louis Pasteur's dictum that "chance favors only the prepared mind." In other words, to benefit from serendipity in science one must understand the known in order to recognize the significance of the unknown.[19] It is a major form of creativity.[20]

The relationship between research and serendipity has been well expressed by Norman Cousins.[21]

The best research laboratory is a serendipitous arena—a place where unplanned but significant things can happen. Most people have yet to understand that research cannot be expected to go forward in a straight line from theory to materialization. Creative research is full of detours, and those who have their eyes fixed only on a clearly defined objective may miss important signs along the way. Edward Jenner, . . . Sir Alexander Fleming, . . . and Ignatz Philip Semmelweis . . . have demonstrated . . . that the powers of observation may represent the most important ingredient in 'luck.' The imaginative researcher must be prepared to spot and pounce upon happy surprises.

A modern research scientist has put serendipity in more prosaic terms. "If you do not find the activity you want, study the activity you get; it is probably more interesting than what you had expected."[22] The restriction of serendipitous learning in health education has been deplored because it may result in a rigid adherence to prescribed learning objectives.[23] Serendipity has gained considerable prominence in medicine. A MEDLINE computerized search of the years 1966 to 1983 has yielded this word in the title of thirty-six articles in medical or medically related journals.[24] All described accidental discoveries. Seven were general reviews of fortuitous events in medicine. The others each related to a specific individual event: twelve to diagnosis, five to other aspects of disease, four to pharmacology, and eight to a variety of other medical topics. Such prominence given to serendipity may overshadow the importance of other forms of discovery, such as discovery by design or intention and by intuition or imagination.[25] Its significance in psychiatric discoveries has been negated.[26] Although serendipity has been called "the happy accident,"[27] it may be a crippling neurotic symptom that impairs the ability of the serendipidist to learn by unconsciously deflecting him from his aim to that of aimless dilettantism.[28]

1. OED: IX:p. 492.
2. Rossman, R. E.: The history and significance of serendipity in medical discovery: *Trans. Stud. Coll. Physicians*, 33:104–120, 1965.
3. Halacy, D. S., Jr.: *Science and Serendipity. Great Discoveries by Accident*: Philadelphia, Macrae Smith, 1967.
4. Dale, H.: Accident and opportunism in medical research: *Br. Med. J.*, 2:451–455, 1948.
5. Ochsner, A.: The influence of serendipity on medicine: *J. Med. Assoc. State Alabama*, 15:357–366, 1946.
6. Cooper, I. S.: Surgical occlusion of the anterior choroidal artery in Parkinsonism: *Surg. Gynecol. Obstet.*, 99:207–219, 1954.
7. Hald, J., Jacobsen, E. & Larsen, V.: The sensitizing effect of tetraethyliuramdisulphide (Antabuse) to ethylalcohol: *Acta Pharmacol.*, 4:285–296, 1948.
8. Vogl, A.: The discovery of the organic mercurial diuretics: *Am. Heart J.*, 39:881–883, 1950.
9. Howard, J. E.: Serendipity in clinical investigation: *J.A.M.A.*, 207:736–739, 1969.
10. Jefferson, G.: Man as an experimental animal: *Lancet*, 268:59–61, 1955.
11. Laughlin, V. C.: The Princes of Serendip: *J. Am. Inst. Homeopathy*, 12:228–234, 1947.
12. Walpole, H. *The Letters of Horace Walpole, Earl of Oxford*: vol. 12, P. Cunningham, Ed., London, Bickers & Son, 1880, pp. 364–367.
13. Sommer, F. R.: "Travels of the Three Sons of the King of Serendip. A Précis of an Old Tale": T. Benfley translator, in *Old Folklore Series*, D. K. Webb, Ed., vol. 5, Chillicothe, Ohio, Ross County Historical Society, 1959.
14. Chronical and comment: *The Bookman*, April, 1908, pp. 113–114.
15. Fraser, L.: A study of literary geneology: *Mod. Language Notes*, 21:245–247, 1906.
16. Voltaire: *Zadig and Other Romances*: H. I. Woolf, translator, London, George Routledge & Sons, n.d., pp. 1–12.
17. Eco, U.: *The Name of the Rose*: New York, Warner Books, 1984, pp. 16–20.
18. Rossman, R. E.: Serendipity in medical discovery: *Surg. Gynecol. Obstet.*, 124:837–838, 1967.
19. Golin, M.: Serendipity—Big word in medical progress. Does "pure luck" deserve all the credit?: *J.A.M.A.*, 165:2084–2087, 1957.
20. Mednick, S. A.: The associative basis of the creative process: *Psychol. Rev.*, 69:220–232, 1962.
21. Cousins, N., Ed.: *The Physician in Literature*: Philadelphia, W. B. Saunders, 1982, p.1.
22. Racker, E.: Resolution and reconstruction of biological pathways from 1919 to 1984: *Fed. Proc.*, 42:2899–2909, 1983.
23. Styles, M. M.: Serendipity and objectivity. An essay on wild flowers—and not coincidentally, behavioral objectives: *Nursing Outlook*, 23:311–313, 1975.
24. Rodin, A. E. & Key, J. D.: The influence of literary legends on medicine: *Y Med. Inquirer*, 1:8–11, 1985.

25. Blalock, A.: The nature of discovery: *Ann. Surg.*, 144:289–303, 1956.
26. Jeste, D. V. et al.: Serendipity in biological psychiatry—A myth?: *Arch. Gen. Psychiatry*, 36:1173–1178, 1979.
27. McLean, F. C.: The happy accident: *Scientif. Monthly*, 53:61–70, 1941.
28. Evans, W. N.: Serendipity: *Psychoanal. Q.*, 32:165–180, 1963.

Shandy Syndrome

(acucollophalia susannahus, penile slam syndrome, Susannah sash syndrome, toilet seat syndrome, window sash syndrome)

A young male child while urinating may have his penis slammed against the toilet bowl rim if the raised toilet seat falls on it.[1] The result is the "smirk syndrome—nothing very serious, just painful." Such an event has become more generalized than the toilet seat syndrome, the Shandy Syndrome being applied to any sudden compression trauma to the penis.[2] The derivation of this literary eponym[3] is found in Laurence Sterne's *Tristram Shandy*[4] of the mid-eighteenth century.

The chamber-maid had left no ******* *** [chamber pot] under the bed:—Cannot you contrive, master, quoth Susannah, lifting up the sash with one hand, as she spoke, and helping me up into the window-seat, with the other,—cannot you manage, my dear, for a single time, to **** *** ** *** ******* [piss out of the window]? I was five years old.—Susannah did not consider that nothing was well hung in our family,—so slap came the shash down like lightning upon us;—Nothing is left, cried Susannah,—nothing is left—for me, but to run my country.—"

The asterisks in the quote are Sterne's satire of false modesty shown by not using the name of genital organs. This was evident not only in "better circles" three hundred years ago, but also today. The editorial in the April 3rd, 1973, issue of the *Journal of the American Medical Association*[1] is certainly a tongue-in-cheek reaction to undue prudishness: " . . . with diligent search an eponym can be derived so that mention of the penis can be avoided by a prudish mother in polite company." The same tone is apparent in responses to the editorial,[1, 2, 3] one of which supplies the designation of the Shandy Syndrome.[2]

Aside from filial pain and maternal embarrassment, little damage is done to the male organ or to procreation. In Tristram Shandy's case "... Twas nothing,—I did not lose two drops of blood by it—'twas not worth calling in a surgeon, had he lived next door to us. . . ."[4]

1. Editorial: Small slam: *J.A.M.A.*, 224:1414, 1973.
2. Webb, H. B.: To the Editor: *J.A.M.A.*, 226:1571, 1973.
3. Raleigh, R. R. R.: To the Editor: *J.A.M.A.*, 226:1571, 1973.
4. Sterne, L.: *The Life and Opinions of Tristram Shandy Gentleman*: Book V., New York, Random House, 1950, pp. 391–392.

Sherlock Holmes Method

The eponym Sherlock Holmes Method has been applied to the use of intentional experiments in ethology (the scientific study of animal behavior). This research method consists of single intentional provocations which lead to a specific reaction which is then studied.[1] Such provocations are contrary to the usual investigative methods for animal behavior, which consist of repeated and frequent observations of stereotypic behavior of a species in the absence of any intervention. The results of the latter method do not necessarily indicate intelligence. There is good evidence of intelligence, however, if an intentional and unusual provocation results in a novel response that cannot be explained by prior conditioning or habit.

A justification for applying the name of the master detective to this method of behavioral investigation is found in "A Scandal in Bohemia".[2] Holmes had gained false entry into the home of Irene Adler by posing as an injured nonconformist clergyman. Watson then threw a smoke bomb into the room through a window and yelled, "Fire." She reacted immediately to this intentional provocation by running to a sliding panel behind which she had hidden the photograph which could compromise the king of Bohemia. As Irene Adler indicated in a subsequent letter to Holmes, "You really did it very well. You took me in completely. Until after the alarm of fire, I had not a suspicion."

In the case of the ethologist, such planned provocation can result in evidence of animal intelligence and, in the case of Sherlock Holmes, in the solution to a mystery. In the latter, however, it is the detective who demonstrated intelligence rather than the subject who acted instinctively. Therefore, the ethological eponym, the Sherlock Holmes Method, is not quite congruent with the fictional episode from which it was derived.

Conan Doyle did provide Holmes with some insight into the behavior of animals. The detective concluded that it was the cabman who had entered the house with Drebber, the murder victim, from the fact that the cab tracks wandered in a way which indicated that no one was in control of the horse.[3] In "The Sign of the Four,"[4] he used the instinctive behavior of a dog, Toby, to follow the tracks of Tonga, the murderer from the Andaman Islands, who had inadvertently stepped into creosote.

More widely acknowledged is the inference which Holmes derived from the fact that the dog kept in the stables did not bark during the night when the race horse, Silver Blaze, was kidnapped.[5] Obviously the midnight visitor was well known to the dog, thus pointing the finger at Jack Straker. An example of the use of this episode as a metaphor is found in a history of the English Channel in discussing the English Civil War of 1642.[6] "Few historians have recognized that what the Navy could have done and did not do, like Sherlock Holmes's dog that did not bark, was the decisive factor of the story." More medical is the comparison of the barkless dog with the enigma of why every premature infant does not develop retrolental fibroplasia.[7] In these instances, the connotation is that something which does not happen may be as significant as something which does happen.

The lack of response by the mute dog to provocation is an example of conditioned behavior resulting in no reaction. It does not fulfill the definition of the Sherlock Holmes Method because Straker did not plan to provoke the dog. The derivation of such an eponym is yet a further attestation to the caliber of Conan Doyle as a writer and to the extent to which Sherlock Holmes has permeated many aspects of our society and even academia and medicine.[8]

1. Dennett, D. C.: Intentional systems in cognitive ethology: The "panglossian paradigm" defended: *Behavioral Brain Sci.*, 6:343–390, 1983.
2. Doyle, A. C.: "A Scandal in Bohemia": *Strand Mag.*, 2:61–75, 1891.
3. Doyle, A. C.: *A Study in Scarlet. The Reminiscences of John H. Watson, M.D.*: London, Ward, Lock & Co., 1888.
4. Doyle, A. C.: "The Sign of the Four": *Lippincott's Monthly Mag.*, 17:3–11, 1899.
5. Doyle, A. C.: "The Adventure of Silver Blaze": *Strand Mag.*, 4:645–660, 1892.
6. Williamson, J. A.: *The English Channel. A History*: London, Collins, 1959, p. 235.
7. Howell, M. & Ford, P.: *The Beetle of Aphrodite and Other Medical Mysteries*: New York, Random House, 1985, p. 234–235.
8. Key, J. D. & Rodin, A. E.: The Permeation of Medicine by a Literary Character: Arthur Conan Doyle's Consulting Detective, Mr. Sherlock Holmes: *Baker Street Misc.*, No. 42, Spring, 1985, pp. 11–17.

Sherlock Holmes Test

The HemoQuant test for fecal occult blood is also called the Sherlock Holmes Test. It consists of removing iron from heme to yield fluorescing porphorins which are then purified by extraction with solvents and assayed fluorometrically.[1] It is quantitative, and heme specific, without false-positive and false-negative reactions,[2] unlike the long-established guaiac test.[3]

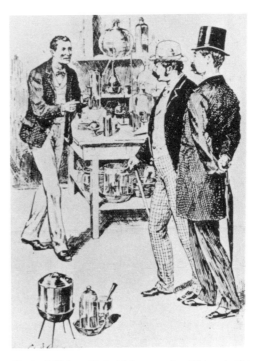

Sherlock Holmes Test Holmes meeting Watson in the chemical laboratory of St. Bartholomew Hospital.[5] (by Hutchinson, 1891)

Sherlock Holmes is Conan Doyle's master detective, who was endowed with considerable medical knowledge, including chemistry.[4] When he was first seen at the St. Bartholomew's chemistry laboratory by his more stoic companion-to-be, Doctor Watson, Holmes cried excitedly, "I've found it!. . . . I have found a reagent which is precipitated by haemoglobin and nothing else. . . . Don't you see that it gives us an infallible test for blood stains. . . . The old guaiacum test was very clumsy and uncertain."[5] Guaiac, derived from the resin of a tropical American tree,[6] is indeed old in respect to medicine. It was described by Fracastorius in the sixteenth century as a treatment for syphilis.[7]

The HemoQuant test appears to fulfill the qualities of the test for blood described by Sherlock Holmes in 1887, almost a century before. He did not, however, use the test in any of his sixty adventures.[8]

1. Schwartz, S.: et al.: The "HemoQuant test": A specific and qualitative determination of heme (he-

moglobin) in feces and other materials: *Clin. Chem.*, 29:2061–2067, 1983.

2. Ahlquist, D. A. et al.: HemoQuant test for occult blood: The Sherlock Holmes test?: *Mayo Clin. Proc.*, 59:766–768, 1984.

3. Markman, H. D.: Errors in the guaiac test for occult blood: *J.A.M.A.*, 202:846–847, 1967.

4. Rodin, A. E. & Key, J. D.: *Medical Casebook of Doctor Arthur Conan Doyle. From Practitioner to Sherlock Holmes and Beyond*: Malabar, Florida, Robert E. Krieger, 1984.

5. Doyle, A. C.: *A Study in Scarlet*: London, Ward, Lock, Bowden, 1891.

6. Harrar, E. S. & Harrar, J. G.: *Guide to Southern Trees*: New York, Dover Publications, 1946, pp. 387–389.

7. Fracastorius, H.: *Contagion, Contagious Diseases and Their Treatment*: W. C. Wright translator, New York, G. P. Putnam's Sons, 1930, pp. 235–237.

8. Rodin, A. E. & Key, J. D.: The scientific Holmes. A survey of science, medicine and deduction in the 60 tales: *Sherlock Holmes Rev.*, 1:81–86, 116–122, 1987.

Sherlockitis

The term sherlockitis designates an common type of addictive commitment to all matters relating to Conan Doyle's master detective, Sherlock Holmes.[1] It includes all events, descriptions, and minutiae found in the fifty-six short stories and four novels in which he is featured.[2] Sherlock Holmes aficionados have elevated these writings to the point of calling them the Canon and the Sacred Writings. The suffix "itis" is used in the eponym because "clinical characteristics are trance-like phases alternating with periods of feverish activity" as seen in virus infections.[1]

The Holmesian mystique has permeated medicine to a considerable degree. Approximately fifty papers dealing with the fictional detective have appeared in various national, regional, state, specialty, and general medical journals from 1966 to 1982.[3] Many of these articles treat Holmes and Watson as actual historical figures. Some focus on the considerable medical content of these adventures, and some on the usefulness in modern-day medicine of the techniques and deductive methods of the sleuth, including acute observation and ratiocination. The latter has been called Sherlockian Ability in referring to the diagnosis of occupational calluses.[4]

Sherlockitis could be considered, in some cases, as a type of monomania, a form of insanity in which the patient is irrational on one subject only. Conan Doyle, in his autobiography, refers to "what the South Americans now call 'Sherlock-holmitos,' which means clever little deductions, which often have nothing to do with the matter at hand but impress the reader with a general sense of power."[5] Sigmund Freud himself has been called the Viennese detective in a comparison with Sherlock Holmes.[6]

1. Hench, P. S.: On Violence at Meiringen: in *Exploring Sherlock Holmes*, E. W. McDiarmid & T. C. Blegen, Eds., La Crosse, Wisconsin, Sumac Press, 1957, p. 117.
2. Baring-Gould, W. S., Ed.: *The Annotated Sherlock Holmes. The Four Novels and the Fifty-Six Short Stories Complete by Sir Arthur Conan Doyle*: 2nd. ed., 2 Vols., New York, Clarkson N. Potter, 1967.
3. Key, J. D. & Rodin, A. E.: Permeation of medicine by a literary legend: Arthur Conan Doyle's consulting detective, Mister Sherlock Holmes: *Baker St. Misc.*, No. 42, Spring, 1985, pp. 11–17.
4. Ronchese, F.: Knuckle pads and similar-looking disorders: *Giornale Ital. Dermatol.*, 107:1227–1236, 1966.
5. Doyle, A. C.: *Memories and Adventures*: London, Hodder & Stoughton, 1924, p. 107.
6. Shepherd, M.: *Sherlock Holmes and the Case of Dr. Freud*: London, Tavistock Publications, 1985.

Sick Santa Syndrome

There is an increased incidence of infectious disease in individuals who assume the role of Santa Claus during the Yuletide season—December to mid-January.[1] The symptoms are those of a generalized and relatively mild communicable disease, including low-grade fever, myalgia, sinusitis, nasal congestion, painful swallowing, decreased appetite, and cervical lymphadenopathy. Infectious agents include mycoplasma, streptococci, and the viruses of influenza, coryza, mumps, and measles. These are transmitted by respiratory droplets and saliva to those "playing" Santa Claus while "ho, ho, hoing, hugging, listening, reassuring, and winking done face to face."

1. Dembert, M. L.: Sick Santa syndrome: *J.A.M.A.*, 256:3216–3217, 1986.

Sirenomelia

(mermaid deformity, sympodia)

Fusion of the lower extremities is called sirenomelia.[1] The anatomical abnormality may be due to fusion of the soft tissues with one set of bones, reduced number of bones, or none at all. In the majority of instances, it is associated with the major congenital abnormalities of cau-

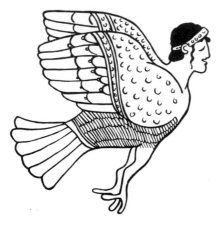

(A)

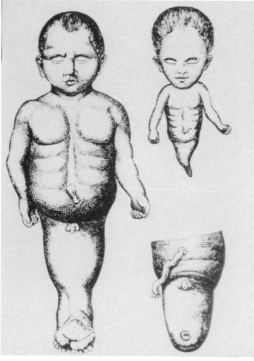

(B)

Sirenomelia A. The classic siren, part woman, part bird, from a 5th century B.C. vase.[11] (by permission, Dover Pubns., Inc.) **B.** Three variants of sirenomelia.[10]

dal dysplasia, which includes anomalies of the lumbar spine and sacrum, imperforated anus, and agenesis of the kidneys, urinary tract, and genital organs, but not of the gonads.[2] There is usually absence of one umbilical artery. The complex thus represents a severe form of caudal developmental regression.[3] It has also been found in association with anencephaly.[4]

In Greek mythology, a siren was a fabulous monster, part woman, part bird, who lured sailors to their destruction by enchanting singing.[5] They were muses of the sea and death. They are best known from Homer's *Odyssey*, in which Ulysses (Odysseus) was sorely tempted by the spell of their enchanting singing.[6] Fortunately, he had been forewarned by Circe, the daughter of the sun. He stuffed the ears of his men with wax, but not of his own because he wanted to listen to their song. Ulysses had enough wisdom, however, to have his men lash him to the mast so that he would not change the course of the ship. The Argonauts, on their way home from seeking the golden fleece, were also sorely tempted by the sirens.[7] Orpheus, who had been taught by his parents, Apollo and Calliope, to play the lyre to perfection, overcame their seductive singing by his own more melodious and persuasive song.

Sirens were confused with mermaids in the English literature of the fourteenth century.[5] Mermaids occurred in European folklore as legendary beings, half human, half fish, who were long lived but mortal, had no souls, and often sang.[8] They were considered as dangerous to man, bringing floods and other disasters.[9] Therefore, designation as mermaid deformity is more appropriate than sirenomelic deformity on the basis of both mythological sources and morphological structure.

In medieval times, congenital anomalies were considered to be due to a visit by an incubus or a merman, who impregnated the woman.[1] In the nineteenth century, concepts were somewhat more enlightened, the anomaly being attributed to fusion of the legs by intrauterine compression during early gestation.[10] Today, etiological classifications of anomalies include abnormal genes, maternal drug ingestion, and intrauterine infections.

1. Bloch, B.: Sirenomelia (sympodia or mermaid deformity): *S. Afr. Med. J.*, 52:196–200, 1977.
2. Duhamel, B.: From the mermaid to anal imperforation: The syndrome of caudal regression: *Arch. Dis. Child.*, 36:152–155, 1961.
3. Young, I. D. et al.: Etiological heterogenicity in sirenomelia: *Pediatr. Pathol.*, 5:31–43, 1986.
4. Schwaibold, H. et al.: Sirenomelia and anencephaly in one of dizygotic twins: *Teratology*, 34:243–247, 1986.
5. Gayley, p. 57.
6. Homer, chap. XII.
7. Gayley, p. 232.
8. *Encyclopaedia Britannica*: VI:808.
9. Magalini, S. I. & Scrascia, E.: *Dictionary of Medical Syndromes*: 2nd ed., Philadelphia, J. B. Lippincott, 1981, p. 543.
10. Gould, G. M. & Pyle, W. L.: *Anomalies and Curiosities of Medicine*: Philadelphia, W. B. Saunders, 1896, p. 270.
11. Huber, R.: *Treasury of Fantastic and Mythological Creatures*: New York, Dover, 1981, 5:3.

Sisyphus Reaction

A type of coronary-prone individual who is more likely to undergo sudden death is characterized by a strong commitment to hard work without experiencing any sense of accomplishment or satisfaction.[1] This differs from the Type A personality in which there is a sense of emotional fulfillment with achievement.[2] Individuals with the Sisyphean variant of Type A have feelings of psychological uncertainty,[3] which can lower the threshold for electrical conduction disturbances in the heart with resultant undampened autonomic nerve discharges and sudden death.[4]

Such a psychological orientation has been named after Sisyphus, the king of Cornith in Greek mythology. He observed the abduction by Jupiter (Zeus) of Aegina, and was indiscreet enough to tell her father, the river god, Asopus.[5] The angry king of the gods condemned Sisyphus to Hades. After several attempts to escape, he was given eternal punishment—forever rolling a huge stone up a hill, only to have it roll back down each time it almost reached the top. As described by Odysseus:

And Sisyphus I saw in bitter pains, forcing a monstrous stone along with both his hands. Tugging with hand and foot, he pushed the stone upward along a hill. But when he thought to heave it on clear to the summit, a mighty power would turn it back; and so once more down to the ground it would tumble. Again he strained to push it back; sweat ran down from his limbs, and from his head a dust cloud rose.[6]

The common denominator is the ever-present sense of frustration, whether induced by the gods or by one's own personality. An example is the report of two young males with severe coronary artery disease, and the same emotional predicament: One had a wife and a fiancee, and the other two fiancees, in each case both visiting the patient in the hospital. The Sisyphus Pattern is a prognostic global personality assessment procedure to determine if a person fits the Sisyphus description.[1] Freud stated that in treating hysterical individuals, "The physician will not be spared the depressing feeling of being faced by a Sisyphean task."[8] The context is that of an impossible task, as was Sysiphus's punishment in Hades.

Albert Camus has titled a collection of essays as *The Myth of Sisyphus and Other Essays*.[9] In the preface he equates this myth with the need "to wonder whether life has a meaning." In the essay itself, Sisyphus is considered as everyman, the absurd hero who is penalized by accomplishing nothing as "the price that must be paid for the passions of this earth." On a less philosophical plane, Sisyphus has also been invoked for the frustrating inability to keep the doctorate degree for nursing in a prominent and permanent academic light.[10]

The adjective sisyphean is used in general for a task that requires continual redoing.[11] It is a common theme in literature, one example occurring in Dostoevsky's novel *Memoirs from the House of the Dead* (1861–1862).[12] In this fictional account of his own penal servitude in Siberia, he comments that "if it were desired to crush and destroy a man completely and punish him with the most frightful possible penalty, which would make even the most terrible criminal quail and fill him with dread, it would suffice to give the penal work the most completely and utterly useless and nonsensical character."

1. Bruhn, J. G. et al.: Psychological predictors of sudden death in myocardial infarction: *J. Psychosomat. Res.*, 18:187–191, 1974.
2. Friedman, M. & Rosenman, R. H.: Association of specific overt behavior pattern with blood

and cardiovascular findings. Blood cholesterol level, blood clotting time, incidence of arcus senilis, and clinical coronary artery disease: *J.A.M.A.*, 169:1286–1296, 1959.

3. Engel, G. L.: Psychological stress, vaso-depressor (vasovagal) syncope: *Ann. Int. Med.*, 59:403–412, 1978.
4. Wolf, S.: Psychosocial forces in myocardial infarction and sudden death: *Circulation*, 39/40(Suppl. IV):74–81, 1969.
5. Gayley, p. 73.
6. Homer.
7. Gizzi, M. S. & Gitler, B.: Coronary risk factors: The contemplation of bigamy: *J.A.M.A.*, 256: 1138, 1986.
8. Brueer, F. & Freud, *S. E.*, Vol. II, *Studies on Hysteria*, p. 263.
9. Camus, A.: *The Myth of Sisyphus and Other Essays*: J. O'Brien translator, New York, Random House, 1959.
10. Lancaster, L. A.: Doctoral education in nursing, the Sisyphian concept, and Pandora's box: *Crit. Care Nursing*, 4:6–17, 1984.
11. Espy, pp. 37–38.
12. Dostoevsky, F.: *Memoirs from the House of the Dead*: J. Coulson translator, Oxford, England, Oxford University Press, 1983, p. 24.
13. Huber, R.: *Treasury of Fantastic and Mythological Creatures*: New York, Dover, 1984, p. 5, no. 3.

Sleeping Beauty Syndrome

A child after being unconscious for some time due to severe head injury awakens in the strange and frightening atmosphere of an intensive care unit, often with complete immobilization and tubes and wires attached to parts of the body.[1] The child may react with a psychic emergency reaction manifested as a feigned-death response which can simulate an organic coma state. This can be misleading as to the degree of recovery and delay rehabilitation efforts.

This feigned-death state has been named after "Sleeping Beauty." the fairy tale which first appeared as "La Belle au Bois Dormant" by Charles Perrault, a seventeenth century French writer and critic.[2] It then became one of the fairy tales of the Grimm brothers, Jacob and Wilhelm, in the early nineteenth century.[3] It is a story of romance in which a magic spell is cast upon a beautiful princess, Rosamond, by a wise woman (witch) who was angry because she was not invited to a feast celebrating her birth. She ordained that in her fifteenth year Rosamond would prick her finger on a spindle and fall asleep for one hundred years. This came to pass, and all the inhabitants of the castle fell asleep. With the passage of time the castle became hidden by a dark wood of thorns. After a hundred years a prince penetrated the woods and kissed her. All awoke and the prince and princess were married.

The Sleeping Beauty Syndrome actually includes two periods of unconsciousness, one traumatic and the other psychological in origin. It is much more a horror story than a nursery tale. In another vein, "Sleeping Beauty" has been equated with escape from adolescence by passivity, or by retreat into abnormal states such as schizophrenia, use of drugs, delinquency, or joining a religious cult.[4] The use of narcolepsis as a diagnostic and therapeutic tool has been compared to "La Belle au Bois Dormant."[5]

The story of "Sleeping Beauty" has been used allegorically to discuss some women who do not have orgasms.[6] The finger prick is the onset of menses when her parents warn her of the dangers of sexuality, and the one-hundred-year sleep a state of fantasizing in which she dreams of a prince with a magical kiss (his penis).

1. Todorow, S.: Recovery of children after severe head injury: *Scand. J. Rehab. Med.*, 7:93–96, 1975.
2. Benét, pp. 92, 775.
3. Grimm, J. & Grimm, W.: "Sleeping Beauty": in *Grimm's Fairy Tales*, Garden City, New York, n.d., pp. 205–210.
4. Bruch, H.: The Sleeping Beauty: Escape from change: in *The Course of Life: Psychoanalytic Contributions Toward Understanding Personality Development*, Vol. II, *Adolescence and Youth*, S. I. Greenspan & G. H. Pollock, Eds., Adelphia, Maryland, National Institute for Mental Health, 1980, pp. 431–444.
5. Cornet, C., Sylva, P. & Szafran, A. W.: La narroanalyse La Belle au Bois Dormant: *Psychiatr. Belgica.*, 80:91–100, 1980.
6. Kerr, C.: TA and sex therapy for women. Nonorgasmic scripts: *Transact. Anal. J.*, 6:28–36, 1976.

Snowman Heart

(snowman sign)

In type one total anomalous pulmonary return, the anomalous pulmonary veins unite to form a common trunk that enters the superior vena cava or azygos vein.[1] The result is two enlargements of the heart shadow as seen on x-ray. The lower one is due to right atrial and ventricular enlargement, and the smaller upper one to widening of the superior mediastinum by the anomalous pulmonary vein. A similar appearance may occur in infants with right-sided enlargement of the heart resulting from a left-to-right shunt and mediastinal enlargement by abundant thymus tissue.[2]

The widened mediastinum represents the head of a snowman and the increased cardiac diameter, the body. The snowman is a popular winter creation in many countries. He was immortalized by Hans Christian Andersen's story of the snowman who fell in love with a large black stove he saw through a window.[3] He daydreamed about it happily until he melted in warmer weather. Only then was it revealed that it was the old poker of his beloved black stove that had held him together. This anthropomorphized romantic tale has no relationship to the hemodynamics of the Snowman Heart, except for an imaginative physical similarity to the character.[4]

1. Schwischuk, L. E.: *Plain Film Interpretation in Congenital Heart Disease*: Philadelphia, Lea and Febiger, 1970, pp. 83–93.
2. Eisenberg, p. 278.
3. Andersen, H. C.: "The Snowman": in *The Complete Fairy Tales and Stories*, E. C. Haugaard translator, New York, Doubleday, 1974, pp. 718–722.
4. Vaisrub, p. 116.

Snow White—Cinderella Theme

Fathers play a greater role than generally thought in the feminine identification of their daughters.[1] A basic problem is the ever-present triangle of father, daughter, and mother, with the young child adoring her father. This type of Jocasta-Oedipus conflict should normally be resolved by the father in developing a "desexualized affection" and an acceptance of her femaleness in adolescence.

The second marriages of the fathers of Snow White[2] and Cinderella[3] were two women who proved to be wicked, and who were greatly jealous of the beauty of their step-daughters. Snow White was sent to the woods to be killed. She was rescued by dwarfs to the dismay of the stepmother, who then bound her with new lace so tightly that it took Snow White's breath away and she fell as dead. Cinderella was relegated to a menial existence of doing the lowest and dirtiest of housework. Each of these downtrodden girls was rescued by a prince—a symbol for the daydreams of women.

The fathers of Snow White and Cinderella were weak individuals who could not contribute anything to the feminine development of their daughters. The fictional women married quite well in the end—in spite of their father's neglect. It is suggested that the absence of a father leads to considerable fantasizing of a loving and protective father.[1] Other examples given of inappropriate relationships between father and daughter are King Lear and his daughter Cordelia (see Electra and Lear Complexes).[1]

Another aspect of the daughter/mother relationship has been labeled as the Snow White Syndrome.[4] This refers to a family in which the mother is envious of the budding beauty of her own daughter whom she considers as a rival. If the mother's envy is excessive, the daughter fears that "If she surpasses her mother . . . she will arouse her mother's envy and insecurity." The end result is that the daughter grows up with a fear that she will not be liked if she becomes too successful. The Snow White fairy tale has also been interpreted as a depiction of some problems of female development and as a symbolic description of development in both sexes.[5] Snow White's dwarfs can be considered as symbols of the creative power of the unconscious or as phallic characters.

A pastiche of the Snow White story has been written with the nurse as the downtrodden Snow White, the doctor as the wicked witch, Sleepy as the intern, and Grumpy as the hospital administrator.[6] The spell which the witch doctor placed on the nurse was finally broken by Prince Medicare, who "wanted Snow White to develop into the beautiful and competent nurse he knew was buried underneath fatigue and harassment." This is indeed a sad commentary on the relationship between some doctors and nurses.

1. Kestenbaum, C. J.: Fathers and daughters: The father's contribution to feminine identification in girls as depicted in fairy tales and myths: *Am. J. Psychoanal.*, 43:119–127, 1983.
2. Grimm, W. & Grimm, J.: "Snow-White": in *Grimm's Fairy Tales*, Garden City, New York, Junior Deluxe Editions, n.d., pp. 219–231.

3. Perrault, C.: *Cinderella or the Little Slipper*: New York, Henry Z. Walch, 1971.
4. Cohen, B.: *The Snow White Syndrome. All About Envy*: New York, Macmillan, 1986.
5. Arnold, H. M.: Snow White & the Seven Dwarfs: *Perspect. Psychiatr. Care*, 17:218–222, 236, 1979.
6. Ward, V. S.: Snow White and the seven missing dwarfs—A fantasy: *Colorado Nurse*, 66:17–19, 1966.

Somniferous

Somniferous is defined as anything that induces sleep, such as drugs.[1] Chloral derivatives and barbiturates are prime examples, but more prominent now are the benzodiazepines.[2] Somnus (Sleep, Hypnos) was the son of Night (Nox) and the brother of Thanatos (Death).[3] These gods lived in subterranean darkness, one bringing mortals fair dreams, and the later closing forever their eyes (see Hypnosis).

1. Stein, p. 1356.
2. Gilman, pp. 339–371.
3. Gayley, pp. 54, 176.

Sphincter

A sphincter is a circular band of voluntary or involuntary muscle which encircles an orifice of the body or of one of its hollow organs, and thus controls the flow of liquids or solids.[1] The word is derived from the Sphinx of Greek mythology, which was a hybrid monster, usually described as having the head of a woman and the winged body of a lion.[2] The Sphinx asked a riddle of all travelers who passed by:[3] "What animal is it that in the morning goes on four feet, at noon on two, and in the evening on three?" Those who could not provide the correct answer were squeezed to death by the embrace of the Sphinx, and thus the similarity to the contraction of sphincters. It was Oedipus who provided the correct answer when challenged. "Man, who in childhood creeps on hands and knees, in manhood walks erect, and in old age goes with the aid of a staff." The Sphinx then threw herself down from the rock and died.

Freud equated the child's question as to where babies come from with a distorted version of the riddle of the Sphinx, although he did not clearly explain the reasoning behind this assumption.[4] He considered this to be one of the first problems which is of concern to the child.[5]

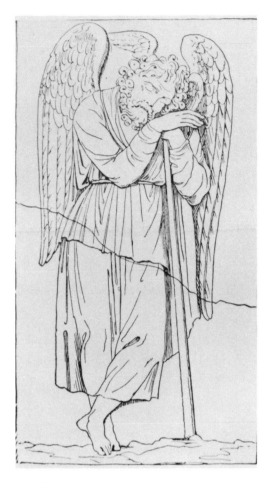

Somniferous Somnos sleeping.[3]

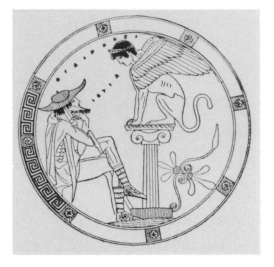

Sphincter Oedipus responding to the riddle of the sphinx.[3, p. 261]

Neuroses and phobias may develop with inappropriate answers. In a mechanical allusion, the riddle of the Sphinx has also been invoked for the mystery and uncertainty of the role of the lower esophageal sphincter in the occurrence of sliding hiatus hernias of the stomach.[6]

Diel has given a universal interpretation of the Riddle of the Sphinx.[7]

The riddle concerns every human being personally. The answer is "myself." Each man, to a different degree, is the victim of the perverse spirit (blinding vanity). "To solve the riddle" thus becomes synonymous with the central statement of the myth: "Know thyself." It is the meaning of the smile of the Sphinx, both mysterious and ironic.

1. Stein, p. 1369.
2. Haubrich, pp. 226–227.
3. Gayley, pp. 261–262.
4. Tourney, G.: Freud and the Greeks: A study of the influence of classical Greek mythology and philosophy upon the development of Freudian thought: *J. Hist. Behavior. Sci.*, 1:67–85, 1965.
5. Freud: *S.E.*, Vol. IX, pp. 135–136.
6. Ingelfinger, F. J.: The sphincter that is a sphinx: *N. Engl. J. Med.*, 284:1095–1096, 1971.
7. Diel, p. 133.

Stentorial Snoring

The very loudest and most obnoxious type of snoring is called stentorial snoring.[1] Snoring occurs in over 50% of the population, and may be a risk factor for such conditions as hypertension and heart disease.[2] One study has shown that people who snore have a smaller pharyngeal cross-sectional area than do nonsnorers.[3] Stentor was a Greek hero of the Trojan war[4] whose voice was, according to Homer, as loud as that of fifty men together.[5] " . . . then stood the white-armed goddess Hera and shouted in the likeness of great-hearted Stentor with voice of bronze, whose cry was as loud as the cry of fifty other men."

The word stentorian means very large or powerful in sound.[6] A stentor is one who has a "loud mouth." Stentors are also ciliated protozoa that have mouths shaped like trumpets.[7] On a similar basis, a trumpet-shaped plant has been called a stentor, as has the platyrrhine monkey of the South American genus *Mycetes*.[8] An interesting allusion to snoring is found in Shakespeare's *Tempest*.[9] Sebastian tells Antonio that "Thou dost snore distinctly; there's meaning in thy snores." This suggests both loud snores and inflections in its sound.

Another eponym for a powerful voice is Boanerges, or the "sons of thunder," as referred to by Christ for the two sons of Zebedee whom he chose as preachers and healers of the sick.[10] It is used for a loud and noisy orator or speaker.[11]

1. Snoring can harm your health and ruin your marriage: Here is how it can be stopped: *Mayo Clin. Health Lett.*, 3:1, 1985.
2. Norton, P. G. & Dunn, E. V.: Snoring as a risk factor for disease: An epidemiological survey: *Br. Med. J.*, 291:630–632, 1985.
3. Bradley, T. D. et al.: Pharyngeal size in snorers, nonsnorers and patients with obstructive sleep apnea: *N. Engl. J. Med.*, 315:1327–1331, 1986.
4. Schmidt, p. 254.
5. Homer: *The Iliad*: New York, Random House, 1950, Book V, p. 97.
6. Stein, p. 1393.
7. Espy, p. 39.
8. OED: X:915.
9. Shakespeare, *The Tempest*: II, i.
10. NT: Mark 3:14–17.
11. Hendrickson, p. 332.

Straw Peter Syndrome

(hyperactive child syndrome, minimal brain

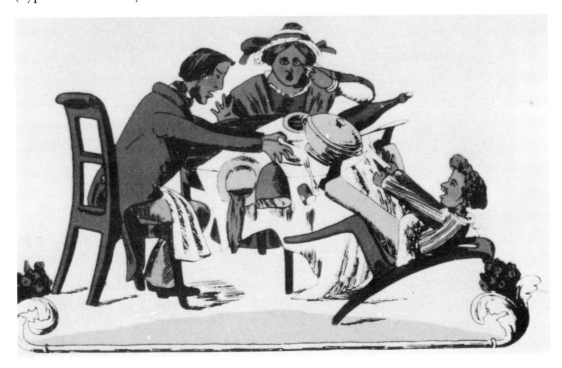

Straw Peter Syndrome   Fidgety Philip fidgeting.[7, p. 44]

dysfunction [damage], sloveny Peter,[1] struw-welpeter syndrome)

The syndrome of minimal brain damage (dysfunction) is characterized by a type of hyperkinesis in which the child constantly moves about, touching and handling objects without any discernible purpose.[2] Other behavioral activities include short attention span, impulsiveness, aggressive acts, sexual displays, and learning difficulties. The cause of such manifestations appears to be heterogeneous.[3] There are proponents of no, minimal, and major brain damage,[4] of hereditary factors,[5] and of delayed physiological development of the brain.[6] Estimated incidence varies from four to twenty percent of all school children.

Struwwelpeter, the origin of the eponym, is the main character of a German children's book written in the nineteenth century by Heinrich Hoffman, a pediatrician.[7] The name has been translated as Straw Peter or Slovenly Peter, but more accurately as Shaggy-headed Peter. He and his friends were involved in many frenetic and cruel activities, all described in verse form. Peter "never has once combed his hair" and "his nails are never cut." Cruel Frederick tore wings off flies, killed birds, broke chairs, and whipped Mary. Fidgety Philip "won't sit still;/He wriggles and giggles,/And then, I declare,/Swings backwards and forwards,/And tilts up his chair, . . . See the naughty, restless child/Growing still more rude and wild,. . . ."

The syndrome is a composite of the activities of Straw Peter, Cruel Frederick, and Fidgety Philip. There is an excellent relationship between these fictional characters and the medical condition. Their stories, and that of others in the book, are essentially moralistic, as are most children stories. The picaresque nature of Dr. Hoffman's verses appealed to the waggish nature of Mark Twain, who published his own translation from the German.[8]

Punishment for misbehavior is included in *Struwwelpeter*. Conrad the thumb-sucker is threatened by his mother, with "The great tall tailor [who] always comes/ To little boys who suck their thumbs;/ And ere they dream what he's about,/ He takes his great sharp scissors out,/ And cuts their thumbs clean off. . . ."[7] It has been suggested that exposure as a child to such *Struwwelpeter* stories may have contributed to Dylan Thomas's subconscious preoccupation with fears of loss of penis and castration.[9] Striking images of scissors and tailors are found in his poems.[10] In one of his early stories, which is filled with sexual symbols and activities, there is "a child who had cut off his double thumb."[11] Freud considered thumbsucking to be a manifestation of infantile sexuality, and one that could lead to masturbation.[12] Conrad in *Struwwelpeter* is given as an example of thumb-sucking in a footnote to this section by the editor of Freud's collected works.

1. Magalini, S. I. & Scrascia, E.: *Dictionary of Medical Syndromes*: 2nd. ed., Philadelphia, J. B. Lippincott, 1981, p. 780.
2. Pincus, J. H. & Glaser, G. H.: The syndrome of "minimal brain damage" in childhood: *N. Engl. J. Med.*, 275:27–35, 1966.
3. Strother, C. R.: Minimal cerebral dysfunction: A historical overview: *Ann. N.Y. Acad. Sci.*, 205:6–17, 1973.
4. Benton, A. L.: Minimal brain dysfunction from a neuropsychological point of view: *Ann. N.Y. Acad. Sci.*, 205:29–37, 1973.
5. Vandenberg, S. G.: Possible hereditary factors in minimal brain dysfunction: *Ann. N.Y. Acad. Sci.*, 205:223–230, 1973.
6. Editor: 'Hyperactive child' syndrome recognized 100 years ago?: *J.A.M.A.*, 202:28–29, 1967.
7. Hoffman, H.: *Struwwelpeter. Merry Stories and Funny Pictures*: New York, Grolier Society, n.d.
8. Hoffmann, H.: *Slovenly Peter (Der Struwwelpeter)*: Mark Twain translator, New York, Harper & Bros., 1935.
9. Neill, M.: Dylan Thomas's "Tailor Age": *Notes and Queries*, Feb., 1970, pp. 59–63.
10. Ferris, P.: *Dylan Thomas*: New York, Dial Press, 1977, pp. 40–41.
11. Thomas, D.: "The Mouse and the Woman": in *Dylan Thomas. The Collected Stories*, New York, New Directions, 1984, pp. 72–86.
12. Freud: "The Manifestations of Infantile Sexuality": *S.E.*, Vol. VII, pp. 179–183.

Syphilis

(French disease, lues, Neopolitan disease,[1] syphilitic[2])

There is still controversy as to whether syphilis was present in Europe before the return of Columbus to Spain from the Americas in 1493.[3] Infection with the spirochete of syphilis (*Treponema pallidum*) is still a major venereal disease because of the development of resistance of the

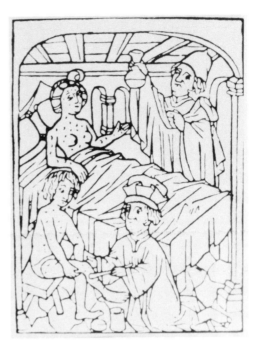

Syphilis Treatment of syphilis with mercury ointment.[31] (woodcut, 1497/8) (by permission, U.S. Department of the Army)

organism to antibiotics, of more liberal sexual mores, and of the decrease in use of condoms since the availability of oral contraceptives.[4] The use of condoms has, however, increased since the AIDS epidemic.

Syphilis was named after a poem written by Hieronymus Fracastorius (Giorolama Fracastoro) in 1525.[5] Fracastorius was born in Verona in 1483, became a renowned physician, and died of apoplexy in 1553. He is best known for his *Treatise on Contagion*,[6] which was almost modern in its concept of the spread of infection;[7] and for his lengthy poem, *Poetical History of the French Disease*, more commonly called Syphilus[8] The hero, Syphilus, was a shepherd whose flock was dying in the parched land from extreme heat and thirst. He cried out against the sun in anger and persuaded others to no longer worship him.

Th' all-seeing Sun no longer could sustain
These practices, but with enrag'd Disdain
Darts forth such pestilent malignant Beams,
As shed Infection on Air, Earth and Streams;
From whence this Malady its birth receiv'd,
And first th' offending *Syphilus* was griev'd, . . .
He first wore Buboes dreadful to the sight,
First felt strange Pains and sleepless past the Night: . . .
From him the Malady receiv'd its name,
The neighboring Shepherds catcht the spreading Flame.

In the sixteenth century, syphilis did not have the connotation of immorality, primarily because of the belief in the astrological causation of diseases.[9] Although there were many names for the disease before Fracastorius's poem, Syphilis became very popular in short order, possibly because of its hissing, sibilant sound. There is controversy over Fracastorius's source for the name Syphilus. Suggested derivations are from the Greek,[10] or from Sypilus,[11] one of the seven sons of Niobe, queen of Thebes. Sypilus and Niobe were slain by the arrows of Diana and Apollo, who reacted in anger to Niobe's boasting of her sons' beauty and her ridicule of Leto, Apollo's mother.[12] An analogy has been suggested between the arrows of Apollo and the unseen viruses implied by Fracastorius in his book on contagion.[9] Another possible derivation is from Thypalus, a scribal error for Priapus, the Greek god of gardens and the phallus.[13] An eponym for syphilis is Cupid's Disease, used primarily by prostitutes.[14]

Syphilis occurs in many fictional works. It has been suggested as the cause of skin lesions in the Summoner, the Cook and the Wife of Bath in Chaucer's *Canterbury Tales* of the fourteenth century.[15] Such a premise could only be valid if syphilis existed in Europe before Columbus's voyage of 1492. Shakespeare's plays contain more definite references to syphilis, although using the terms of his time: Neopolitan disease, malady of French, goujeers.[16] In Defoe's *Moll Flanders* of 1722,[17] the antiheroine caught syphilis from a baronet who might have sown "the contagion in the lifeblood of his posterity."[18] It has been suggested that syphilis is a major theme of Joyce's *Ulysses*,[19] there being frequent mention of signs and symptoms that occur in this disease and of a whorehouse.[20]

Rabelais dedicated his *Gargantua* of 1534 to the "Most noble and illustrious drinkers, and you thrice precious pockified [syphilitic] blades."[21] In Book One, chapter IV of *Gargantua*, it is noted that "his said preceptor died of the French pox, which was in the year one thousand four hundred and twenty." This predates, at least fictionally, Columbus's return from America. A passage in Shakespeare's *Timon of Athens*[22] is suggestive of syphilis. Timon is speaking to two prostitutes. "Consumptions sow/In hollow bones of man; strike their sharp shins/And mar men's spurring..down with the nose/Down with it flat; take the bridge away. . . ." This description fits well with that of syphilitic osteitis and its saddle-nose deformity. References to syphilis are also found in the writings of Donne and Ibsen. It has been claimed that the minds of writers, artists, poets, and musicians were stimulated by the presence of early general paresis of tertiary syphilis.[23]

Descriptions of syphilis have even been suggested as occurring in the Bible, particularly in Leviticus.[24] An example quoted from Deuteronomy is contained in Moses' warning about the dangers of disobedience to the laws.[25] "The Lord will strike you with madness, blindness and confusion . . . the Lord will smite you within your knees and on your legs, from the sole of your foot to the crown of your head with malignant sores." There can, however, be many interpretations other than syphilis. Saint's names given to syphilis are St. Mevius, St. Sementius, St. Regius, and St. Evagrius.[24] More vulgar terms were used for syphilis in eighteenth and nineteenth century England—fireship (syphilitic woman), peppered, running horse or nag.[26] A more respectable term still used today is lues (luetic), which is of Greek origin, meaning a contagious disease.[27]

Diagnoses of syphilis have been made on bones dating to pre-Columbian America and the Old World.[28] Such a diagnosis on this type of material is, however, open to considerable question.[29] Several cranial specimens unearthed in Florida have lesions which resemble the early stages of tertiary syphilis that precede gummatous necrosis.[30] There has yet to be a definitive settlement of the dispute over which direction syphilis first crossed the Atlantic Ocean.

1. Dennie, C. C.: *A History of Syphilis*: Springfield, Illinois, Charles C Thomas, 1962.
2. OED: X:389–390.
3. Fleming, W. L.: Syphilis through the ages: *Med. Clin. North Am.*, 48:587–611, 1964.
4. Robbins, S. L. et al.: *Pathologic Basis of Disease*: 3rd ed., Philadelphia, W. B. Saunders, 1984, pp. 335–338.
5. Barnett, C. F., Jr.: Hieronymus Fracastorius: Namer of syphilis: *New Physician*, 13:117–118, 1964.
6. Fractastorius, H.: *Hieronymus Fracastorius. Contagion, Contagious Diseases and Their Treatment*: W. C. Wright translator, New York, G. P. Putman's Sons, 1930.
7. Singer, C. & Singer, D.: The scientific position of Girolamo Fracastoro (1478?–1553) with especial reference to the source, character and influence of the theory of infection: *Ann. Med. Hist.*, 1:1–34, 1917.
8. Fracastorius, H.: A poetical history of the French disease: in R. H. Major, *Classic Descriptions of Disease*, 3rd ed., Springfield, Illinois, Charles C Thomas, 1947, pp. 39–42.
9. Montgomery, D. W.: Hieronymus Fracastorius. The author of the poem called Syphilis: *Ann. Hist. Med.*, 11:406–413, 1930.
10. Hendrickson, G. L.: The "syphilis" of Girolamo Fracastoro with some observations on the origin and history of the word "syphilis": *Bull. Inst. Hist. Med.*, 2:515–546, 1934.
11. Glickman, F. S.: Syphilus: *J. Am. Acad. Dermatol.*, 12:593–596, 1985.

12. Bulfinch, pp. 136–140.
13. Graziani, R.: Fracastoro's 'Syphilis' and Priapus: *Clio Med.*, 16:93–99, 1981.
14. Sacks, O.: Cupid's disease: *MD Mag.*, 31:54–55, 1987.
15. Mandel, S.: Chaucer's vivid medical word pictures (reflections of yore afflictions): *Intern. J. Dermatol.*, 22:329–331, 1983.
16. Kail, A. C.: Medicine in Shakespeare. The Bard and the body 3. Venereal disease—"the pox": *Med. J. Aust.*, 2:445–449, 1983.
17. Schneck, J. M.: Daniel Defoe's *Moll Flanders* and congenital syphilis: *N.Y. State J. Med.*, 78:2104–2105, 1978.
18. Defoe, D.: *The Fortunes and Misfortunes of the Famous Moll Flanders*: New York, Collectors Ed., Pocket Books, 1951, p. 245.
19. Hall, V. & Waisbren, B. A.: Syphilis as a major theme of James Joyce's *Ulysses*: *Arch. Int. Med.*, 140:963–965, 1980.
20. Joyce, J.: *Ulysses*: New York, Random House, 1986.
21. Rabelais: *Gargantua*: in *The Works of Rabelais*, Urquhart & Motteux translators, London (published for the Trade), n.d.
22. Shakespeare, *Timon of Athens*: IV:iii.
23. Walker, pp. 277–280.
24. Rosebury, T.: *Microbes and Morals. The Strange Story of Venereal Disease*: New York, Viking Press, 1971, p. 31.
25. OT: Deuteronomy 28:28–35.
26. Bloch, pp. 45–46.
27. Skinner, p. 257.
28. Steinbock, R. T. & Sterart, T. D.: *Paleopathological Diagnosis and Interpretation. Bone Diseases in Ancient Populations*: Springfield, Illinois, Charles C Thomas, 1976, pp. 136–137.
29. Brothwell, D. & Sandison, A. T.: *Diseases in Antiquity*: Springfield, Illinois, Charles C Thomas, 1967, 583–584.
30. Iscan, M. Y. & Miller-Shaivitz, P.: Prehistoric syphilis in Florida: *J. Florida Med. Assoc.*, 72:109–113, 1985.
31. Schreiber, W.: Syphilis treatment through the ages: *Med. Bull. U.S. Army, Eur.*, 40:21–31, 1983.

Syringe

Syringes have long been used in medicine, from as early as the beginning of the seventeenth century.[1] The origin of the syringe is uncertain.[2] The hypodermic type was not introduced until 1845 in Europe and 1878 in America.[3] Syringes is the plural of the name Syrinx, who was an Arcadian nymph in Greek mythology.[4] One day, as Syrinx was returning from the chase with Diana, she was in turn chased by Pan, the hoofed and horned god of woods and fields. He overtook her at the bank of a river and she called to the water nymphs for help.[5] As Pan embraced her, Syrinx changed into a tuft of reeds. When he sighed, the air going through the reeds produced such a lovely melody that he made a musical instrument out of them.

The flow of air or fluid through the hollow tube (pipe) of the syringe may be the origin of its name from the nymph.[6] Also named after Syrinx are the reed mouth organ (pan-pipes), and the vocal organ of birds. Of similar derivation is the name of some tumors with empty structures, the syringoma and syringadenoma of sweat glands; and of abnormal dilatations of the ventricles of the brain and the central canal of the spinal cord—syringobulbia, syringoencephalomyelia, syringomeningocele, syringomyelia, syringomyelocele.[7] Syrinx is a rarely used synonym for fistula, and syringotomy for its excision.

Syringa is the name of mock-orange because its stems were used for pipe-stems (*Philadelphus coronarius*), and of a lilac (pipe-tree).[1] An anatomical use is the name syringe for the tubular elephant's trunk.[8]

1. OED: X:390–391.
2. Boraker, D. K.: The syringe: *Med. Herit.*, 2:341–348, 1986.
3. Garrison, F. H.: *An Introduction to the History of Medicine*: 4th ed., Philadelphia, W. B. Saunders, 1960, pp. 159, 251, 656.
4. Stein, pp. 1443–1444.
5. Bulfinch, pp. 41–42.
6. Espy, p. 301.
7. Stedman, pp. 1400–1401.
8. Editors of the American Heritage Dictionaries: p. 239.

T

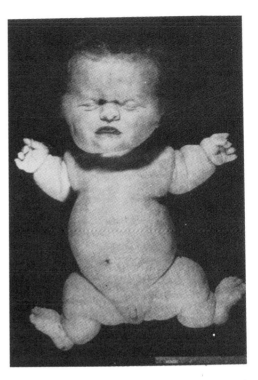

Thanatophoric Dwarf   Dwarf with very small chest.[5] (by permission, *Am. J. Obstet. Gynecol.*)

Thanatophoric Dwarf

(thanatophilic dysplasia)

Described in 1967 was a variety of short-limbed dwarfism which was labeled as thanatophoric.[1] It is distinguished from other types of dwarfism by a large head, firm skull bones, prominent forehead, hypertelorism, saddle nose, very short limbs, small thorax, and hypoplastic, atelectatic lungs. Because of the latter, most of these infants survive for only a few hours or days.[2] They have some features in common with achondroplastic dwarfs—narrow thorax, short limbs, prominent forehead, and saddle nose.[3] Their extremities, however, are bowed, abducted, and short, with disorganized endochondrial ossification.

Neurological abnormalities can include cloverleaf skull deformity, megalencephaly, displacement of basal ganglia, and fiber tract abnormalities.[4] Inheritance is that of a dominant lethal mutation with an incidence of about 1/100,000. Chromosomes are normal. It occurs more frequently in males,[5] and has been reported in twins.[6] Another type of dwarfism with marked respiratory distress at birth is asphyxiating thoracic dysplasia, which has short ribs and microscopic cysts of the liver and kidneys.[7]

The designation of a dwarf as thanatophoric refers to Thanatos, the personification of death in Greek mythology.[8] Thanatophoric can be defined as leading to death,[9] as does its namesake. Dwarfism at birth has become a complex

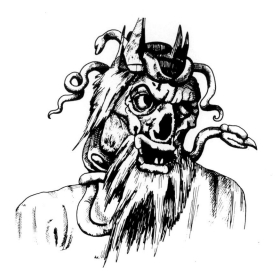

Thanatos Death personified.[18] (from an engraving by Albrecht Dürer, 1513) (by permission, Dover Pubns., Inc.)

subject, there being over 55 distinct syndromes, many with subtypes (see Thanatos).[7]

1. Maroteaux, R. et al.: Le nanisme thanatophore: *Presse Med.*, 75:2519–2524, 1967.
2. Kaufman, R. L. et al.: Thanatophoric dwarfism: *Am. J. Dis. Child.*, 120:53–57, 1970.
3. Nissenbaum, M. et al.: Thanatophoric dwarfism. Two case reports and survey of the literature: *Clin. Pediatr.*, 16:690–697, 1977.
4. Wongmongkolrit, T. et al.: Neuropathological findings in thanatophoric dysplasia: *Arch. Pathol. Lab. Med.*, 107:132–135, 1983.
5. Thompson, B. H. & Parmley, T. H.: Obstetric features of thanatophoric dwarfism: *Am. J. Obstet. Gynecol.*, 109:396–401, 1971.
6. Sato, D. et al.: Thanatophoric dysplasia of identical twins: *Acta Pathol. Jpn.*, 31:895–902, 1981.
7. Sillence, D. O. et al.: Neonatal dwarfism: *Pediatr. Clin. North Am.*, 25:453–483, 1978.
8. Stedman, p. 1436.
9. Gayley, p. 54.

Thanatos

(thanatism[1])

Thanatos is defined in psychotherapy as the death principle.[2] Freud indicated that "We may suppose that the final aim of the destructive instinct is to reduce living things to an inorganic state. For this reason we also call it the death instinct."[3] He differentiated this from the "instinct of self-preservation and of the preservation of the species. . . ." (which he called Eros).

The death instinct may be expressed not only in self-destruction, but also in homicidal intent, as illustrated by Cain.[4] It has been proposed that "The tendency to destructiveness and self-destructiveness is universal because the maternal filicidal impulse is universal. . . ."[5] This is the basis for the catastrophic death complex which has its beginnings in infancy.

Thanatos was the Greek mythological figure who was the personification of death. He and his brother Somnus (Sleep, Hynpnos) lived in subterranean darkness.[6] The inevitability of death is related to another Greek deity, Ananke, who was the personification of compelling necessity, the ultimate fate.[7] The need for such a goddess of destiny was recognized by Freud.[8] "If we are to die ourselves, and first to lose in death those who are dearest to us, it is easier to submit to a remorseless law of nature, to the sublime Ananke, than to a chance which might perhaps have been escaped." An Anankastic Syndrome is described in "Ananke," a short story by Stanislow Lem, a Polish medical graduate and science fiction writer.[9] It is a severe psychiatric complex of compulsive neuroses.

Thanatopsy is a synonym for autopsy, and the thanatophidia are a group of venomous snakes.[1] The term thanatophobia has been used for obsession with death and for sudden attacks of anxiety about imminent dissolution.[5] This has been expressed in milder tones by poets such as Keats.[10] "When I have fears that I may cease to be/ Before my pen has glean'd my teeming brain . . . then on the shore/ Of the wide world I stand alone, and think/ Till love and fame to nothingness do sink." In nineteen of twenty-nine poems by another poet, John McCrae, death is considered more benignly, often as a friend who brings an end to pain through peaceful sleep.[11] This is also well exemplified by Shakespeare in Macbeth's comment about the murdered King Duncan. "Duncan is in his grave; After life's fitful fever, he sleeps well."[12] Novelists may also exhibit a death instinct, as in the works of Dickens,[13] or depict a struggle with death, as in Tolstoy's *The Death of Ivan Ilyich*.[14]

The Thanatos Syndrome[15] is the title of a novel by Walker Percy, a physician/author. It is applied to a syndrome induced by the illegal addition of heavy sodium (high molar 24) to the water supply of a city in Louisiana. The result is degeneration of neurons in the cerebral neocortex with regression to a primitive, primate state in which psychological and emotional problems vanish. Sexual behavior is open and aggressive, behavior in general is placid, and speech consists of two-word sentences. Crime disappears, and psychiatrists are bereft of patients. The noble intentions of the perpetrators crumble when some who are not exposed to the illicit water take sexual advantage of complacent children. The use of the eponym Thanatos Syndrome may be applicable, in the sense of death of the neocortex, or more likely, to the death of all that makes humanity "human," including both the evil and the humanistic.

A Foundation of Thanatology was established in 1967 "for scientific and humanistic inquiries into death, loss, grief, bereavement and recovery from bereavement."[16] The official journal of this organization appeared in 1971 and was named *Journal of Thanatology*. In 1977, the title was changed to *Advances in Thanatology*.[17] Its scope was modified to emphasize the publication of clinical, theoretical, and research material from various disciplines which "represents an advance or is of heuristic value in explaining and understanding dying, death and bereavement."

1. OED: XI:245–246.
2. Stedman, p. 1436.
3. Freud, S.: *Outline of Psychoanalysis*: New York, Norton, 1949.
4. Szondi, L.: *Thanatos and Cain*: M. W. Webb translator, *Am. Imago*, 21:52–63, 1964.
5. Rheingold, J. C.: *The Mother, Anxiety, and Death. The Catastrophic Death Complex*: Boston, Little, Brown & Co., 1967, pp. 48, 202–203.
6. Gayley, p. 54.
7. *Encyclopaedia Britannica*: I:340.
8. Freud, S.: *Beyond the Pleasure Principle*: S.E., Vol. 18, p. 45.
9. Lem, S.: "Ananke": in *More Tales of Prix the Pilot*, New York, Harcourt Brace Jovanovich, 1982.
10. Keats, J.: Sonnet: in *The Poetical Works of John Keats*, H. B. Forman, Ed., New York, Thomas Y. Crowell, 1895, p. 376.
11. Rodin, A. E.: John McRae, poet-pathologist: *Can. Med. Assoc. J.*, 88:204–205, 1963.
12. Shakespeare, *Macbeth*: III,ii.
13. Manheim, L. F.: Thanatos: The death instinct in Dickens' later novels: *Psychoanal. Rev.*, 47:17–31, 1960–61.
14. Tolstoy, L.: *The Death of Ivan Ilyich*: L. Solotaroff translator, Toronto, Bantam Books, 1981.
15. Percy, W.: *The Thanatos Syndrome*: New York, Farrar, Straus, Giroux, 1987.
16. Foundation of Thanatology. New organization established: *J.A.M.A.*, 205:35, 1968.
17. Editorial: *Adv. Thanatol.*, 4:1, 1977.
18. Huber, R.: *Treasury of Fantastic and Mythological Creatures*: New York, Dover, 1981, 14:1.

Traviata Beauty

Young women dying of tuberculosis may have a certain ethereal, languorous beauty.[1] This is caused by their heightened color, produced by fever, and their somewhat emaciated state. The source of the eponym is *La Traviata*, the name of a Verdi opera, which was premiered in Venice in 1853.[2] It means the "lost one," who is Violetta Valery, a young courtesan

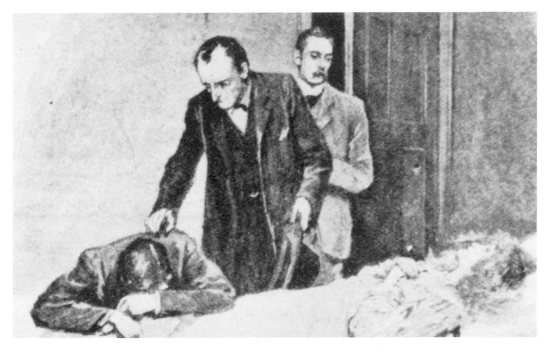

Traviata Beauty   Holmes and Watson consolling the missing three-quarter whose wife has just died of tuberculosis.[8] (by Paget)

who dies of tuberculosis. The opera was adapted from Alexander Dumas's drama *The Lady of the Camillas* (*La Dame aux Camélias*) of 1848.[3] "Among the invalids at the hotel there was a lovely young girl, the same age as Ma'amselle Marguerite, suffering from the same complaint, and bearing such strong resemblance to her that . . . they were called twin sisters." Dumas himself feel deeply in love with a courtesan who left him to return to her life of luxury.[4] He was baffled by the fact that she looked like a saint but behaved like a sinner (see Madonna-Harlot Syndrome).

Another operatic victim of tuberculosis is Mimi of Leoncavall's *La Bohème*.[5] In the nineteenth century, tuberculosis became "in fashion."[6] Thoreau remarked in his journal that "Decay and disease are often beautiful, like . . . the hectic glow of consumption."[7] In one of Conan Doyle's short stories "The Missing Three-Quarter,"[8] a soccer player was eventually found by Sherlock Holmes at the bedside of his beautiful wife, who was in the terminal stage of tuberculosis. Romanticization of tuberculosis decreased considerably with the development of specific antitubercular agents about the mid-twentieth century.[9] Prior to then, quackery ran rampant with spurious cures.[10] St. Pantelon is known as the saint against all wasting diseases, including tuberculosis.[11]

1. Dudzinski.
2. Ewen, D.: *Encyclopedia of the Opera*: New York, Hill & Wang, 1963, pp. 515–517.
3. Dumas, A.: *The Lady of the Camellias. A Drama in Four Acts*: adapted by M. McCarthy, in *La Traviata*, Boston, Little, Brown, 1983.
4. Barnes, A. C.: *La Traviata*: *J.A.M.A.*, 208:93–96, 1969.
5. Ewen, D.: *Encyclopedia of the Opera*: New York, Hill & Wang, 1963, pp. 52–54.
6. Dubos, R. J.: Microbiology in fable and art: *Bacterial. Rev.*, 16:145–151, 1952.
7. Thoreau, H. D.: *The Heart of Thoreau's Journals*: O. Shepard, Ed., Boston, Houghton Mifflin, 1927.
8. Doyle, A. C.: "The Missing Three-Quarter": *Strand Mag.*, 28:122–135, 1904.
9. Waksman, S. A.: *The Conquest of Tuberculosis*: Berkeley, California, University of California Press, 1964.
10. Smith, B.: Gullible's Travails: Tuberculosis and quackery 1890–1930: *J. Contemp. Hist.*, 20:733–756, 1985.
11. Ohry, A. & Ohry-Kossoy, K.: St. Giles, St. Francis et al.: Medical patron saints: *Adler Museum Bull.*, 18:18–22, 1986.

Tweedledum and Tweedledee Syndrome

Some patients with systematized hallucinations may project such a strong semblance of reality that they create in those around them a strong conviction of the correctness of their hallucinations.[1] This could be called folie á deux—delusions of two individuals.[2] Tweedledum and Tweedledee are two small, fat brothers whom Lewis Carroll's Alice met when she went through the looking glass.[3] They were mirror images of each other and alternated phrases and sentences in carrying on the same inane conversation with Alice. Being found much earlier in an eighteenth century epigram the names of these identical individuals were not original with Carroll.[4]

The literary name for this syndrome is attractive because of the iteration of the names, but their insanity was mental rather than hallucinatory. The phrase Tweedledum and Tweedledee has been used more appropriately to indicate nonsensical discussion, as applied to a debate on the financing of the British National Health Service.[5] Many other Lewis Carroll characters also spoke nonsense, as, for example, Jabberwocky.

1. Roe, P.: Eponymous disorders: *Lancet*, 2:794, 1978.
2. Dudzinski.
3. Carroll, pp. 229–232.
4. Hendrickson, p. 312.
5. Russell, W.: Tweedledum and Tweedledee debate on NHS finance: *Br. Med. J.*, 291:151, 1985.

U

Ulysses Complex

The Ulysses Complex has three phases: (1) the absence of the father, which is related to the Oedipus Complex; (2) the attempt at paternal identification by superego and further ego formation; and (3) the final phase of a dynamic, ego-strengthening parental-filial affection.[1] It can also be looked at as "a son's reciprocal search for his estranged father to recomplete the trinity of relationships with his mother."

Ulysses (Odysseus) is the hero of Homer's *Odyssey*.[2] After leaving his wife, Penelope, and his infant son, Telemachus, he spent many years traveling to Troy, at the battle of Troy, and returning home.[3] After growing up, Telemachus went out to search for Ulysses, but was unsuccessful. When the son returned home he was disturbed by all the suitors of his mother. Finally, after twenty years, Ulysses came home, and an excellent relationship developed between them.

The Ulysses saga and the life of James Joyce, as projected in his novel of 1922, *Ulysses*,[4] have been considered to be quite similar, possibly because of Bloom's wandering in Dublin.[5] The Homeric substructure of the *Odyssey* cannot, however, be considered as equivalent to the Dublin of 1904, as depicted in Joyce's novel.[6] Another interpretation is that Joyce and his book are not examples of the Ulysses or Oedipus Complexes, but of the search for his preoedipal mother.[5]

1. Santiago, L. P. R.: The Ulysses complex: *Am. Imago*, 28:158–186, 1971.

2. Homer.
3. Gayley, pp. 318–345.
4. Joyce, L.: *Ulysses*: New York, Random House, 1986.
5. Liegner, E. & Motycka, R.: James Joyce's *Ulysses* Revisited: matricide and the search for the mother: *Psychoanal. Rev.*, 68:561–579, 1981–2.
6. Kenner, J.: *Dublin's Joyce*: Boston, Beacon Press, 1956, pp. 179–193.

Ulysses Syndrome

False-positive results of laboratory, radiological, and even clinical examinations may lead to mental and physical disorders.[1] An example is the mistaking of a normal variant in a bone radiograph as abnormal, with resultant surgery followed by complications. Another example is the anguish and expenses incurred by a young woman who was told that her newborn died because of her syphilis, based on a false-positive test.[2] A contributing factor is poor communication between different hospitals and investigations.[3] Five similar instances have been reported from Spain.[4] The situation is aggravated by the large number of meaningless abnormal and borderline results obtained with clinical laboratory screening profiles.[5]

The consequences of overinterpretation of diagnostic procedures was named after Homer's Ulysses (Odysseus) because of his long journey to Troy, his many adventures, and his final return home.[6] False-positive results can cause considerable unnecessary wandering of the patient in the health care system, as did Ulysses in the days of Troy. However, the fit between the syndrome and the Greek hero is somewhat stretched.

The request of a schizophrenic patient, while nonpsychotic, to be given an experimental antipsychotic drug, but his refusal to take it when he was psychotic, has been termed a Ulysses Contract. The similarity is to Ulysses's instruction of his crew, while he was competent, to disregard his deranged requests to set him free when exposed to the singing of the sirens.[7] This situation presents both legal and ethical issues. The eponym Medical Odyssey has been used for the experience of a patient who had undergone prolonged medical investigation at many different centers for a mysterious illness.[8] He was angry, not because of the long period of time before diagnosis, but because of being addressed and treated as would be a child.

Homer's *Odyssey* and *Iliad* have many references to medicine, such as the treatment of wounds by debridement, and the infliction of a deadly plague on King Agamemnon's army by Apollo. Among the many medications is one that brings forgetfulness of every sorrow.[9] The latter may well have been the first tranquilizing drug.

1. Rang, M.: The Ulysses syndrome: *Can. Med. Assoc. J.*, 106:122–123, 1972.
2. Campos, F.-J., & Mercado-Rodriguez, U.: The Ulysses syndrome: *Can. Med. Assoc. J.*, 113:493, 1975.
3. Hansen, N. E. et al.: Odysseus-Syndromet—Et Kulturmedicinsk Problem: *Ugeskr. Laeger*, 141: 2877–2881, 1979.
4. Rodriguez, U. M.: El Síndrome de Ulises: *Rev. Clin. Esp.*, 164:127–128, 1982.
5. Korvin, C. C.: Laboratory screening—A critical survey (Part II): *Can. Med. Assoc. J.*, 105:1157–1161, 1971.
6. Gayley, pp. 318–345.
7. Winston, M. E. et al.: Can a subject consent to a 'Ulysses contract'?: *Hastings Center Rep.*, 12:26–28, 1982.
8. Katz, J.: *The Silent World of Patient and Doctor*: New York, The Free Press, 1984, p. 211.
9. Sieben, R.: The Homeric concept and practice of medicine: *Stanford Med. Bull.* 20:130–136, 1962.

Uraniscus

Uraniscus is a seldom used medical term for the hard palate.[2] Its combining form, urano-, occurs in several words, such as uranoplasty, an operation for cleft palate.[2] The derivation is from Uranus, the Greek god of the heavens.[3] Thus, the palate—the roof of the mouth—is likened to the heavens—the roof of the world. The relationship is physical rather than behavioral, Uranus being noted for hating his many children and confining them in Tartarus (the underworld) immediately after their birth. Both a distant planet and a radioactive element are also named after Uranus.[4]

1. Thomas, p. 1806.
2. Dirckx, p. 61.
3. Bulfinch, p. 499.
4. Espy, p. 15.

V

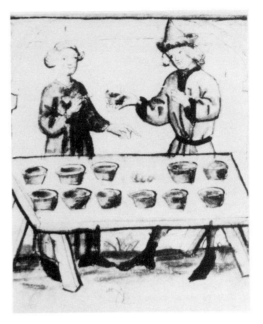

Vampirism Diagnoses being made from observing blood drawn for patients.[29, p. 61] (from 15th century German Manuscript) (by permission, The British Library).

Vampirism

Vampirism is an uncommon condition characterized by the ingestion of blood, by necrophilic activity which may or may not include sexual activity, and by necrosadism.[1] It may occur as ingestion of blood of others or of oneself (autovampirism). The latter is manifested by drawing and drinking one's own blood.[2] It has been suggested that such activity occurs in individuals functioning at a primitive mental and emotional level, and that it has some of the dynamics of schizophrenia.[3] It may also be a "projection of oral sadism left over from the early infant-mother relationship."[4] Drinking of blood may occur in sadomasochism, blood rituals, fetishism, psychosis, and drug intoxication.[5] Vampirism may be associated with cannibalism.[6]

The vampire is a popular and old superstition which is primarily a Slavic legend, but is best known throughout Europe and Asia.[7] The tradition is, however, worldwide and of considerable antiquity. There appeared to be an epidemic of vampirism in the seventeenth and eighteenth centuries in Hungary, Moravia, and Galicia. The word vampire was first used in English in 1734. It is related to the Magyar vampir, the Bulgarian vapir, and the Russian upuir.[8]

Vampires of legend are characterized by the need to drink fresh blood, and by having an abnormal interest in death and the dead. The terms necrophilia, thanatophilia, and thanatomania could therefore be applied to vampires.

They were considered to be evil spirits that were not let into the nether world, but must return to the grave during daylight.[9] Another related belief is that anyone born with a caul will become a vampire, although its presence is otherwise considered as a good omen and lucky charm. The ancient magical belief in blood as life is related to the reviving of vampires by blood sucking. The spirits in the *Odyssey* of Homer were restored by drinking blood.[10]

The popularity of the vampire myth was greatly enhanced by Stoker's novel of 1897, *Dracula*,[11] especially in the United States where it has become the subject of many pastiches and several movies. The Dracula story has been related to the psychological effect of surgical trauma on children. They fear subconsciously that the surgeon is trying to alleviate his own misery of losing sexual battles by castrating them or emptying their body of its contents.[12] The novel *Dracula* has been analyzed as "covert treatment of perverted sexuality,"[13] but Stoker as being largely unaware of such sexual content. Some supportive examples for this statement are that the vampire attacks in the novel are always on members of the opposite sex; and the blood taken by female vampires equates to the emission of semen. A psychobiological study of Dracula and his creator has been used as the basis for discussion of object-relations psychology.[4]

There is thought to be some connection between vampires and werwolves (werewolves) in some countries (see Lycanthropy).[8] In fact, porphyria, a rare genetic defect in the formation of the heme of hemoglobin, has been suggested as the cause of physical changes in both.[14] Although both may have excess hair, the skin of vampires is white rather than red, the teeth long, sharp and curved, the breath fetid, and the strength remarkable.[15] At times children born with harelips, odd birthmarks, or natal teeth have been persecuted as vampires.

Psychic vampirism is a term used for the drawing and absorbing of physical, nervous, and psychic energy by one person from another.[16] The flow of such vital energy is claimed to be the basis for the healing power of "natural" healers and touch-healers. It is also presumed to occur during sexual activity.

Dracula is not the only literary vampire, there being others such as *Le Vampire*, a play by Dumas.[17] A short story of 1819 was titled "The Vampyre; a Tale by Lord Byron," although it was written not by Byron, but by John Polidori, who was his traveling physician.[18] Even Doctor Watson, the somewhat dull-witted foil of Sherlock Holmes, was familiar with vampires, both literary and factual.[19] "But surely . . . the vampire was not necessarily a dead man? A living person might have the habit. I have read . . . of the old sucking the blood of the young in order to retain their youth."[20] Holmes, always the pragmatist, ridiculed any such possibility.

A more recent musical play, *Little Shop of Horrors*,[21] was first performed in 1982. It features a plant that arrived on earth from outer space during an eclipse of the sun. It is "An anthropomorphic cross between a Venus flytrap and an avocado" and has a huge, nasty-looking pod which is shark-like when open. Not only does it (he) speak, but also requires human blood to survive and grow—which it eventually does to so enormous a size that it engulfs both hero and heroine.

The eponym Medical Vampire has been applied to physicians who withdraw blood excessively or when not indicated.[22] A relatively minor example is removal of more blood than needed for laboratory tests. The prime example is "bloodletting," which was practiced extensively for two thousand years as treatment for the majority of illnesses. The rational was removal of excess humors, considered by Hippocrates to be an abnormal state that is the cause of all disease.[23] Benjamin Rush was a fervent believer in its efficacy. He carried out bloodletting to the extreme during the 1793 yellow fever epidemic in Philadelphia.[24] Copious bleeding was used on George Washington in 1799 for a severe laryngotracheitis, and undoubtedly contributed to his death.[25] Bloodletting diminished during the nineteenth century to be replaced in part by the counter-irritation principle of therapy—based on the assumption that cures occur with remedies which in themselves give rise to symptoms different from those of the disease.[26] This is the reverse of one of the principles of homeopathic therapy, which also arose in the nineteenth century. It has been suggested that bulimia (binge eating followed by induced vomiting) represents the modern psychological equivalence of purging by the copious bloodletting in previous centuries.[27]

The medical extravagance of bloodletting was not overlooked by Voltaire in the eighteenth century.[28] "With the aid of medicines and blood lettings, Candide's illness became serious." Bloodletting also provided blood from which to make a diagnosis based upon taste, smell, heat, clotting, and the presence of impurities.[29] Shakespeare did not neglect bloodletting. When the Duke of York realizes that his forces are inferior to those of King Henry IV he compares the situation with bloodletting. "Briefly to this end: we are all diseased;/ And with our surfeiting and wanton hours/ Have brought ourselves into a burning fever,/ And we must bleed for it: of which disease/ Our late king, Richard, being infected, died./ . . . To diet rank minds stick of happiness/ And purge the obstructions which begin to stop/ Our very veins of life. . . ."[30] (see Lasthénie de Ferjol Syndrome).

In a more general sense, the word vampire is applied to anyone who preys upon his fellow man; that is, a "blood sucker."[31] The common notion that certain lunatic behavior coincides with the full moon has been called the Transylvania Effect,[32] undoubtedly after the geographical origin of Dracula. Such a proposed effect has been attributed to the hot and humid weather that is associated with the full moon (see Lunacy).[33]

1. Prins, H.: Vampirism—A clinical condition: *Br. J. Psychiatry*, 146:666–668, 1985.
2. McCully, R. S.: Vampirism: Historical perspective and underlying process in relation to a case of auto-vampirism: *Nerv. Ment. Dis.*, 139:440–452, 1964.
3. Kayton, L.: The relationship of the vampire legend to schizophrenia: *J. Youth Adolesc.*, 1:303–314, 1972.
4. Henderson, J.: Exorcism, possession, and the Dracula cult. A synopsis of object-relations therapy: *Bull. Menninger Clin.*, 40:603–628, 1976.
5. Hemphill, R. E. & Zabow, T.: Clinical vampirism. A presentation of 3 cases and a re-evalua-

tion of Haigh, the 'acid-bath murderer': *South Afr. Med. J.*, 63:278–281, 1983.

6. Benezech, M. et al.: Cannibalism and vampirism in paranoid schizophrenia: *J. Clin. Psychiatry*, 42:290, 1981.

7. Summers, M.: *The Vampire. His Kith and Kin*: New Hyde Park, New York, University Books, 1960.

8. Hill, D.: *The History of Ghosts, Vampires and Werewolves*: Memphis, Ottenheimer, 1973, p. 19.

9. Hoyt, O.: *Lust for Blood. The Consuming Story of Vampires*: New York, Stein and Day, 1984.

10. Homer.

11. Stoker, A.: *Dracula*: New York, Modern Library, n.d.

12. Shuster, S.: Dracula and surgically induced trauma in children: *Br. J. Med. Psychol.*, 46:259–270, 1973.

13. Bentley, C. F.: The monster in the bedroom: Sexual symbolism in Bram Stoker's *Dracula*: *Lit. Psychol.*, 22:27–34, 1972.

14. Vampires: Rare disease may have spurred myths: *Albuquerque Tribune*, May 31, 1985, A-16.

15. Iveson-Iveson, J.: When fantasy meets reality: *Nursing Mirror*, 156:18–20, 1983.

16. Walker, pp. 230–231.

17. Twitchell, J. B.: *The Living Dead. A Study of the Vampire in Romantic Literature*: Durham, North Carolina, Duke University Press, 1981.

18. Viets, H. R.: The London editions of Polidori's *The Vampyre*: *Papers Biol. Soc. Am.*, 63:83–103, 1969.

19. Jones, J.: The Carfax Syndrome, Being a Study in Vampirism in the Canon: *Magico Mag.*, 1984.

20. Doyle, A. C.: "The Adventure of the Sussex Vampire": *Strand Mag.*, 67:3–13, 1924.

21. Ashman, H. & Menken, A.: *Little Shop of Horrors*: New York, Samuel French, 1985.

22. Burnum, J. F.: Medical vampires: *N. Engl. J. Med.*, 314:1250–1251, 1986.

23. Hudson, R. P.: *Disease and Its Control. The Shaping of Modern Thought*: Westport, Connecticut, Greenwood Press, 1983.

24. Powell, J. H.: *Bring Out Your Dead. The Great Plague of Yellow Fever in Philadelphia in 1793*: Philadelphia, University of Pennsylvania Press, 1949.

25. Davies, N. E. et al.: William Cobbett, Benjamin Rush, and the death of George Washington: *J.A.M.A.*, 249:912–915, 1983.

26. Schwartz, J. G.: The automation of leeches: *Texas Med.*, 82:27–31, 1986.

27. Cosman, B. C.: Bloodletting as purging behavior: *Am. J. Psychiatr*, 143:1188–1189, 1986.

28. Voltaire: *Candide*: L. Blair translator, New York, Bantam, 1959, p. 82.

29. Jones, P. M: *Medieval Medical Minatures*: Austin, Texas, University of Texas Press, 1984, pp. 60–62.

30. Shakespeare, 2 Henry: IV, i.

31. Benét, p. 1047.

32. Shapiro, J. L. et al.: The moon and mental illness. A failure to confirm the Transylvania

effect: *Percept. Motor Skills*, 30:827–830, 1970.
33. Geller, S. H. & Shannon, H. W.: The moon, weather and mental hospital contacts. Confirmation and explanation of the Transylvania effect: *J. Psychiatr. Nursing*, 14:13–17, 1976

Venereal

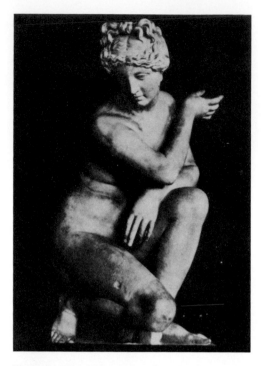

Venereal   Venus, the epitomy of the alluring woman.[12]

Venereal is an adjective that denotes the relationship of a noun to sexual intercourse, as, for example, venereal disease.[1] It is used to specify certain lesions as being associated with syphilis—venereal bubo, collar (dermatitis), sore (chancroid), urethritis, and wart. The noun venery is defined as overindulgence in sexual activities, and so used as early as the fifteenth century;[2] and more specifically for syphilis as lues venerea.[3] Venus was the Greek goddess of love and beauty, being the daughter of Jupiter and Dione.[4] By another account, she arose from the foam of the sea when Uranus was wounded, and thus had also been called Aphrodite (foam-born). She was attended by her son, Cupid. Venus bestowed her sexual favors freely. They were a blessing to only a few; to others they were for treacherous purposes.

The best known representation of Venus is the Greek marble statue Venus de Milo (circa 200 B.C.), found in 1920 on the island of Milos.[5] The word venom was derived from the name Venus, being originally a love potion.[6] Venus has also been used as a generic name for any beautiful woman. William Carlos Williams, the physician-poet, made an interesting comment on the words venereal and Venus in his autobiography.[7] "Only yesterday, reading Chapman's *The Iliad of Homer*, did I realize for the first time that the derivation of the adjective venereal is from Venus! And I a physician practicing medicine for the past forty years. I was stunned!"

A psychological interpretation of Shakespeare's poem of 1593, *Venus and Adonis*[8] suggests that Venus's attempt to seduce the youth Adonis has a subtext of a "preoedipal conflict between an overactive, too-loving mother and her resisting nursing infant." At a deeper level "it becomes the fantasy of an oral rape of a passive infant's mouth by the breast or mouth of his aggressive mother, with results that are ultimately fatal to the infant."[9] Shakespeare referred to the female genitalia as Venus's grove.[10]

Operation Venus is a national "hotline" for information on venereal diseases.[11] Information is provided about treatment centers, clinics, and physicians. It was established in 1976 because of the marked increase in the incidence of venereal diseases and the lack of referral centers in about two thousand counties in the United States.

1. Thomas, p. 1842.
2. OED: XII:94–95.
3. Guenter, B. B.: *Hospital Life in Enlightenment Scotland*: Cambridge, Cambridge University Press, 1986, p. 127.
4. Gayley, pp. 31–32.
5. *Random House Dictionary*: p. 1586.
6. Espy, p. 312.
7. Williams, W. C.: *The Autobiography of William Carlos Williams*: New York, New Directions, 1948, p. 3.
8. Shakespeare, *Venus and Adonis*.
9. Rothenberg, A. B.: The oral rape fantasy and rejection of mother in the imagery of Shakespeare's Venus and Adonis: *Psychoanal. Q.*, 40: 447–468, 1971.
10. Kail, p. 260.
11. Chiappa, J. A.: Operation Venus: *J.A.M.A.*, 236:2173, 1976.
12. Bulfinch, p. 67.

W

Walter Mitty Syndrome

Individuals playing false roles in hospitals include both those pretending illness, the Munchausen Syndrome, and those impersonating physicians, the Walter Mitty Syndrome.[1] Thurber created Walter Mitty, who played many roles in his fantasy life of adventure and heroism, much to the chagrin of his more prosaic and nagging wife.[2]

The Walter Mitty Syndrome is exemplified by one of his daydreams in which he was the surgeon who saved the day.[2] ". . . Mitty saw the man [surgeon] turn pale. 'Coreopsis has set in,' said Renshaw nervously. 'If you would take over, Mitty?' Mitty looked at . . . the grave, uncertain faces of the two great specialists. 'If you wish,' he said." This episode is also depicted in a musical play of the same name.[3] The Walter Mitty phenomenon can also be considered as a split between the ideal and the real. The function of such escapist fiction may be to counterbalance the agony of reality by hilarity.[4]

Walter Mitty has been invoked for situations the reverse of the syndrome, in which physicians become prominent for engaging in nonmedical activities.[5] Examples include Salvador Allende (former president of Chile), Arthur Conan Doyle (creator of Sherlock Holmes), John Keats (poet), Anton Chekov (drama), Alexander Borodin (composer of the opera *Prince Igor*), Leopold Damrosch (conductor), and Richard Gatling (inventor of the Gatling gun). But their activities were not fantasies, as were those of Walter Mitty, although avocations may also help us keep our sanity.

1. Asher, R.: Munchausen's syndrome: *Lancet*, 1: 339–341, 1951.
2. Thurber, J.: "The Secret Life of Walter Mitty": in *The Thurber Carnival*, New York, Harper & Row, 1945, pp. 47–51.
3. Manchester, J. & Shuman, E.: *The Secret Life of Walter Mitty*: New York, Samuel French, 1963.
4. Sewell, E.: Poetry and madness, connected or not?—The case of Holderlin: *Lit. Med.*, 4:41–69, 1985.
5. Kassel, V.: The secret lives of some Drs. Mitty: *Med. Times*, 104:183–186, 1976.

Werther Effect

The eponym Werther Effect was applied in 1974 to the increase in number of suicides which immediately follows the appearance of a suicide story in newspapers.[1] The increased incidence occurs in the area of distribution of the news item. Studies of nationally televised suicide events have also shown a direct relationship between the number of networks carrying such a story and the number of subsequent teenage suicides.[2] Such an increase has been attributed to imitative behavior. Also implicated have been suicides in fictional films shown on television,[3,4] although the statistical basis for such a conclusion has been challenged.[5] Suicide is now the second commonest cause of death in teenagers between the ages of fifteen and nineteen years of age, second only to deaths from accidents.[6] The imitative variety of suicide may, however, be only a part of the overall incidence.[7]

Werther is the main character in a novel by Goethe. *The Sorrows of Young Werther* was published in 1774, consisting of letters to a friend, except for the final denouement.[8] Werther was an artistic, sentimental, and intelligent young man, who had an inclination to speculative thought and fantastic dreams. He retired to the countryside because of a stressful love triangle. There he met Charlotte and fell deeply in love with her. She, however, was engaged to Albert. Even after she married Albert, Werther continued to see her frequently and became rabidly obsessed with her. He was devastated when her husband ordered Charlotte not to see him again. Werther then wrote a letter to her which

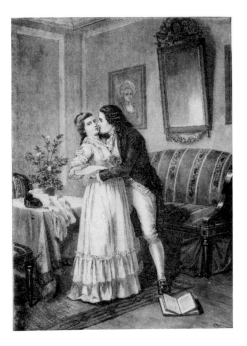

Werther Effect   Werther being rejected by Charlotte.[22]

began with "It is all over, Charlotte: I am resolved to die." And he did by means of shooting himself in the head, his last words being "... the clock strikes twelve. I say amen. Charlotte, Charlotte! farewell, farewell!"

The novel became quite popular throughout Europe and was blamed for leading impressionable adolescents to suicide.[7] Although this was never proven, the book was banned in Leipzig, Copenhagen, and Milan in fear of its negative influence. Quite suggestive of the validity of such a cluster effect is a recent series of suicides in the United States. On March 11, 1987, four teenagers committed suicide in New Jersey by carbon monoxide after locking themselves in a running car in a closed garage.[9] The event received national newspaper and television coverage. On March 13, two more teenagers committed suicide in Illinois by the same method.[10] This was repeated in Chicago by individual teenagers on March 14, 17, and 18.[11] The imitative nature of such copycat suicides is apparent from the actions of a young couple who were rescued on March 17 while attempting the same suicide method by breaking into the garage where the original four had committed suicide.[12] Some experts, however, consider that parents with emotional problems and who abuse drugs or alcohol have a greater importance in teenager suicide.[13] Imitative suicides would then be much more likely to occur in adolescents who are so preconditioned. Studies since the March, 1987, copycat suicides have failed to show significant increased rates after a deliberate overdose of a drug in a British television soap opera,[14] and after three American televised films depicting suicides.[15]

Over the last thirty years, teenage suicides have increased from about a third of all cases to an equal incidence with older age groups.[16] The attractions of suicide for adolescents include perceptions that it is a glamorous way to die, a means of getting attention, a feeling that there will never be an end to their problems; and the lack of understanding of the finality of their action. They may even feel that they are only imagining the staging of their own death. This has been called the Tom Sawyer Syndrome,[16] presumably because Mark Twain's character decided not to reveal he was alive after being presumed drowned.[17] However, suicidal people do plan and carry out their own deaths, unlike the Tom Sawyer story.

Suicide also occurs in fictional works other than "Werther." The romantic concept of such a tragedy is frequent.[18] An example is Shakespeare's Romeo Montague, who was a teenager. He poisoned himself because he though Juliet Capulet dead; to be followed by Juliet's suicide with his dagger when she found him dead (see Romeo Error).[19] In Puccini's opera *Madame Butterfly*, Cio Cio San, a geisha girl, commits suicide when her husband returns home with a new wife after a three-year absence.[20] Suicide is also featured in many novels as, for example, Dreiser's *Sister Carrie*, Wharton's *The House of Mirth*, and Jack London's *Martin Eden*.[21]

1. Phillips, D. P.: The influence of suggestion on suicide: Substantive and theoretical implications of the Werther effect: *Am. Sociol. Rev.*, 39:340–354, 1974.
2. Phillips, D. P. & Carstensen, L. L.: Clustering of teenage suicides after television news stories about suicide: *N. Engl. J. Med.*, 315:685–689, 1986.
3. Gould, M. S. & Shaffer, D.: The impact of suicide in television movies. Evidence of imitation: *N. Engl. J. Med.*, 315:690–694, 1986.
4. Ostroff, R. B. & Boyd, J. H.: Television and suicide: *N. Engl. J. Med.*, 316:876–877, 1987.
5. Marks, A.: Television and suicide: *N. Engl. J. Med.*, 316:877, 1987.
6. Chapman, A. H. et al.: *Textbook of Psychiatry. An Interpersonal Approach*: 2nd ed., Philadelphia, J. B. Lippincott, 1976, pp. 290–293.
7. Eisenberg, L.: Does bad news about suicide beget bad news?: *N. Engl. J. Med.*, 315:705–707, 1986.
8. Goethe, J. W. von: "The Sorrows of the Young Werther": O. Falk translator, in *Great German Novels and Stories*, New York, Modern Library, 1933, pp. 1–120.
9. Teens have suicide pact, mother says: *Dayton Daily News and J. Herald*, March 12, 1987, p. 39.
10. 2 More teen-agers die; Suicide cases similar: *Dayton Daily News and J. Herald*, March 14, 1987, p. 2.
11. McQuay, T.: Suicide experts: Point teens to help: *USA Today*, March 17, p. 3A, March 18, p. 4A, 1987.
12. Lyons, C. & McQuay, T.: Copycat suicide fails; 2 other teens die: *USA Today*, March 18, 1987, p. 3A.
13. Whyche, S.: Family: The crucial factor in teen suicide risk: *USA Today*, May 14, 1987, p. 4D.
14. Platt, S.: The aftermath of Angie's overdose: Is

soap (opera) damaging to your health?: *Br. Med. J.*, 294:954–967, 1987.

15. Phillips, D. P. & Paight, D. J.: The impact of televised movies about suicide: *N. Engl. J. Med.*, 317:809–811, 1987.

16. Wilentz, A.: Teen suicide. Two death pacts shake the country: *Time*, 129:12–13, March 23, 1987.

17. Twain, M. (Clemens, S. L.): *The Adventures of Tom Sawyer*: Chicago, Spencer Press, 1953.

18. Feggetter, G.: Suicide in opera: *Br. J. Psychiatry*, 136:552–557, 1980.

19. Shakespeare, *Romeo and Juliet*: V.

20. Ewen, D.: *Encyclopedia of the Opera*: new ed., New York, Hill & Wang, 1963, pp. 279–281.

21. Spangler, G. M.: Suicide and social criticism: Durkheim, Dreiser, Wharton and London: *Am. Q.*, 31:496–516, 1979.

22. Brewer, 4:236.

References

The following list of references are those which are used for at least five different eponyms. In the text they are indicated by the author's last name or abbreviated title.

Anson, B., Ed.: *Morris's Anatomy*: 12th ed., New York, McGraw-Hill, 1966.

Benét, W. R.: *The Reader's Encyclopedia*: 2 vols. 2nd ed., New York, Thomas Y. Crowell, 1965.

Berkow, R., Ed.: *The Merck Manual of Diagnosis and Therapy*: 14th ed., Rathway, New Jersey, Merck Sharp & Dome Research Laboratory, 1982.

Bloch, I.: *Ethnological and Cultural Studies of the Sex Life in England Illustrated as Revealed in Its Erotic and Obscene Literature and Art*: R. Deniston translator, New York, Falstaff Press, 1934.

Boase, W.: *The Folklore of Hampshire and the Isle of Wight*: Totowa, New Jersey, Rowman & Littlefield, 1976.

Boycott, R.: *Batty, Bloomers and Boycott. A Little Etymology of Eponymous Words*: New York, Peter Bedrick, 1982.

Braunwald, E. et al.: *Harrison's Principles of Internal Medicine*: 7th ed., New York, McGraw-Hill, 1987.

Brewer, E. C.: *Character Sketches of Romance, Fiction and the Drama*: 4 vols., New York, Selmar Hess, 1882.

Bulfinch, T.: *The Age of Fables or Beauties of Mythology*: revised ed., J. L. Scott, Ed., Philadelphia, David McKay, 1898.

Campbell, R. J.: *Psychiatric Dictionary*: 5th ed., New York, Oxford University Press, 1981.

Carroll, L. (Dodgson, C. L.): *Alice's Adventures in Wonderland* and *Through the Looking Glass*: in M. Gardner, Ed., *The Annotated Alice*, New York, Bramhall House, 1960.

Chapman, A. H.: *Textbook of Clinical Psychiatry*: 2nd ed., Philadelphia, J. B. Lippincott, 1976.

Ciardi, J.: *A Browser's Dictionary and Native's Guide to the Unknown American Language*: New York, Harper & Row, 1980.

Diel, P.: *Symbolism in Greek Mythology. Human Desires and Transformations*: V. Stuart et al. translators, Boulder, Colorado, Shambhala, 1980.

Dirckx, J. H.: *The Language of Medicine. Its Evolution, Structure and Dynamics*: 2nd ed., New York, Praeger, 1983.

Dodgson, C. L. (pseudonym Lewis Carroll): *Alice's Adventures in Wonderland*, and *Througfh the Looking-Glass*: with ninety-two illustrations by John Tenniel, new ed. in one vol., New York, Macmillan, 1885.

Dudzinski, W.: Literary Originals of some syndromes and pathological symptoms (Polish): *Pol. Tyg. Lek.*, 35:1197–1201, 1980.

Durham, R. H.: *Encyclopedia of Medical Syndromes*: New York, Harper & Row, 1965.

Editors of The American Heritage Dictionaries: *Word Mysteries & Histories From Quiche to Humble Pie*: Boston, Houghton Mifflin, 1986.

Eisenberg, R. L.: *Atlas of Signs in Radiology*: Philadelphia, J. B. Lippincott, 1984.

Encyclopaedia Britannica: Micropaedia: 10 vols., 15th ed., Chicago, Encyclopaedia Britannica, 1974.

Espy, W. R.: *Thou Improper, Thou Uncommon Noun*: New York, Clarkson N. Potter, 1978.

Ferner, H., Ed.: *Pernkopf Atlas of Topography and Applied Human Anatomy*: Baltimore, Urban & Schwarzenberg, 1980.

Freedman, A. M. et al.: *Comprehensive Textbook of Psychiatry—II*: 2 vols., 2nd ed., Baltimore, Williams & Wilkins, 1975.

Freud, S.: *The Standard Edition of the Complete Psychological Works of Sigmund Freud*: vols. I–XXIV, J. Strachey translator, London, Hogarth Press, 1975.

Gayley, C. M.: *The Classic Myths in English Literature and in Art*: new ed., Boston, Ginn & Co., 1939.

Gilman, A. G. et al., Eds.: *Goodman and Gilman's The Pharmacological Basis of Therapeutics*: 7th ed., New York, Macmillan, 1985.

Guirand, F.: *Greek Mythology*: D. Ames translator, Middlesex, England, Paul Hamlyn, 1964.

Guirand, F., Ed.: *New Larousse Encyclopedia of Mythology*: new ed., R. Aldington & D. Ames translators, Middlesex, England, Paul Hamlyn, 1968.

Haubrich, W. S.: *Medical Meanings. A Glossary of Word Origins*: San Diego, Harcourt Brace Jovanovich, 1984.

Hendrickson, R.: *The Dictionary of Eponyms. Names That Became Words*: New York, Stein & Day, 1985.

Homer: *The Odyssey of Homer*: A. Pope translator, New York, Heritage Press, 1942.

Index of NLM Serial Titles: National Library of Medicine, 5th ed., NIH Pub. No. 84-3124, U.S. Dept. Health & Human Services, 1984.

Jaeger, E. C.: *A Source-Book of Medical Terms*: Springfield Illinois, Charles C Thomas, 1953.

Jung, C. G. et al.: *Man and His Symbols*: New York, Dell, 1968.

Kail, A. C.: *The Medical Mind of Shakespeare*: Balgowlah, Australia, Williams & Wilkins, 1986.

Kolb, L. C. & Brodie, H. K. H.: *Modern Clinical Psychiatry*: 3rd ed., Philadelphia, W. B. Saunders, 1982.

Levin, S.: *Adam's Rib: Essays on Biblical Medicine*: Los Altos, California, Geron-X, 1970.

Murphy, E. L.: The saints of medicine: *J. Irish Med. Assoc.*, 43:257–265, 1985.

(NT) New Testament: in *The Holy Bilble Containing the Old and New Testaments*, Grand Rapids Michigan, Zondervan Publishing House, 1969.

Ober, W. B.: *Boswell's Clap and Other Essays. Medical Analyses of Literary Men's Afflications*: Carbondale Illinois, Southern University Press, 1979.

(OED) Murray, J. A. H. et al., Eds.: *The Oxford English Dictionary*: London, Oxford University Press, 1969–1986.

(OT) *The Holy Scriptures According to the Masoretic Text. A New Translation*: new ed., Philadelphia, Jewish Publishing Society of America, 1955.

Paré, A.: *On Monsters and Marvels*: J. L. Pallister translator, University of Chicago Press, 1982.

Partridge, E.: *A Dictionary of Slang and Unconventional English*: 8th ed., P. Beale, Ed., New York, Macmillan, 1984.

Schmidt, J.: *Larousse Greek and Roman Mythology*: S. Benardete, Ed., S. O'Halloran translator, New York, McGraw-Hill, 1980.

Shakespeare, W.: *The Annotated Shakespeare*: 2 vols. A. L. Rowse, Ed., New York, Clarkson N. Potter, 1978.

Shelley, M. W.: *Frankenstein or, The Modern Prometheus*: London, Lackington, Hughes, Harding, Major & Jones, 1818.

Skinner, H. A.: *Origin of Medical Terms*: Baltimore, Williams & Wilkins, 1961.

Stedman, T. L.: *Illustrated Stedman's Medical Dictionary*: 24th ed., Baltimore, Williams & Wilkins, 1982.

Stein, J., Ed.: *The Random House Dictionary of the English Language*: unabridged ed., New York, Random House, 1967.

Thomas, C. L., Ed.: *Taber's Cyclopedic Medical Dictonary*: 15th ed., Philadelphia, F. A. Davis, 1985.

Thurston, S. J. & Attwater, D., Eds.: *Butler's Lives of the Saints*: 4 vols., 2nd complete ed., Westminister, Maryland, Christian Classics, 1956.

Vaisrub, S.: *Medicine's Metaphors: Messages & Menaces*: Oradell, New Jersey, Medical Economics, 1977.

Walker, B.: *Encyclopedia of Metaphysical Medicine*: London, Routledge & Kegan Paul, 1978.

Weekley, E.: *An Etymological Dictionary of Modern English*: 2 vols., New York, Dover, 1967.

Williams, C.: *Saints. Their Cults and Origins*: New York, St. Martin's Press, 1980.

Index

An asterisk* after a page number indicates the first page of a literary medical eponym which serves as a main heading in the encyclopedia. The eponyms in which only the first letter of each work is capitalized are those that are not literary but named after actual persons. First letters of words in eponyms named after inanimate objects are capitalized.

granulomatous disease, chronic 116
Great Expectations (Dickens) 165
"Great Keinplatz Experiment, The"
  (Doyle, A.C.) 106
Great Ormand Street Sick Children's
  Hospital 219
greed 162–163, 214
griffins 44, 52
Griselda Complex 83*, 189
guaicum 287
Guild of St. Luke, SS. Cosmas and
  Damian 84*
guilt feelings 10, 26, 29, 86, 99, 172,
  180, 190, 214
Gulliver's Travels (Swift) 137

–H–

Hades 159, 199, 215, 253, 291
hair (see bezoar, hirsutism) 124, 258
hallucinations 137, 147, 200, 212, 312
halo effect 149
hamartoma 251
Hamlet (Shakespeare) 62, 86, 91, 199
Hamlet-Gertrude Complex 86*, 189
Hansen's Disease (see Lazarus Illness)
Happy Puppet Syndrome xii, 87*
Harlequin Color Change 89*
Harlequin Fetus 90*
Harpies 109
hashish 24, 137
hatter's shakes 147
head injury 293
health care 45, 96, 208
health care costs 80, 138, 169–170,
  238–239
health care, administration 161, 268,
  296
health care systems (see Medical
  Nemesis) 238–239, 268, 312
Health Service Corps 242
heart anomalies 62, 294–295
heart disease 76, 209, 291
Heart's Reason, The (Mallea) 204
Hebephrenia 91*
Heir of the Oedipus Complex 190
Helen of Troy 77, 177
Helios 141
hemangioma 227
Hemera 71, 92, 183
Hemeralopia 92*

hemlock 143
hemoglobin 287, 318
HemoQuant Test 287
hemorrhage 126
hemorrhoids 78
Henry V (Shakespeare) 74
Henry IV (Shakespeare) 74, 75, 132,
  320
Hera 41, 91
Heracles (see Hercules)
Hercules 91, 125, 126, 239
Hercules Morbus 272
heredity 239–240
Hermaphrodite 55, 92*
Hermes (see Mercury) 95*
Hermes Syndrome 96
hernia 85
hiatus hernia 298
Hippocrates 13, 31, 229, 277, 319
Hippolytus 220
hirsutism 68, 213
Hitler, Adolph 225
Hodgkin's Disease 20
Hogarth, William 152, 202
Holmesian Technique 97*
Holmes, Sherlock 32, 96, 142, 172,
  286, 287, 311, 319
Homage to the Red Queen 262
homeopathy 320
Homeric Laughter syndrome 88
homicide 38, 57, 86, 126, 168, 204
homosexuality 57, 120, 138, 213
Hospital, The (Wilde, Joseph) 13
hospitals 7, 238, 315
House of Mirth, The (Wharton) 327
Huckleberry Finn Syndrome 98*
Humbert Complex 139
humors 319
Humpty Dumpty Complex 103
Humpty Dumpty Etymology 100*
Humpty Dumpty Phenomenon 101*
Humpty Dumpty Syndrome 101*
Hunchback of Notre Dame, The (Hugo,
  Victor) 250
Hunter-Hurler disease 82
Hunting of the Snark (Carroll, Lewis)
  31
Huxley, Aldous 34
hybrids (see Chimera)
hydronephrosis 161

hydrophobia 274
Hygeia (Hygiea) 13, 103*
Hygiene 103*
Hymen 104*
hymenotomy 104
hyperactive child syndrome 299
hyperactivity 276, 300
hypercalcemia (see calcium excess)
Hyperion 141
hypersomnia 221, 222, 256, 263–264
hypertelorism 202, 307
hypertension 147, 280, 298
hypertrichosis (see Esau Lady) 135
Hypnos 105, 297
Hypnosis 105*, 151, 152
hypochondriasis 174, 223
hypoglycemia 35, 218
hypopituitarism 218
hypothalamus dysfunction 89, 197
hypoventilation 197, 221, 222
hyssop 131
hysteria 172
hysteria, mass 143, 274

–I–

Icarus Complex 108*
Icarus, or the Future of Science (Russell, Bertrand) 109
Idiot, The (Dostoevski) 273
ignis sacer 266
Iliad, The (Homer) 316, 322
immortality 137, 172, 246
imposture syndrome 174
impotency 195
incest 33, 119, 142, 188–190
incubus 182–183, 290
Infant Esau 69
infanticide 67, 125
infectious mononucleosis 19, 256
inferiority feeling 77
infidelity 204
insanity 141–143
Insurance Hebephrenia 92
inverse cerebral steal 264
Inverted Oedipus Complex 190
Invisible Man, The (Wells) 138
Invisible Man Syndrome 138
Io 27
Iris 109*
Isis 110*

Isis Revisited (Blavatsky, H.) 110
Isle of Wight 19, 226
Ixon 41

–J–

jabberwocky 20, 201, 313
Jack the Ripper 148
Jacob 68, 121
Jairus 129
Janiceps Twins 112*
Janus 112, 113*
Janus-faced 81, 114
Janusian Thinking 113
Jason 150
J.B. (McLeash) 117
jealousy 134–135, 204
Jean-Baptiste Grandjean, Anne 94
Jekyll-and-Hyde Syndrome 114*
Jenner, Edward 280
Jesus (Christ) 128–129, 160, 172
Jews 160, 168
Job's Comforters (boils) 116, 118
Job's Disease 116
Job's Syndrome 116*
Job's Tears 118
Job's Ward 117
Jocasta (queen of Thebes) 119, 125, 188
Jocasta Complex 119*, 150, 189, 212, 295
Jocasta-Oedipus Conflict 295
John (king of England) 143
John the Baptist, Saint 69, 275
Johnson, Samuel 68
Jones-Elliot, Annie 68
Jones, James 225
Joppa 130
Joseph 90
Joseph and the Amazing Technicolor Dreamcoat (Rice & Webber) 121
Joseph Complex 120*, 189
Joseph Fantasy 121
Judah 194
Judith (Giraudoux) 180
Jung, Carl 8, 18, 67, 77, 95, 169, 215
Juno 109
Jupiter (see Zeus)

–K–

Kalevala (Finnish) 191

syringoma 306
syringomyelia 306
Syrinx 305

−T−

Tales of Mother Goose (Perrault) 45
talion fear 181
Talley's Folly (Wilson) 103
Talmud 281
Tamar 194
Tamora 29
Tantalos 154
tarantulism 274
Tartarus (underworld) 316
technology, medical 78, 154, 194, 242
Telesphorus 13
television 171, 191, 325–326
Tempest, The (Shakespeare) 298
teratogenesis 43, 52
thanatophilia 317
Thanatophoric Dwarf 307*
thanatopsy 309
Thanatos 105, 297, 307, 308*
Thanatos Syndrome, The (Percy, Walker) 309
Thaumus 109
Theosophy 110
Theseus 220, 238
Thetis 8
Thomas, Dylan 301
Thomas, Saint (erysipelas) 272
thoracic dysplasia 307
Thoreau, Henry D. 311
Through the Looking Glass (Carroll) 18–19, 260–261
Thucydies syndrome 270
thumb-sucking 300
Thyestes Complex 29
thymus gland 23, 295
Timon of Athens (Shakespeare) 303
Tiny Alice (Albee) 180
Tiresias 94
Titans 28, 239, 277
Titus Andronicus (Shakespeare) 29
toilet seat syndrome 284
Tom o' Bedlam 7
Tom Sawyer 99
Tom Sawyer Syndrome 326
Tragedy of Coriolanus, The (Shakespeare) 190

Tragical History of Doctor Faustus, The (Marlowe) 77
Transylvania effect 320
Traviata, La (Verdi) 310
Traviata Beauty 310*
Treatise on Contagion (Fracastorius) 302
Treves, Frederick, Doctor 251
tribadism 275
trichobezoars 258
trichotillomania 258
Trilby. A Novel (du Maurier) 106
Tristram Shandy (Sterne, Lawrence) 284
Troilus and Cressida (Shakespeare) 66
Trojan War 262, 298
truancy 98–99
tuberculosis 181, 310–312
Twain, Mark (Clemens, Samuel) 196
Tweedledum and Tweedledee 18, 20, 312
Tweedledum and Tweedledee Syndrome 312*
Twelfth Night (Shakespeare) 15
twins 43, 102
typhoid fever 74
Typhon, 43
typhus 132, 226
typist tendinitis 207

−U−

Ulysses (Joyce) 303, 314
Ulysses (Odysseus) 66, 262, 290, 291
Ulysses Complex 314*
Ulysses Contract 315
Ulysses Syndrome 315*
umbilicus 12, 38–39
unconsciousness 294
Under Western Eyes (Conrad) 17
Uraniscus 316*
Uranus 316, 322
uroscopy 54

−V−

vaccines 162
Vaisrub, Samuel 230
Valentine, Saint 272
vampire 106, 126, 317–320
Vampire, Le (Dumas) 319
Vampirism 317, 318